Fluid, Electrolyte and Acid-Base Disorders

Alluru S. Reddi

Fluid, Electrolyte and Acid-Base Disorders

Clinical Evaluation and Management

Second Edition

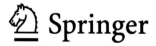

Alluru S. Reddi, MD, PhD
Professor of Medicine
Chief, Division of Nephrology and Hypertension
Rutgers New Jersey Medical
Newark, NJ
USA

ISBN 978-3-319-60166-3   ISBN 978-3-319-60167-0   (eBook)
DOI 10.1007/978-3-319-60167-0

Library of Congress Control Number: 2017954276

Printed on acid-free paper

This Springer imprint is published by Springer Nature
The registered company is Springer International Publishing AG
The registered company address is: Gewerbestrasse 11, 6330 Cham, Switzerland

Preface

Like the previous edition, the second edition of *Fluid, Electrolyte and Acid–Base Disorders* provides a clear and concise understanding of the fundamentals of these clinical problems that are encountered daily in our practice. Most of the chapters have been updated and expanded. Six pertinent new chapters have been added. Also, some new study questions have been discussed.

Similar to the first edition, each chapter begins with pertinent basic physiology followed by its clinical disorders. Cases for each fluid, electrolyte, and acid–base disorder are discussed with answers. In addition, board-type questions with explanations are provided for each clinical disorder to increase the knowledge of the physician.

The revision of the book would not have been possible without the help of many students, house staff, and colleagues, who made me understand nephrology and manage patients appropriately. I am grateful to all of them. I am extremely thankful and grateful to my family for their immense support and patience. I extend my thanks to Gregory Sutorius of Springer New York for his continued support, help, and advice. Finally, I am thankful to many readers for their constructive critique of the previous edition and also expect such a positive criticism from readers of the current edition of the book.

Newark, NJ, USA   Alluru S. Reddi

Contents

Part I

Physiologic Basis and Management of Fluid, Electrolyte and Acid-Base Disorders

Body Fluid Compartments

Water is the most abundant component of the body. It is essential for life in all human beings and animals. Water is the only solvent of the body in which electrolytes and other nonelectrolyte solutes are dissolved. An electrolyte is a substance that dissociates in water into charged particles called *ions*. Positively charged ions are called *cations*. Negatively charged ions are called *anions*. Glucose and urea do not dissociate in water because they have no electric charge. Therefore, these substances are called *nonelectrolytes*.

Terminology

The reader should be familar with certain terminology to understand fluids not only in this chapter but the entire text as well.

Units of Solute Measurement

It is customary to express the concentration of electrolytes in terms of the number of ions, either milliequivalents/liter (mEq/L) or millimoles/L (mmol/L). This terminology is especially useful when describing major alterations in electrolytes that occur in response to a physiologic disturbance. It is easier to express these changes in terms of the number of ions rather than the weight of the ions (milligrams/dL or mg/dL).

Electrolytes do not react with each other milligram for milligram or gram for gram; rather, they react in proportion to their chemical equivalents. Equivalent weight of a substance is calculated by dividing its *atomic weight* by its *valence*. For example, the atomic weight of Na^+ is 23 and its valence is 1. Therefore, the equivalent weight of Na^+ is 23. Similarly, Cl^- has an atomic weight of 35.5 and valence of 1. Twenty-three grams of Na^+ will react with 35.5 g of Cl^- to yield 58.5 g of NaCl. In other words, one Eq of Na^+ reacts with one Eq of Cl^- to form one Eq of NaCl. Because the

© Springer Science+Business Media LLC 2018
A.S. Reddi, *Fluid, Electrolyte and Acid-Base Disorders*,
DOI 10.1007/978-3-319-60167-0_1

electrolyte concentrations of biologic fluids are small, it is more convenient to use *milliequivalents* (mEq). One mEq is 1/1,000 of an Eq. One mEq of Na^+ is 23 mg.

So far, we have calculated equivalent weights of the monovalent ions (valence = 1). What about divalent ions? Ca^{2+} is a divalent ion because its valence is 2. Since the atomic weight of Ca^{2+} is 40, its equivalent weight is 20 (atomic weight divided by valence or 40/2 = 20). In a chemical reaction, 2 mEq of Ca^{2+} (40 g) will combine with 2 mEq of monovalent Cl^- (71 g) to yield one molecule of $CaCl_2$ (111 g).

Nonelectrolytes, such as urea and glucose, are expressed as mg/dL. To simplify the expression of electrolyte and nonelectrolyte solute concentrations, *Système International* (SI) units have been developed. In SI units, concentrations are expressed in terms of *moles* per liter (mol/L), where a molar solution contains 1 g molecular or atomic weight of solute in 1 L of solution. On the other hand, a *molal* solution is defined as 1 g molecular weight of solute in a kilogram of solvent. A *millimole* (mmol) is 1/1000 of a mole. For example, the molecular weight of glucose is 180. One mole of glucose is 180 g, whereas 1 mmol is 180 mg (180,000 mg/1000 = 180 mg) dissolved in 1 kg of solvent. In body fluids, as stated earlier, the solvent is water.

Conversions and Electrolyte Composition

Table 1.1 shows important cations and anions in plasma and intracellular compartments. The table illustrates expression of electrolyte concentrations in mEq/L (conventional expression in the United States) to other expressions because ions react

Table 1.1 Normal (mean) plasma and intracellular (skeletal muscle) electrolyte concentrations

Electrolyte	Mol wt	Valence	Eq wt	Concentrations			Intracellular concentration
				mg/dL	mEq/dL	mmol/L	mEq/L
Cations							
Na^+	23	1	23	326	142	142	14
K^+	39	1	39	16	4	4	140
Ca^{2+a}	40	2	20	10	5	2.5	4
Mg^{2+}	24	2	12	2.5	2	1.0	35
Total cations	–	–	–	354.5	153	149.5	193
Anions							
Cl^-	35.5	1	35.5	362	104	104	2
HCO_3^{-b}	61	–	22	55	25	25	8
$H_2PO_4^- HPO_4^{2-}$	31	1.8	17	4	2.3	1.3	40
SO_4^{2-}	32	2	16 $\cdot$	1.5	0.94	0.47	20
Proteins	–	–	–	7,000	15	0.9	55
Organic acids[c]	–	–	–	15	5.76	5.5	68
Total anions	–	–	–	7,437.5	153	137.17	193

[a]Includes ionized and bound Ca^{2+}
[b]Measured as total CO_2
[c]Includes lactate, citrate, etc.

Table 1.2 Conversion between conventional and SI units for important cations and anions using a conversion factor

Analyte	Expression of conventional units	Conventional to SI units (multiplication factor)	SI to conventional units (multiplication factor)	Expression of SI units
Na$^+$	mEq/L	1	1	mmol/L
K$^+$	mEq/L	1	1	mmol/L
Cl$^-$	mEq/L	1	1	mmol/L
HCO$_3^-$	mEq/L	1	1	mmol/L
Creatinine[a]	mg/dL	88.4	0.01113	µmol/L
Urea nitrogen	mg/dL	0.356	2.81	mmol/L
Glucose	mg/dL	0.055	18	mmol/L
Ca^{2+}	mg/dL	0.25	4	mmol/L
Mg^{2+}	mg/dL	0.41	2.43	mmol/L
Phosphorus	mg/dL	0.323	3.1	mmol/L
Albumin	g/dL	10	0.1	g/L

[a]1 mg creatinine = 0.0884 mmol/L

mEq for mEq, and not mmol for mmol or mg for mg. Furthermore, expressing cations in mEq demonstrates that an equal number of anions in mEq are necessary to maintain electroneutrality, which is an important determinant for ion transport in the kidney. It is clear from the table that Na$^+$ is the most abundant cation, and Cl$^-$ and HCO$_3^-$ are the most abundant anions in the plasma or extracellular compartment. The intracellular composition varies from one tissue to another. Compared to the plasma, K$^+$ is the most abundant cation, and organic phosphate and proteins are the most abundant anions inside the cells or the intracellular compartment. Na$^+$ concentration is low. This asymmetric distribution of Na$^+$ and K$^+$ across the cell membrane is maintained by the enzyme, Na/K–ATPase.

Some readers are familiar with the conventional units, whereas others prefer SI units. Table 1.2 summarizes the conversion of conventional units to SI units and vice versa. One needs to multiply the reported value by the conversion factor in order to obtain the required unit.

Osmolarity Versus Osmolality

When two different solutions are separated by a membrane that is permeable to water and not to solutes, water moves through the membrane from a lower to a higher concentrated solution until the two solutions reach equal concentration. This movement is called *osmosis*. Osmosis does not continue indefinitely but stops when the solutes on both sides of the membrane exert an equal *osmotic force*. This force is called *osmotic pressure*.

The osmotic pressure is the colligative property of a solution. It depends on the number of particles dissolved in a unit volume of solvent and not on the valence, weight, or shape of the particle. For example, an atom of Na$^+$ exerts the same osmotic pressure as an atom of Ca^{2+} with a valence of 2. Osmotic pressure is expressed as *osmoles* (Osm). One *milliosmole* (mOsm) is 1/1000 of an osmole, which can be calculated for each electrolyte using the following formula:

$$mOsm/L = \frac{mg/dL \times 10}{Mol\,wt.}$$

Osmolarity refers to the number of mOsm in 1 L of solution, whereas *osmolality* is the number of mOsm in 1 kg of water. However, osmolality is the preferred physiological term because the colligative property depends on the number of particles in a given weight (kg) of water.

The osmolality of plasma is largely a function of Na^+ concentration and its anions (mainly Cl^- and HCO_3^-) with contributions from glucose and urea nitrogen. Since each Na^+ is paired with a univalent anion, the contribution from other cations such as K^+, Ca^{2+}, and Mg^{2+} to the osmolality of plasma is generally not considered. Therefore, the plasma osmolality is calculated by doubling Na^+ and including the contribution from glucose and urea nitrogen (generally expressed as blood urea nitrogen or BUN), as follows:

$$Osmolality\,(mOsm/kg\,H_2O) = 2[Na^+] + \frac{Glucose}{18} + \frac{BUN}{2.8}$$

where 18 and 2.8 are derived from the molecular weights of glucose and urea, respectively. Because serum glucose and urea concentrations are expressed as mg/dL, it is necessary to convert these concentrations to mOsm/L by dividing the molecular weights of glucose (180) or urea nitrogen (28) by 10. Normal serum values are $Na^+ = 142$ mEq/L, glucose = 90 mg/dL, and urea nitrogen = 12 mg/dL. The serum osmolality, therefore, is:

$$mOsm/kg\,H_2O = 2[142] + \frac{90}{18} + \frac{12}{2.8} = 284 + 5 + 4 = 293$$

The normal range is between 280 and 295 mOsm/kg H_2O (some use the value 285 ± 5 mOsm/kg H_2O). Inside the cell, the major electrolyte that contributes to the osmolality is K^+.

Total Osmolality Versus Effective Osmolality

The term *total serum* or *plasma osmolality* should be distinguished from the term *effective* osmolality or *tonicity*. Tonicity is determined by the concentration of those solutes that remain outside the cell membrane and cause osmosis. Na^+ and glucose remain in the extracellular fluid compartment (see the following text) and cause water movement. These solutes are, therefore, called *effective osmolytes* and thus contribute to plasma tonicity. Mannitol, sorbitol, and glycerol also behave as effective osmolytes. On the other hand, substances that can enter the cell freely do not maintain an osmotic gradient for water movement. Urea can penetrate the membrane easily and therefore does not exert an osmotic force that causes water movement. For this reason, urea is referred to as an *ineffective osmolyte*. Urea, therefore, does not contribute to tonicity. Ethanol and methanol also behave like urea. The contribution of urea is thus not included in the calculation of effective osmolality. Effective osmolality is calculated using the following equation:

$$\text{Effective osmolality}\,(\text{mOsm}\,/\,\text{kg}\;H_2O) = 2[Na] + \frac{\text{glucose}}{18}$$

The normal range for effective osmolality is between 275 and 290 mOsm/kg H_2O.

Isosmotic Versus Isotonic

The term *isosmotic* refers to identical osmolalities of various body fluids, e.g., plasma versus cerebrospinal fluid. However, when discussing osmolalities of solutions used clinically to replace body fluid losses, the terms *isotonic, hypotonic,* or *hypertonic* are used. A solution is considered isotonic if it has the same osmolality as body fluids. When an isotonic solution is given intravenously, it will not cause red blood cells to change in size. However, a hypotonic solution will cause red blood cells to swell, and a hypertonic solution will cause red blood cells to shrink. Isotonic solution that is commonly used to replace loss of body fluids is 0.9% NaCl (normal saline).

Body Fluid Compartments

As stated, the major body fluid is water. In a lean individual, it comprises about 60% of the total body weight. Fat contains less water. Therefore, in obese individuals the water content is 55% of the total body weight. For example, a 70 kg lean person contains 42 L of water ($70 \times 0.6 = 42$ L). This total body water is distributed between two major compartments: the *extracellular fluid* (ECF) and *intracellular fluid* (ICF) compartments. About one-third (20%) of the total amount of water is confined to the ECF and two-thirds (40%) to the ICF compartment (Fig. 1.1). The ECF compartment, in turn, is divided into the following subdivisions:

1. Plasma
2. Interstitial fluid and lymph
3. Bone and dense connective tissue water
4. Transcellular (cerebrospinal, pleural, peritoneal, synovial, and digestive secretions)

Of these subdivisions, the plasma and interstitial fluids are the two most important because of constant exchange of fluid and electrolytes between them. Plasma and interstitial fluid are separated by the capillary endothelium. Plasma circulates in the blood vessels, whereas the interstitial fluid bathes all tissue cells except for the formed elements of blood. For this reason, Claude Bernard, the French physiologist, called

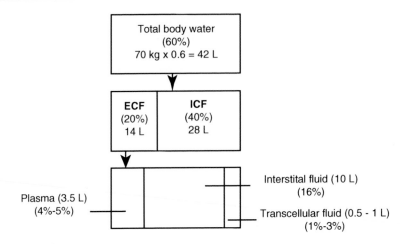

Fig. 1.1 Approximate distribution of water in various body fluid compartments: *ECF* extracellular fluid, *ICF* intracellular fluid. A 70 kg lean man has 42 L of water, assuming the total body water content is 60% of the body weight ($70 \times 0.6 = 42$ L)

the interstitium "the true environment of the body" (*milieu interieur*). Figure 1.1 summarizes the distribution of water in various body fluid compartments.

Water Movement Between ECF and ICF Compartments

In a healthy individual, the ECF and ICF fluids are in osmotic equilibrium. If this equilibrium is disturbed, water moves from the area of lower solute concentration to the area of greater solute concentration in order to reestablish the osmotic equilibrium. The following *Darrow–Yannet* diagram illustrates this point (Fig. 1.2). Let us assume that a lean male weighs 70 kg and the osmolality in both ECF and ICF compartments is 280 mOsm/kg H_2O. His total body water is 60% of the body weight; therefore, the total body water is 42 L. Of this amount, 28 L are in the ICF and 14 L are in the ECF compartment. What happens to osmolality and water distribution in each compartment if we add 1 L of water to the ECF? Initially, this additional 1 L of H_2O would not only increase the ECF volume but it would also decrease its osmolality from 280 to 261 mOsm/kg H_2O (total ECF mOsm ($280 \times 14 = 3{,}920$ mOsm)/new ECF water content (15 L) $= 3{,}920/15 = 261$ mOsm). Since the ICF osmolality is higher than this new ECF osmolality, water will move into the ICF until a new osmotic equilibrium is reached. As a result, the ICF volume also increases. The net result is an increase in volume and a decrease in osmolality in both compartments. These changes are shown in Fig. 1.2.

Thus, addition of 1 L of water to ECF decreases the final osmolality to 273 mOsm/kg H_2O (total body mOsm ($280 \times 42 = 11{,}760$)/new total body water (43 L) $= 11{,}760/43 = 273$ mOsm) and increases water content in the ICF by 0.72 L and ECF by 0.28 L (ICF mOsm ($280 \times 28 = 7{,}840$)/new osmolality (273) $= 7{,}840/273 = 28.72$ L). It should be noted that these changes are minimal in

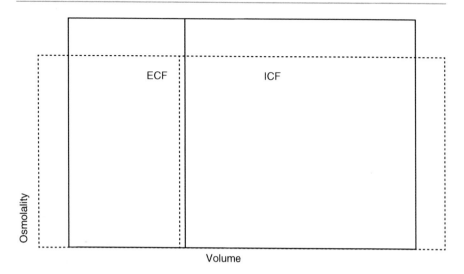

Fig. 1.2 Darrow–Yannet diagram showing fluid and osmolality changes in the ECF and ICF compartments following addition of 1 L of water to the ECF. Initial state is shown by a *solid line* and final state by a *dashed line*. Width represents the volume of the compartments, and height represents osmolality

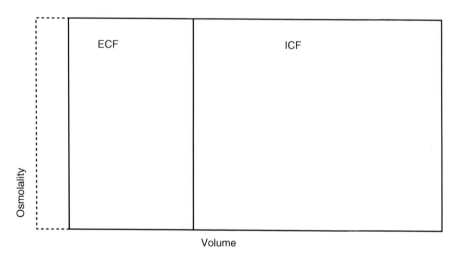

Fig. 1.3 Darrow–Yannet diagram showing volume change following addition of 1 L of isotonic NaCl

an individual with normal renal function, since the kidneys compensate for these changes by excreting excess water in order to maintain fluid balance.

Let us use another example. What would happen if 1 L of isotonic (0.9%) saline is added instead of pure water to ECF? Since 0.9% saline is isotonic, it does not cause water movement. Therefore, body osmolality does not change. However, this isotonic saline will remain in the ECF compartment and cause its expansion, as shown in Fig. 1.3. Healthy individuals excrete saline to maintain normal ECF volume.

Study Questions

Case 1 A 28-year-old type 1 diabetic male patient is admitted to the hospital for nausea, vomiting, and abdominal pain. His weight is 60 kg and the initial laboratory values are:

Na^+ = 146 mEq/L
K^+ = 5 mEq/L
HCO_3^- = 10 mEq/L
BUN = 70 mg/dL
Glucose = 540 mg/dL

Question 1 Calculate this patient's plasma osmolality and explain his fluid shift.

Answer Plasma osmolality is calculated by using the following formula:

$$\text{Plasma osmolality} = 2[\text{Plasma Na}^+] + \frac{\text{Glucose}}{18} + \frac{\text{BUN}}{2.8}$$
$$= 2[146] + \frac{540}{18} + \frac{70}{2.8} = 347 \text{ mOsm / kg H}_2\text{O}$$

Because plasma osmolality is elevated, water initially moves out of cells, i.e., from the ICF to the ECF compartment, and causes expansion of the latter until a new steady state is reached. The patient receives insulin and normal saline. Repeat blood chemistry shows:

Na^+ = 140 mEq/L
K^+ = 4.2 mEq/L
HCO_3^- = 20 mEq/L
BUN = 40 mg/dL
Glucose = 180 mg/dL

Question 2 Does increase in BUN contribute to fluid shift?

Answer No. Although BUN contributes 14 mOsm to plasma osmolality, no fluid shift will occur on its account. The lack of fluid shift is due to its ineffectiveness as an osmole, i.e., urea crosses the cell membrane easily and does not establish a concentration gradient.

Question 3 Calculate this patient's plasma tonicity (effective plasma osmolality).

Answer Tonicity is a measure of the osmotically active particles from Na^+ and glucose. Therefore, the serum concentration of BUN is not included in the calculation. The plasma tonicity is:

$$2[140]+\frac{180}{18} = 290 \text{ mOsm / kg } H_2O$$

Case 2 A 30-year-old patient with AIDS (acquired immunodeficiency syndrome) is admitted for weakness, weight loss, fever, nausea, vomiting, and mental irritability. His blood pressure is low. The diagnosis of Addison's disease (a disease caused by deficiency of glucocorticoid and mineralocorticoid hormones produced by the adrenal cortex) is made. Admitting laboratory values are as follows:

Na^+ = 120 mEq/L
K^+ = 6.2 mEq/L
Cl^- = 112 mEq/L
HCO_3^- = 14 mEq/L
BUN = 70 mg/dL
Glucose = 60 mg/dL

Question 1 Explain the fluid shift in this patient.

Answer This patient lost Na^+ than water from the ECF compartment due to mineralocorticoid (aldosterone) deficiency. As a result of low serum Na^+, his plasma osmolality is low. Decreased plasma osmolality causes water to move from the ECF to the ICF compartment. The net result is the contraction of ECF volume and a transient increase in ICF volume and reduction in osmolality in both compartments, as shown in Fig. 1.4.

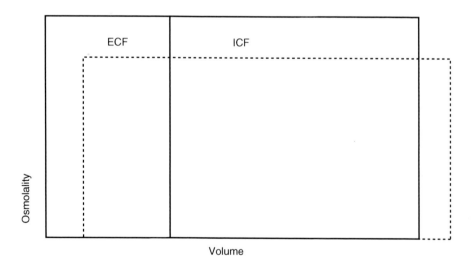

Fig. 1.4 The net result in this patient is the contraction of ECF volume and a transient increase in ICF volume and reduction in osmolality in both compartments. Initial state is represented by *solid line* and final state by *dashed line*

Case 3 A patient on maintenance hemodialysis three times a week for kidney failure is admitted with shortness of breath and a weight gain of 22 lbs. He missed two
treatments (last treatment 6 days ago). His last weight after hemodialysis was 50 kg.
His serum chemistry is as follows:

	After dialysis	On admission
Na^+	140 mEq/L	135 mEq/L
K^+	3.6 mEq/L	5.8 mEq/L
HCO_3^-	28 mEq/L	18 mEq/L
Cl^-	100 mEq/L	106 mEq/L
BUN	40 mg/dL	120 mg/dL
Creatinine	8 mg/dL	12 mg/dL
Effective osmolality	290 mOsm/kg H_2O	282 mOsm/kg H_2O

Question 1   Calculate the following after dialysis and on admission.

(A) Total body water
(B) ICF volume
(C) ECF volume
(D) Total body effective osmoles
(E) ICF effective osmoles
(F) ECF effective osmoles
(G) Serum glucose concentration

Answer After Dialysis

(A) Total body water comprises 60% of body weight. Of this, 40% is in the ICF and
     20% is in the ECF compartment. Total body water (0.6×50 kg) = 30 L
(B) ICF volume (0.4×50 kg) = 20 L
(C) ECF volume (0.2×50 kg) = 10 L
(D) Total body effective osmoles (290×30 L) = 8,700 mOsm/kg H_2O
(E) ICF effective osmoles (290×20 L) = 5,800 mOsm/kg H_2O
(F) ECF effective osmoles (290×10 L) = 2,900 mOsm/kg H_2O
(G) Serum glucose concentration = 180 mg/dL

   Note that only Na^+ and glucose are used to calculate the effective osmolality.
Since Na^+ concentration is 140 mEq/L, its contribution is 280 mOsm. The remaining
10 mOsm are contributed by glucose (1 mOsm = 18 mg or 10 mOsm = 180 mg/dL).
   On Admission

(A) Total body water (0.6×60 kg) = 36 L (The gain of 22 lbs is equal to gaining
     10 kg. Therefore, the body weight on admission is 60 kg.)
(B) ICF volume (0.4×60 kg) = 24 L
(C) ECF volume (0.2×60 kg) = 12 L
(D) Total body effective osmoles (280×36 L) = 10,080 mOsm/kg H_2O

(E) ICF effective osmoles $(280 \times 24 \text{ L}) = 6,720 \text{ mOsm/kg H}_2\text{O}$
(F) ECF effective osmoles $(280 \times 12 \text{ L}) = 3,360 \text{ mOsm/kg H}_2\text{O})$
(G) Serum glucose concentration = 216 mg/dL (1 mOsm = 18 mg or 12 mOsm = 216 mg/dL)

Case 4 In a patient who has been vomiting and has no fluid intake and no blood pressure changes, the volume of all the body fluid compartments:

(A) Increases proportionately
(B) Does not change
(C) Decreases proportionately
(D) Decreases only in the ECF compartment
(E) Increases only in the ICF compartment

The answer is C This patient is dehydrated. In dehydration, water is lost initially from the ECF compartment. This causes an increase in plasma $[\text{Na}^+]$ and thus osmolality. As a result, water moves from the ICF to the ECF compartment to maintain isotonicity between the two compartments. The net result is a decrease in the volume of both the ICF and ECF compartments.

Suggested Reading

1. Arroyo JP, Schweickert AJ. Back to basics in physiology. Fluids in the renal and cardiovascular systems. Amsterdam: Academic; 2013.
2. Fanestil DD. Compartmentation of body water. In: Narins RG, editor. Clinical disorders of fluid and electrolyte metabolism. 5th ed. New York: McGraw-Hill; 1994. p. 3–20.
3. Yoshika T, Iitaka K, Ichikawa I. Body fluid compartments. In: Ichikawa I, editor. Pediatric textbook of fluids and electrolytes. Baltimore: Williams and Wilkins; 1990. p. 14–20.

Interpretation of Urine Electrolytes and Osmolality

2

Measurement of urine Na^+, Cl^-, and K^+ is rather common in hospitalized patients, and these urine electrolytes are useful in the diagnostic evaluation of volume status, hyponatremia, acute kidney injury (AKI), metabolic alkalosis, hypokalemia, and urine anion gap (urine net charge). A spot urine sample is generally adequate for determination of these electrolytes. In addition, urine creatinine is determined to calculate the fractional excretion of Na^+, K^+, or other electrolytes. Also, urine osmolality is helpful in the differential diagnosis of hyponatremia, polyuria, and AKI. Table 2.1 summarizes the clinical applications of urine electrolytes and osmolality.

Table 2.1 Clinical applications of urine electrolytes and osmolality

Electrolyte	Use
Na^+	To assess volume status
	Differential diagnosis of hyponatremia
	Differential diagnosis of AKI
	To assess salt intake in patients with hypertension
	To evaluate calcium and uric acid excretion in stone formers
	To calculate electrolyte-free water clearance
Cl^-	Differential diagnosis of metabolic alkalosis
K^+	Differential diagnosis of dyskalemias
	To calculate electrolyte-free water clearance
Creatinine	To calculate fractional excretion of Na^+, renal failure index, and hypokalemia
	To assess the adequacy of 24 h urine collection
Urine osmolality	Differential diagnosis of hyponatremia
	Differential diagnosis of polyuria
	Differential diagnosis of AKI
Urine anion gap	To distinguish primarily hyperchloremic metabolic acidosis between distal renal tubular acidosis and diarrhea
Electrolyte-free-water clearance	To assess the amount of water excretion (without solutes) only in the management of hypo- and hypernatremia

AKI acute kidney injury

© Springer Science+Business Media LLC 2018
A.S. Reddi, *Fluid, Electrolyte and Acid-Base Disorders*,
DOI 10.1007/978-3-319-60167-0_2

Certain Pertinent Calculations

Fractional Excretion of Na$^+$ (FE$_{Na}$) and Urea Nitrogen (FE$_{Urea}$)

Urine Na$^+$ excretion is influenced by a number of hormonal and other factors. Changes in water excretion by the kidney can result in changes in urine Na$^+$ concentration [Na$^+$]. For example, patients with diabetes insipidus can excrete 10 L of urine per day. Their urine [Na$^+$] may be inappropriately low due to dilution, suggesting the presence of volume depletion. Conversely, increased water reabsorption by the kidney can raise the urine [Na$^+$] and mask the presence of hypovolemia. To correct for water reabsorption, the renal handling of Na$^+$ can be evaluated directly by calculating the FE$_{Na}$, which is defined as the ratio of urine to plasma Na$^+$ divided by the ratio of urine (U$_{Cr}$) to plasma creatinine (P$_{Cr}$), multiplied by 100.

$$FE_{Na}(\%) = \frac{\text{Quantity of Na}^+ \text{ excreted}}{\text{Quantity of Na}^+ \text{ filtered}}$$

$$= \frac{U_{Na} \times P_{Cr}}{P_{Na} \times U_{Cr}} \times 100$$

The FE$_{Na}$ is the excreted fraction of filtered Na$^+$. The major use of FE$_{Na}$ is in patients with AKI. Patients with prerenal azotemia have low (<1%) FE$_{Na}$ compared to patients with acute tubular necrosis (ATN), whose FE$_{Na}$ is generally high (>2%). When ATN is superimposed on decreased effective arterial blood volume due to hepatic cirrhosis or congestive heart failure, the FE$_{Na}$ is <2% because of the intense stimulus to Na$^+$ reabsorption. Similarly, patients with ATN, due to radiocontrast agents or rhabdomyolysis have low FE$_{Na}$ for unknown reasons.

It was shown that FE$_{Na}$ in children with nephrotic syndrome is helpful in the treatment of edema with diuretics. In these patients, FE$_{Na}$ <0.2% is indicative of volume contraction, and >0.2% is suggestive of volume expansion. Therefore, patients with FE$_{Na}$ >0.2% can be treated with diuretics to improve edema.

The FE$_{Na}$ is substantially altered in patients on diuretics. In these patients, the FE$_{Na}$ is usually high despite hypoperfusion of the kidneys. In such patients, the FE$_{Urea}$ may be helpful. In euvolemic subjects, the FE$_{Urea}$ ranges between 50% and 65%. In a hypovolemic individual, the FE$_{Urea}$ is <35%. Thus, a low FE$_{Urea}$ seems to identify those individuals with renal hypoperfusion despite the use of a diuretic.

Fractional Excretion of Uric Acid (FE$_{UA}$) and Phosphate (FE$_{PO4}$)

Uric acid excretion is increased in patients with hyponatremia due to syndrome of inappropriate antidiuretic hormone (SIADH) secretion or syndrome of inappropriate antidiuresis (SIAD) and cerebral salt wasting. As a result, serum uric acid level in both conditions is low (<4 mg/dL). Since serum uric acid levels are altered by volume changes, it is better to use FE$_{UA}$. In both SIADH and cerebral salt wasting,

FE_{UA} is >10% (normal 5–10%). In order to distinguish these conditions, FE_{PO4} is used. In SIADH, the FE_{PO4} is <20% (normal <20%), and it is >20% in cerebral salt wasting.

Urine Potassium (U_K) and Urine Creatinine (U_{Cr}) Ratio

In a healthy individual, determination of urine [K^+] reflects the amount of daily dietary K^+ intake. When dietary K^+ intake is reduced, the urinary excretion of K^+ falls below 15 mEq or mmol/day. Since a 24-h urine collection is not feasible all the time, the excretion of urinary K^+ can be obtained from a random urine sample to evaluate dyskalemias (hypo- or hyperkalemia) by calculating U_K/U_{Cr} ratio. In a hypokalemic patient with transcellular distribution, extrarenal (gastrointestinal) loss, or poor dietary intake of K^+, the U_K/U_{Cr} ratio is <15 mmol K^+/g creatinine or <1.5 mmol K^+/mmol creatinine (1 mg creatinine = 88.4 μmol/L or 0.0884 mmol/L). This ratio is >200 mmol K^+/g creatinine or >20 mmol K^+/mmol creatinine in a patient with hypokalemia and normal renal function, which is suggestive of renal loss.

In a patient with chronic hyperkalemia due to K^+ secretion defect, the U_K/U_{Cr} ratio is also low. In such cases, a 24-h urine collection is needed to quantify daily K^+ excretion.

Urine Anion Gap

Urine anion gap (U_{AG}) is an indirect measure of NH_4^+ excretion, which is not routinely determined in the clinical laboratory. However, it is measured by determining the urine concentrations of Na^+, K^+, and Cl^- and is calculated as [Na^+] + [K^+] − [Cl^-]. In general, NH_4^+ is excreted with Cl^-. A normal individual has a negative (from 0 to − 50) U_{AG} ($Cl^- > Na^+ + K^+$), suggesting adequate excretion of NH_4^+. On the other hand, a positive (from 0 to + 50) U_{AG} ($Na^+ + K^+ > Cl^-$) indicates a defect in NH_4 excretion. The U_{AG} is used clinically to distinguish primarily hyperchloremic metabolic acidosis due to distal renal tubular acidosis (RTA) and diarrhea. Both conditions cause normal anion gap metabolic acidosis and hypokalemia. Although the urine pH is always >6.5 in distal RTA, it is variable in patients with diarrhea because of unpredictable volume changes. The U_{AG} is always positive in patients with distal RTA, indicating reduced NH_4^+ excretion, whereas, it is negative in patients with diarrhea because these patients can excrete adequate amounts of NH_4^+. Also, positive U_{AG} is observed in acidoses that are characterized by low NH_4^+ excretion (type 4 RTA).

In situations such as diabetic ketoacidosis, NH_4^+ is excreted with ketones rather than Cl^-, resulting in decreased urinary [Cl^-]. This results in a positive rather than a negative U_{AG}, indicating decreased excretion of NH_4^+. Thus, the U_{AG} may not be that helpful in situations of ketonuria. Table 2.2 summarizes the interpretation of urinary electrolytes in various pathophysiologic conditions.

Table 2.2 Interpretations of urine electrolytes

Condition	Electrolyte (mEq/L)	Diagnostic possibilities
Hypovolemia	Na^+ (0–20)	Extrarenal loss of Na^+
	Na^+ (>20)	Renal salt wasting
		Adrenal insufficiency
		Diuretic use or osmotic diuresis
Acute kidney injury	Na^+ (0–20)	Prerenal azotemia
	Na^+ (>20)	Acute tubular necrosis (ATN)
	FE_{Na} (<1%)	Prerenal azotemia
		ATN due to contrast agent rhabdomyolysis
	FE_{Na} (>2%)	ATN
		Diuretic use
Hyponatremia	Na^+ (0–20)	Hypovolemia
		Edematous disorders
		Water intoxication
	Na^+ (>20)	SIADH
		Cerebral salt wasting (CSW)
		Adrenal insufficiency
	↑FE_{UA} (>10%)	SIADH and CSW
	↑FE_{PO4} (>20%)	CSW
Metabolic alkalosis	Cl^- (0–10)	Cl^--responsive alkalosis
	Cl^- (>20)	Cl^--resistant alkalosis
Hypokalemia (U_K/U_{Cr} ratio)	<1.5 mmol K^+/mmol creatinine	Extrarenal, cellular shift, or poor dietary intake of K^+
	>20 mmol K^+/mmol creatinine	Renal loss of K^+
U_{AG}	Positive (from 0 to +50)	Distal renal tubular acidosis
	Negative (from 0 to −50)	Diarrhea (U_{AG} is negative in normal subject)

SIADH syndrome of inappropriate antidiuretic hormone

Electrolyte-Free Water Clearance

Electrolyte-free-water clearance ($T^e_{H_2O}$) is the amount of water present in the urine that is free of solutes, i.e., the amount of water excreted in the urine. Determination of $T^e_{H_2O}$ is helpful in the assessment of serum [Na^+] in hypernatremia and hyponatremia. For example, hypernatremia may not improve despite volume replacement because the exact amount of free water that is reabsorbed or excreted is not known.

In order to quantify how much electrolyte-free water is being reabsorbed or excreted, the following formula can be used:

$$T^e_{H_2O} = V\frac{\left[U_{Na} + U_K\right]}{\left[P_{Na}\right]} - 1,$$

where V is the total urine volume, and P_{Na} is the plasma [Na$^+$]. $T^e_{H_2O}$ can be positive or negative. Positive $T^e_{H_2O}$ means that less water was reabsorbed in the nephron segments, resulting in hypernatremia. On the other hand, negative $T^e_{H_2O}$ indicates that the nephron segments reabsorbed more water with resultant hyponatremia.

Urine Specific Gravity Versus Urine Osmolality

Clinically, estimation of specific gravity is useful in the evaluation of urine concentration and dilution. It is defined as the ratio of the weight of a solution to the weight of an equal volume of water. The specific gravity of plasma is largely determined by the protein concentration and to a lesser extent by the other solutes. For this reason, plasma is about 8–10% heavier than pure distilled water. Therefore, the specific gravity of plasma varies from 1.008 to 1.010 compared to the specific gravity of distilled water, which is 1.000. Urine specific gravity can range from 1.001 to 1.035. A value of 1.005 or less indicates preservation of normal diluting ability, and a value of 1.020 or higher indicates normal concentrating ability of the kidney.

Osmolality measures only the number of particles present in a solution. On the other hand, the specific gravity determines not only the number but also weight of the particles in a solution. Urine specific gravity and urine osmolality usually change in parallel. For example, a urine specific gravity of 1.020–1.030 corresponds to a urine osmolality of 800–1,200 mOsm/kg H_2O. Similarly, the specific gravity of 1.005 is generally equated to an osmolality < 100 mOsm/kg H_2O. This relationship between the specific gravity and osmolality is disturbed when the urine contains an abnormal solute, such as glucose or protein. As a result, the specific gravity increases disproportionately to the osmolality. In addition to these substances, radiocontrast material also increases the specific gravity disproportionately.

Measurement of urine specific gravity or osmolality is useful in the assessment of volume status, in the differential diagnosis of AKI, polyuria (urination of 3–5 L/day), and hyponatremia. A volume-depleted individual with normal renal function is able to concentrate his or her urine, and, therefore, the specific gravity or osmolality will be greater than 1.020 or 800 mOsm/kg H_2O, respectively. Table 2.3 shows approximate urine osmolalities in various clinical situations.

Table 2.3 Urine osmolalities in various clinical conditions

Condition	Approximate osmolality (mOsm/Kg H_2O)	Comment
Normal	50–1,200	Normal urine dilution and concentration
AKI–prerenal azotemia	>400	Increased water reabsorption by nephron segments
AKI–acute tubular necrosis	<400	Injured tubules cannot reabsorb all the filtered water
SIADH	>200	Excess water reabsorption by distal nephron
Hydrochlorothiazide treatment	>200	Inability to dilute urine
Furosemide	~300 (isosthenuria)	Inability to concentrate and dilute urine
Osmotic diuresis	>300 (usually urine osmolality>plasma osmolality)	Excretion of excess osmoles
Central diabetes insipidus (DI)	≤100	Lack of ADH
Nephrogenic DI	<300	ADH resistance
Psychogenic polydipsia	~50	Decreased medullary hypertonicity

ADH antidiuretic hormone, *AKI* acute kidney injury, *SIADH* syndrome of inappropriate antidiuretic hormone secretion

---

Study Questions

Case 1 A 60-year-old male patient with congestive heart failure (CHF) is admitted for chest pain. He is on several medications, including a loop diuretic. The patient develops acute kidney injury following cardiac catheterization with creatinine increase from 1.5 to 3.5 mg/dL. His urinalysis shows many renal tubular cells and occasional renal tubular cell casts, suggesting ATN.

Question 1 What would his FE_{Na} be?

Answer In ATN, the FE_{Na} should be >2%. However, in a patient with CHF, there is increased Na^+ reabsorption in the proximal tubule. Despite ATN, such a patient excretes less Na^+ in the urine and the FE_{Na} is usually <1%. Other conditions of ATN with low FE_{Na}(<1%) are contrast agents and rhabdomyolysis.

Question 2 How does FE_{urea} help in this patient?

Answer The patient is on a loop diuretic. In order to know the volume status in a patient on diuretic, FE_{Na} may not be that helpful. Instead, FE_{urea} distinguishes volume contraction from volume expansion. In volume contracted patient due to diuretics, FE_{urea} is <35%.

Case 2 A 20-year-old female patient is admitted for weakness, dizziness, and fatigue. Her serum K^+ is 2.8 mEq/L and HCO_3^- is 15 mEq/L. An arterial blood gas revealed a nonanion gap metabolic acidosis. Her urine pH is 6.5.

Question 1 Discuss the clinical application of U_{AG}.

Answer Two major causes of nonanion gap metabolic acidosis with hypokalemia are diarrhea and distal RTA. The urine pH is always >6.5 in distal RTA and mostly acidic in diarrhea unless the patient is severely volume depleted. In this patient, determination of the U_{AG} will distinguish diarrhea from distal RTA.

The U_{AG} is an indirect measure of NH_4^+ excretion. It is calculated as the sum of urinary $[Na^+]$ plus $[K^+]$ minus $[Cl^-]$. Normal U_{AG} is zero to negative, suggesting adequate excretion of NH_4^+. In patients with distal RTA, NH_4^+ excretion is decreased, and the U_{AG} is always positive. In metabolic acidosis caused by diarrhea, the U_{AG} is negative. Thus, the U_{AG} is helpful in the differential diagnosis of hyperchloremic metabolic acidosis. Upon questioning, the patient admitted to laxative abuse.

Case 3 A 32-year-old male patient is referred for evaluation of hypokalemia. His serum $[K^+]$ is 3.1 mEq/L. He is not on any diuretic. His blood pressure is normal.

Question 1 How does U_K/U_{Cr} ratio help in the evaluation of hypokalemia in this patient?

Answer If the U_K/U_{Cr} ratio is <1.5 mmol K^+/mmol creatinine, the cause for his hypokalemia is either poor dietary intake, cellular shift, or extrarenal loss of K^+. On the other hand, if the ratio is >20 mmol K^+/mmol creatinine, the patient has renal loss of K^+. Thus, the U_K/U_{Cr} ratio distinguishes renal from extrarenal loss of K^+, which is helpful in the management of hypokalemia.

Suggested Reading

1. Kamel KS, Halperin ML. Intrarenal urea cycling leads to a higher rate of renal excretion of potassium: an hypothesis with clinical implications. Curr Opin Nephrol Hypertens. 2011;20:547–54.
2. Kamel KS, Ethier JH, Richardson RMA, et al. Urine electrolytes and osmolality: when and how to use them. Am J Nephrol. 1990;10:89–102.
3. Harrington JT, Cohen JJ. Measurement of urinary electrolytes-indications and limitations. N Engl J Med. 1975;293:1241–3.
4. Schrier RW. Diagnostic value of urinary sodium, chloride, urea, and flow. J Am Soc Nephrol. 2011;22:1610–3.

Renal Handling of NaCl and Water

3

The kidneys filter about 180 L of plasma daily. Most of this plasma must be reclaimed in order to maintain fluid and electrolyte homeostasis. The protein-free ultrafiltrate is modified in composition as it passes through various segments of the nephron to form urine. Sodium (Na^+) and its anion chloride (Cl^-) are the major determinants of the extracellular fluid (ECF) volume, and both ions are effectively reabsorbed. Water reabsorption follows Na^+ reabsorption in order to maintain normal osmolality in the ECF compartment. The proximal tubule is the major site of reclamation, whereas the other segments reclaim to a variable degree.

Proximal Tubule

The proximal tubule, as a whole, reabsorbs about 60–70% of the filtered NaCl and water and thus plays a major role in the maintenance of ECF volume. For the purpose of clear understanding, the proximal tubule can be arbitrarily divided into two zones of reabsorption. Reabsorption of Na^+, glucose, amino acids, lactate, and HCO_3^- occurs primarily in the first half (early) of the proximal tubule, while Cl^- is predominantly reabsorbed in the second half (late) of the proximal tubule. Reabsorption of Cl^- is coupled with that of Na^+.

Na⁺ Reabsorption

The kidney filters approximately 25,200 mEq (glomerular filtration rate (GFR)×serum Na^+ concentration: 180 L×140 mEq/L=25,200 mEq/day) of Na^+ daily. Of this amount, the proximal tubule reabsorbs 15,120–17,640 mEq (60–70%). Na^+ is transported across the apical membrane by two basic mechanisms: *passive* and *active*. Passive entry of Na^+ into the proximal tubule occurs down its electrochemical gradient because the luminal Na^+ concentration is approximately

© Springer Science+Business Media LLC 2018
A.S. Reddi, *Fluid, Electrolyte and Acid-Base Disorders*,
DOI 10.1007/978-3-319-60167-0_3

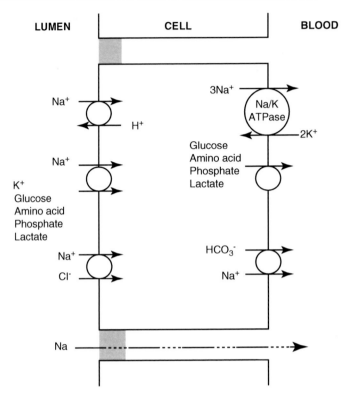

Fig. 3.1 Cellular model for Na$^+$ entry into the first half (early part) of the proximal tubule. Note that many of these mechanisms are also present in the second half (later part) of the proximal tubule. Passive transport of Na$^+$ is indicated by *broken arrow*

140 mEq/L compared to 14–15 mEq/L inside the cell. This gradient is maintained mostly by the action of Na/K-ATPase at the basolateral membrane.

Na$^+$ also moves into the cell by two active mechanisms. One mechanism involves coupling of Na$^+$ with a variety of solutes such as glucose, amino acids, lactate, and phosphate (Fig. 3.1). This cotransport creates a negative potential difference of 4 mV in the tubule, which, in turn, is partly responsible for passive diffusion of Na$^+$ across the membrane. The transport of organic solutes is so avid that they are completely removed from the lumen in the first half of the proximal tubule.

Another active mechanism of Na$^+$ entry is through the Na/H exchanger, which pumps Na$^+$ into and H$^+$ out of the cell. It is this exchanger that is responsible for most H$^+$ secretion and Na$^+$ reabsorption in the proximal tubule. During the process of H$^+$ secretion, HCO$_3^-$ is generated and reabsorbed (see Fig. 3.1). Na/H exchanger is mediated by the NHE3 (sodium–hydrogen exchanger isoform 3) protein. Inhibition of Na/H exchanger by acetazolamide decreases NaCl reabsorption.

Na$^+$ extrusion from the cell into the peritubular capillaries is accomplished by the Na/K-ATPase, which transports three Na$^+$ ions out and two K$^+$ ions into the cell. In this way, the intracellular Na$^+$ concentration in the proximal tubule is maintained around 15–35 mEq/L. In addition, Na$^+$ also exits with Na/HCO$_3$ cotransporter. The organic solutes leave the cell by passive transport mechanisms.

Cl⁻ Reabsorption

The second phase of NaCl reabsorption occurs in the late portion of the proximal tubule. As with Na⁺, reabsorption of Cl⁻ occurs by both *active* and *passive* transport mechanisms. There are no Cl⁻ transporters in the early proximal tubule. Therefore, the concentration of Cl⁻ increases as the filtrate moves along the proximal tubule. Thus, the active transport of Cl⁻ becomes dominant in the late proximal tubule. Cl⁻ entry occurs via Na/Cl cotransport as well as an exchange between the luminal Cl⁻ and cellular anions such as formate, oxalate, sulfate, or HCO_3^-. Although the tubular concentrations of either formate or oxalate are substantially low, they combine with the H⁺ secreted by the Na/H exchanger to form formic acid or oxalic acid in the lumen. These acids are converted into their bases inside the cell, which then return to the tubular lumen via Cl/formate or Cl/oxalate exchangers (Fig. 3.2). Thus, a substantial amount of Na⁺ and Cl⁻ is reabsorbed through Na/H and other exchangers.

Passive Cl⁻ reabsorption occurs via the tight junctions. Because of reabsorption of glucose and amino acids, the lumen becomes slightly negative with the development of an electrical gradient. This lumen-negative voltage favors passive Cl⁻ reabsorption. Paracellular Cl⁻ transport is a major mechanism for Cl⁻ reabsorption. Cl⁻ leaves the cell via Cl⁻ conductance channel and K/Cl cotransporter.

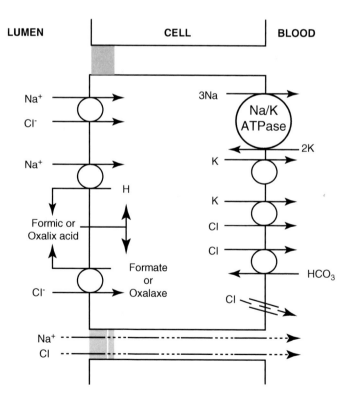

Fig. 3.2 Cellular model for Na⁺ coupled Cl⁻ entry into the second half (later part) of the proximal tubule. Note that many of these transport mechanisms are also present in the first half of the proximal tubule. *Broken arrow* at the basolateral membrane indicates Cl⁻ conductance channel

Thin Limbs of Henle's Loop

The fluid that leaves the proximal tubule and enters the thin descending limb (TDL) of Henle's loop is isosmotic (about 300 mOsm/kg H_2O) to plasma. The TDL is highly permeable to water and relatively less permeable to solutes (Na^+, Cl^-, K^+, and urea). Water, therefore, moves out of the tubule into the surrounding interstitium. The TDL is abundant in aquaporin (AQP)-1 water channel proteins. As a result, the concentration of the tubular fluid increases. In long-looped nephrons, the tubular fluid osmolality increases gradually from 300 to 1,200 mOsm/kg H_2O at the tip of the papilla. The transport characteristics of the thin ascending limb (TAL) of Henle's loop are different from those of the TDL. The TAL is impermeable to water, moderately permeable to urea, and highly permeable to NaCl. Urea diffuses into and NaCl diffuses out of the tubular lumen. Since water does not diffuse out, the tubular fluid is diluted and the osmolality decreases. The decreased osmolality of the tubular fluid creates a large osmolality difference between the tubular lumen and the surrounding medullary interstitium, which has a high osmolality.

Thick ascending limb of Henle's loop

About 30% of the filtered NaCl is reabsorbed into the thick ascending limb of the Henle's loop (TALH). The TALH is virtually impermeable to water but highly permeable to NaCl. This combination of virtually low permeability to water and high reabsorptive rates of NaCl makes the tubular fluid more dilute with a low NaCl concentration. Because the tubular fluid is diluted (hypotonic) in the TALH, it is often referred to as the *diluting segment*. The osmolality of the tubular fluid at the end of the TALH is about half (150 mOsm/kg H_2O) of that of plasma. Both TAL and TALH lack aquaporins.

The reabsorption of NaCl at the apical membrane occurs by a secondary active transport process. The principal transporter, called the Na/K/2Cl cotransporter, transports one Na^+, one K^+, and two Cl^- into the cell (Fig. 3.3). Because of Cl^- movement, the tubular lumen has a positive potential difference as opposed to the negative potential difference in the proximal tubule. Also, the K^+ that enters the cells diffuses back into the tubular lumen via ROMK (renal outer medullary potassium) channels. It is important that K^+ be returned to the tubular lumen for reabsorption of Na^+ via the Na/K/2Cl cotransporter. When this recycling of K^+ is inhibited by blocking ROMK channel, NaCl transport decreases substantially.

Three types of K^+ channels have been identified: a low-conductance 30 pS (picosiemens) channel, an intermediate 70-pS channel, and a high-conductance calcium-activated maxi K^+ channel; the latter participates little to the net K^+ transport. Thus, 30 pS and 70 pS channels make up the ROMK and account for most of the K^+ that diffuses into the lumen in the TALH.

The exit of Cl^- at the basolateral membrane is accomplished by two mechanisms. One involves the exit through conductive Cl^- channel, and this movement is facilitated by the negative intracellular voltage. The second mechanism involves coupling of Cl^- with K^+ and their exit as K/Cl cotransport (see Fig. 3.3). Several

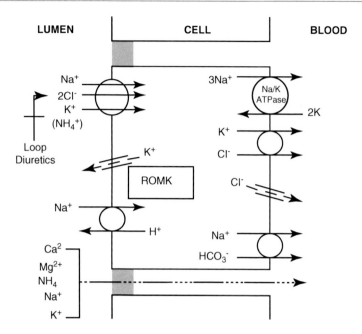

Fig. 3.3 Cellular model for Na/K/2Cl cotransport and for the transport of other cations in the thick ascending limb of Henle's loop. *Broken arrows* indicate diffusion of respective ions through specific conductance channels. *ROMK* renal outer medullary potassium channel. Note that loop diuretics inhibit Na/K/2Cl cotransporter

Cl^- conductance (ClC) channels have been identified. Of these, ClC-ka and ClC-kb are expressed at the basolateral membranes of TALH and TAL. ClC-ks require another protein called *barttin* for their expression in these segments of the nephron. It is the ClC-kb/barttin channel that mediates most of the Cl^- efflux across the basolateral membrane of the TALH.

In addition to NaCl, many cations such as Ca^{2+}, Mg^{2+}, and NH_4^+ are reabsorbed in the TALH. This reabsorption occurs mainly through the tight junctions and intercellular pathways (see Fig. 3.3). The driving force for this paracellular pathway seems to be the positive transepithelial potential difference created by two Cl^- and one Na^+ transport and also by backleak of K^+ into the tubular lumen. Blocking of this K^+ recycling inhibits both Ca^{2+} and Mg^{2+} reabsorption. NH_4^+ can replace K^+ and enter the cell through Na/K/2Cl cotransporter.

Another mechanism for Na^+ transport is the Na/H exchanger (NHE3), which is located in the apical membrane of the TALH. As in the proximal tubule, this mechanism generates HCO_3^- in the TALH and exits via Na/HCO$_3$ cotransporter.

Distal Tubule

In this section, the early and late distal convoluted tubule (DCT) and the connecting tubule (CNT) are discussed together as the distal tubule. The DCT represents the segment of the nephron beyond the macula densa. Both DCT and CNT reabsorb

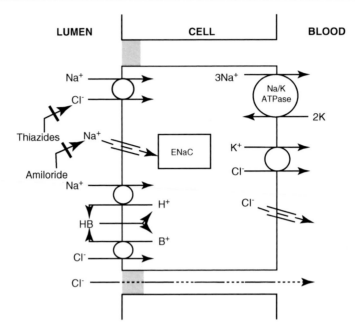

Fig. 3.4 Cellular model for NaCl reabsorption in the distal convoluted tubule cell. Note the thiazide-sensitive Na/Cl cotransporter and amiloride-inhibitable epithelial Na⁺ channel (ENaC). ROMK is not shown in the figure. *Broken arrows* indicate transport through specific conductance channels. Similar mechanisms exist for NaCl transport in the connecting tubule cell. *ENaC* epithelial Na⁺ channel, *B⁻* base, *HB* neutral acid

approximately 10% of the filtered load of NaCl. Na⁺ is actively transported across the apical membrane by three mechanisms (Fig. 3.4). First, NaCl reabsorption occurs by an electroneutral Na/Cl cotransporter, which is inhibited by a thiazide diuretic. Second, Na⁺ enters the cell by an electrogenic epithelial Na⁺ channel (ENaC). The ENaC consists of three homologous subunits (α, β, and γ). All three subunits are required for ENaC activity. This Na⁺ reabsorption via ENaC creates a negative potential difference in the lumen, which drives some Cl⁻ across the paracellular pathway and K⁺ secretion via ROMK channel. Na⁺ transport through ENaC is inhibited by amiloride. Third, NaCl transport involves parallel Na/H exchanger and Cl/base exchanger with the recycling of H⁺ and base. The base exchanged with Cl⁻ appears to be either formate or oxalate. Na⁺ leaves the cell via Na/K-ATPase. It is suggested that Na⁺ reabsorption in the early DCT is largely mediated by Na/Cl cotransporter, while Na⁺ reabsorption in the late DCT is largely mediated by the ENaC. Cl⁻ and K⁺ are transported across the basolateral membrane by Cl⁻ and K⁺ conductance channels. The DCT is impermeable to water.

The mechanisms for NaCl transport in CNT seem to be similar to those of the DCT, except for the ENaC which is the primary Na⁺ transport pathway in CNT. Studies have shown that Na⁺ reabsorption via ENaC is tenfold higher in CNT than in cortical collecting duct. Na⁺ reabsorption facilitates K⁺ secretion via ROMK channel (not shown in Fig. 3.4).

Collecting Duct

The collecting duct is divided into the cortical collecting duct (CCD), the outer medullary collecting duct (OMCD), and the inner medullary collecting duct (IMCD). These segments of the collecting duct help regulate the urinary excretion of Na^+, K^+, H^+, water, and urea. Compared to other parts of the nephron, the collecting duct, on the whole, reabsorbs only 2–3% of the filtered Na^+.

The collecting duct consists of principal and intercalated cells. These cells are morphologically and functionally different. Principal cells are primarily involved in Na^+ reabsorption and K^+ secretion, whereas type A intercalated cells are responsible for H^+ secretion and type B cells for HCO_3^- secretion.

In principal cells, Na^+ enters the cell across the apical membrane through amiloride-sensitive ENaC and is then pumped across the basolateral membrane by Na/K-ATPase (Fig. 3.5). The conductive entry of Na^+ generates a lumen-negative potential difference, and this potential difference causes three important processes to occur: (1) secretion of K^+ into the lumen via low conductance and Ca^{2+}-activated maxi-K ROMK channel, (2) Cl^- reabsorption through paracellular pathway, and (3) H^+ secretion in adjacent type A intercalated cells. The ENaC is inhibited by amiloride. K^+ secretion into the lumen is inhibited by barium and not by amiloride. However, amiloride decreases K^+ secretion indirectly by inhibiting ENaC.

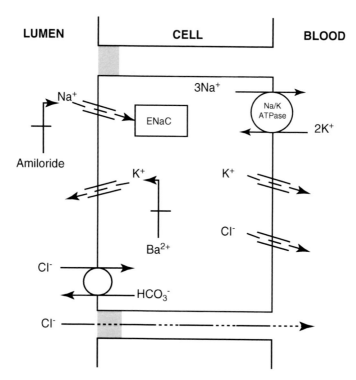

Fig. 3.5 Cellular model for NaCl transport in the principal cell of the cortical collecting duct. *Broken arrows* indicate transport through specific conductive channels. *ENaC* epithelial sodium channel

Cl⁻ reabsorption occurs mainly through the paracellular pathway which is due to the large lumen-negative potential difference generated by Na⁺ transport, as described above. Transcellular Cl⁻ transport mechanism has also been described via an apical Cl/HCO₃ exchanger. The exit of Cl⁻ across the basolateral membrane occurs through Cl⁻ conductive channels (ClC-kb/barttin).

Na⁺ transport in the outer stripe of the outer medulla occurs via ENaC, however, at a much slower rate than in the CCD. The inner stripe of the outer medulla lacks principal cells; as a result, Na⁺ reabsorption does not occur in this segment of the nephron.

The cells of the IMCD function like principal cells of the CCD. These cells reabsorb Na⁺ through ENaC. The transport of Na⁺ creates a negative potential in the lumen, which promotes Cl⁻ reabsorption via the paracellular pathway. The presence of a Na/K/2Cl cotransporter in the basolateral membrane of the IMCD with secretion rather than reabsorption of Na⁺ into the cell is notable.

Water Reabsorption

Proximal Tubule

About 60% of filtered water is reabsorbed in the proximal tubule, which is highly permeable to water. Water reabsorption occurs by transcellular and paracellular pathways with the former being the dominant pathway. Evidence indicates that water reabsorption is secondary to the reabsorption of NaCl. In the early proximal tubule, the rate of solute reabsorption is faster than the rate of water reabsorption, which generates hypotonicity in the lumen and slight hypertonicity in the blood. Although this osmolality gradient is small (3–4 mOsm), it is probably sufficient to promote water reabsorption transcellularly. Water transport also occurs via the tight junctions. Some of the solute that enters the intercellular space through transcellular and paracellular pathways raises the osmolality of the intercellular space, which then drives water across the basement membrane into the interstitium and peritubular capillaries.

Rapid water transport across the proximal tubule is due to AQP-1 water channels, which are expressed in both the apical and basolateral membrane of the proximal tubule cell. It is estimated that the proximal tubule cell contains over 20 million copies of AQP-1.

Water reabsorption follows solute reabsorption throughout the proximal tubule. This reabsorption is isosmotic because the concentration of luminal Na⁺ does not change due to concomitant reabsorption of water. The osmolality of the proximal tubular fluid is similar to that of plasma (285 mOsm). In isosmotic reabsorption, for each 285 mOsm reabsorption of solute, approximately 1 L of water is reabsorbed.

Loop of Henle

As mentioned earlier, the segments of the loop of Henle have different characteristics for water transport. TDL is highly permeable to water because of abundant

AQP-1 water channels. In contrast, the TAL and TALH are impermeable to water and lack water channels. As a result, the osmolality of the tubular fluid declines from TAL to TALH (from 1,000 to 100 mOsm).

Distal Nephron

Water reabsoption is variable in different segments of the distal tubule and is dependent on the presence or absence of ADH. ADH promotes water reabsorption via AQP-2 water channel located in the apical membrane and AQP-3 and AQP-4 water channels located in the basolateral membrane of the principle cell. In the absence of ADH, the segments of the distal nephron reabsorb very little water, resulting in water diuresis (see Chap. 11).

Effect of Various Hormones on NaCl and Water Reabsorption (Transport)

Table 3.1 summarizes the effects of various hormones on NaCl and water reabsorption by the renal tubules. Most of the hormones except aldosterone exert their effects within minutes. The action of aldosterone cannot be observed for at least an hour. Therefore, it seems unlikely that aldosterone plays a significant role in the rapid regulation of NaCl excretion.

Table 3.1 Actions of hormones on NaCl and water reabsorption (transport) by various segments of the nephron

Nephron segment	Hormone	Effect on reabsorption (transport) of	
		NaCl	Water
Proximal tubule	Angiotensin II	↑	↑
	Glucocorticoids	↑	↑
	Atrial natriuretic peptide (ANP)	↓	↓
	Parathyroid hormone	↑	↑
Thick ascending limb	Aldosterone	↑	UK
	ADH	↑	UK
Cortical collecting duct	ADH	↑	↑
	Aldosterone	↑	UK
	Bradykinin	↓	UK
	Digitalis-like factor	↓	UK
	PGE$_2$	↓	UK
Outer medullary collecting duct	ADH	UK	↑
Inner medullary collecting duct	ADH	UK	↑
	Aldosterone	↑	UK
	ANP	↓	↓

UK unknown, *ADH* antidiuretic hormone, ↑ increase, ↓ decrease

Table 3.2 Inherited disorders of NaCl transport mechanisms in segments of the nephron

Segment and involved transporter	Disease	Some clinical features	Inheritance
Thick ascending limb			
Apical Na/K/2Cl cotransporter	Neonatal Bartter syndrome type 1	Hypokalemia, metabolic alkalosis, hypercalciuria, hypotension	AR
Apical K channel (ROMK)	Neonatal Bartter syndrome type 2	Hypokalemia, metabolic alkalosis, hypotension	AR
Basolateral Cl channel (ClC-kb)	Classic Bartter syndrome type 3 (infantile)	Hypokalemia, metabolic alkalosis, hypotension, or normal BP	AR
Basolateral Cl channel (ClC-kb/barttin)	Bartter syndrome type 4	Hypokalemia, metabolic alkalosis, hypotension, sensorineural deafness	AR
Activation of basolateral $Ca^{2}+$-sensing receptor	Bartter syndrome type 5	Salt wasting, hypokalemia, metabolic alkalosis, hypercalciuria	AD
Distal convoluted tubule			
Apical Na/Cl cotransporter	Gitelman syndrome	Hypokalemia, metabolic alkalosis, hypocalciuria, normal to low BP	AR
Apical Na/Cl cotransporter	Gordon syndrome (Pseudohypoaldosteronism type II)	Hyperkalemia, metabolic acidosis, hypertension (responsive to thiazide diuretics)	AD
Cortical collecting duct			
Apical epithelial Na^+ channel (ENaC)	Liddle syndrome	Hypokalemia, metabolic alkalosis, low renin and aldosterone levels, hypertension (responsive to amiloride)	AD
Apical ENaC	Pseudohypoaldosteronism type I	Hyperkalemia, metabolic acidosis, hypotension	AD AR

↑ increase, ↓ decrease, *AD* autosomal dominant, *AR* autosomal recessive, *ROMK* renal outer medullary potassium channel

Disorders of NaCl Transport Mechanisms

Genetic studies have shown that mutations in several genes that encode various transporters in NaCl reabsorption in the nephron induce diseases with different clinical features. Table 3.2 summarizes abnormalities in transporters that involve in NaCl transport and associated disease conditions.

Study Questions

Case 1 A 40-year-old construction worker is brought to the emergency department for a scorpion bite. It is known that scorpion venom contains several inhibitors of ion channels, including K^+ channels. Which one of the following ion movements is mostly affected, if there is K^+ recycling in the thick ascending limb of Henle's loop (TALH)?

(A) HCO_3^-
(B) Ca^{2+} and Mg^{2+}
(C) Phosphate
(D) Cl^-
(E) Glucose

The answer is B K^+ recycling is important for Na/K/2Cl transport in the TALH. If this is selectively poisoned, not only this transport mechanism but also the transport of Ca^{2+} and Mg^{2+} is inhibited. Because of K^+ recycling, the lumen becomes positive. As a result, other positively charged ions (cations) such as Ca^{2+} and Mg^{2+} are transported into the cell passively via the tight junctions. Inhibition of K^+ recycling results in hypocalcemia and hypomagnesemia. Thus, choice B is correct. Reabsorption of HCO_3^-, glucose, and Cl^- alone are not directly connected to K^+ recycling.

Case 2 A healthy individual participates in a hotdog competition and eats dozens of hot dogs. After eating these salt-loaded hot dogs, he drinks 4–5 L of water. His weight increases by 5 kg.

Question 1 How do the kidneys handle Na^+ and water balance?

Answer Excess salt intake causes a transient increase in extracellular volume, which raises cardiac output. Because the sympathetic nervous system and renin-AII-aldosterone system are inhibited, renal blood flow and glomerular filtration rate increase. Also, ADH levels decrease. At the same time, volume overload enhances the secretion of ANP. Because of these hormonal changes, Na^+, Cl^-, and water reabsorption decrease, resulting in enhanced excretion. Increased excretion of Na^+, Cl^-, and water restores euvolemia.

Suggested Reading

1. Gamba G, Wang SL. Sodium chloride transport in the loop of Henle, distal convoluted tubule, and collecting duct. In: Alpern RJ, Moe OW, Caplan M, editors. Seldin and Giebisch's the kidney. Physiology and pathophysiology. 5th ed. San Diego: Academic Press (Elsevier); 2013. p. 1143–79.
2. Martin-Eauclaire M-F, Bougis PE. Potassium channels blockers from the venom of Androctonus mauretanicus. J Toxicol. 2012;2012:103608.
3. Mount DB. Transport of sodium, chloride, and potassium. In: Skorecki K, et al., editors. Brenner & Rector's the kidney. 10th ed. Philadelphia: Elsevier; 2016. p. 144–84.
4. Subramanya AR, Pastor-Solar MM, Reeves WB, et al. Tubular sodium transport. In: Coffman TM, et al., editors. Schrier's diseases of the kidney & urinary tract. 9th ed. Philadelphia: Lippincott Williams & Wilkins; 2013. p. 159–93.

Intravenous Fluids: Composition and Indications

4

This chapter reviews various fluids available for intravenous (IV) administration. The IV fluids can be broadly divided into two categories: *crystalloids* and *colloids*. Crystalloid solutions contain water, electrolytes, and/or glucose, whereas colloids include mostly albumin and blood products. Table 4.1 provides a list of crystalloids and colloids that are available for IV use.

IV solutions can be *isotonic*, *hypotonic*, or *hypertonic*. In general, isotonic solutions are used to treat extracellular fluid (ECF) volume depletion, hypotonic solutions to replace ECF and intracellular fluid (ICF) loss, and hypertonic solutions to correct symptomatic hyponatremia. Hypertonic saline is often used in trauma settings because it decreases the intracranial pressure in patients with head trauma and for patients following burns. It is important to know the composition of commonly used crystalloids and colloids before we understand their indications (Tables 4.2 and 4.3).

Table 4.1 Commonly used crystalloid and colloid solutions

Crystalloids	Colloids
Dextrose in water (D5W) (2.5%, 5%, 10%)	Albumin (5%, 25%)
Sodium chloride (NaCl) (0.225%, 0.33%, 0.45%, 0.9%, 3%, 5%, 7.5%)	Starches (hetastarch 5%, pentastarch 10%)
Ringer's lactate	Dextrans 40 and 70
Plasmalyte A	Blood products (whole blood, packed red blood cells, fresh frozen plasma, cryoprecipitate, platelets, blood substitutes or artificial blood)

© Springer Science+Business Media LLC 2018
A.S. Reddi, *Fluid, Electrolyte and Acid-Base Disorders*,
DOI 10.1007/978-3-319-60167-0_4

Table 4.2 Composition of commonly used crystalloid solutions

Solution	Osmolality (mOsm)	Na+ (mEq/L)	Cl−	K+	Ca²⁺	Lactate	Glucose (g/L)
Normal saline (0.9%)	308ᵃ	154	154	–	–	–	–
D5 normal saline (5% dextrose in 0.9% NaCl)	586	154	154	–	–	–	50
D5water (D5W)	278	–	–	–	–	–	50
D5 0.225% NaCl	355	38	38	–	–	–	50
D5 0.45% NaCl	432	77	77	–	–	–	50
0.45% NaCl	154	77	77	–	–	–	–
3% NaCl	1026	513	513	–	–	–	–
Ringer's lactate	272	130	109	4	3	28	–
Plasma–Lyte Aᵇ	294	140	98	5	–	8	–

ᵃNot corrected for osmotic coefficient, which is calculated as the measured osmolality (using an osmometer) divided by the milliosmoles. For example, the measured osmolality of normal saline is 287 mOsm/kg H_2O. The osmotic coefficient, therefore, is: $287/308 = 0.93$
ᵇContains in addition Mg^{2+} 3 mEq/L, acetate 27 mEq/L, and gluconate 23 mEq/L

Table 4.3 Composition of commonly used colloid solutions other than blood products

Solution	Osmolality (mOsm)	Na+ (mEq/L)	Cl−	Albumin (g/L)	Dextran (g/L)	HES (g/L)	COP (mmHg)
Albumin (5%)	308	154	154	50	–	–	20
Albumin (25%)	308	154	154	250	–	–	100
Dextran-40	310	154	154	–	100	–	68
Dextran-70	310	154	154	–	60	–	70
Hetastarch (HES) (6%)	310	154	154	–	–	60	30

COP colloid oncotic pressure

Crystalloids

Dextrose in Water

Dextrose in water is available as 2.5, 5, 10, and 50% (containing 25, 50, 100, and 500 g dextrose in 1 L of water, respectively) solutions. The dextrose is metabolized to water and CO_2, and the water is distributed between ECF and ICF compartments. In clinical management, the most commonly used solution is 5% dextrose in water, which is usually abbreviated as D5W. This solution provides 170 kcal/L. Pure water causes hemolysis, if given intravenously; therefore, D5W is given to provide pure water. The indications for dextrose in water solutions are shown in Table 4.4.

Sodium Chloride (NaCl) Solutions

NaCl is available as 0.225, 0.45, 0.9, 3, and 5% (containing 38.5, 77,154, 513, and 1250 mEq of Na+ and an equal amount of Cl− in 1 L) solutions. 0.9% NaCl solution

Table 4.4 Indications for dextrose in water (D5W)

1. To replace deficits of total body water in treatment of hypernatremia
2. To provide energy and prevent starvation ketosis
3. To treat hypoglycemia
4. To mix with amino acid solution in total parenteral nutrition
5. *Do not* give D5W to a patient with syndrome of inappropriate antidiuretic hormone because serum [Na$^+$] may become dangerously low
6. *Do not* give D5W alone to expand the ECF volume in a hypovolemic patient or to a patient with hypokalemia

Table 4.5 Indications for NaCl solutions

Isotonic (0.9%) saline
1. To expand ECF volume in a hypovolemic patient
2. To treat hyponatremia in a hypovolemic patient
3. To treat saline-responsive metabolic alkalosis
4. To treat hypernatremia in a patient with hypotension
5. Preferred solution by many physicians in a patient requiring contrast study
6. Preferred solution by many physicians in critically ill patients with shock and ARDS and at times burned patient
7. Use cautiously in patients with Na$^+$ overload such as CHF and liver failure
Hypotonic (0.45%) saline
1. To maintain basic requirements of Na$^+$
2. To treat hypernatremia in a hypovolemic patient who has greater water than solute deficit
3. *Do not* use in a patient with hypotonic hyponatremia
Hypertonic (3%,5%, 7.5%) saline
1. To treat symptomatic hyponatremia
2. To treat trauma patients with head injury
3. To treat hypotension and muscle cramps in hemodialysis patients

ARDS adult respiratory distress syndrome, *CHF* congestive heart failure

is commonly referred to as normal or isotonic saline, whereas 0.225 and 0.45% NaCl are called hypotonic fluids. For example, 1 L of 0.45% saline contains 500 mL of isotonic solution and 500 mL of free water. Therefore, 0.45% NaCl solution provides more free water than 0.9% NaCl solution. Since insensible losses are low in electrolytes, hypotonic solutions are generally considered as true *maintenance* fluids. In general, 3, 5, and 7.5% NaCl are called hypertonic solutions. The indications for NaCl solutions are shown in Table 4.5.

Normal saline is the most commonly used crystalloid worldwide. Infusion of 1 L normal saline to a healthy individual expands intravascular volume by 20%, and the infused volume remains in the vascular space for approximately 30 min. As shown in Table 4.2, normal saline has high Cl$^-$ (154 mEq/L). Recent studies have shown that infusion of solutions containing high Cl$^-$ to critically ill patients has caused some adverse effects such as hyperchloremic metabolic acidosis and acute kidney injury. Balanced electrolyte solutions with low Cl$^-$ concentration, on the other hand, caused less adverse effects compared to normal saline.

Table 4.6 Indications for Ringer's lactate

1. To replace isotonic fluid loss in burns or surgery
2. To correct metabolic acidosis with hypokalemia (infrequently)
3. *Do not* use to expand ECF volume alone, unless the patient has hypokalemia and/or hypobicarbonatemia
4. *Do not* use in a patient with lactic acidosis; however, Ringer's lactate solution does not potentiate lactic acidosis in patients with shock
5. *Do not* use in renal failure patients because of potential development of hyperkalemia
6. Use cautiously in a patient with hepatic failure

Dextrose in Saline

Dextrose in saline is available as D5 0.225, D5 0.45, and D5 0.9% solutions. These fluids provide Na^+, Cl^-, free water, and 170 kcal/L. The indications are similar to those shown in Tables 4.4 and 4.5.

Balanced Electrolyte Solutions

There are a number of "balanced" electrolyte solutions such as Ringer's lactate (also called lactated Ringer's), Ringer's acetate, plasma-lyte 148, normosol R, and isolyte S available for use; however, Ringer's lactate is the most frequently used solution in fluid therapy because of its consideration as *physiologic saline*. Both lactate and acetate are converted to HCO_3^- in the liver. Also, both are vasodilators. Since Ringer's lactate contains less Na^+ than normal saline, it is approximately 10% less effective as a volume expander compared to normal saline. Also, it is not a commended solution in patients with renal failure because of K^+. Table 4.6 shows indications for Ringer's lactate.

Colloids

Albumin

Albumin is the most frequently used colloid in clinical practice. It is extracted from human plasma and is available as 5 or 25% in normal saline. The primary role of albumin is to maintain intravascular oncotic pressure. Albumin stays in the intravascular compartment for at least 16 h before it diffuses into the interstitial space.

Controversy exists regarding the use of albumin as a volume expander. A meta-analysis of 1,419 patients from 30 studies showed higher mortality in critically ill patients. Also, a randomized study (the SAFE Study) showed no survival advantage in critically ill patients with the use of 4% albumin compared to normal saline. Thus, the use of albumin as a volume expander should be individualized. The indications for albumin use are shown in Table 4.7.

Table 4.7 Indications for albumin

1. To expand plasma volume when crystalloids have failed to correct acutely diminished intravascular volume
2. To treat severe edematous patients with nephrotic syndrome resistant to potent diuretic therapy
3. To prevent hemodynamic instability and acute kidney injury following large volume (>5 L) paracentesis
4. To prevent renal impairment and mortality in patients with spontaneous bacterial peritonitis
5. To treat cirrhotic patients with hypoalbuminemia and hypovolemia
6. To treat hepatorenal syndrome with other agents (midodrine, octreotide)
7. To replace plasma volume during plasmapheresis
8. *Do not* use to treat hypoalbuminemia due to malnutrition unless the patient has protein-losing enteropathy
9. *Do not* use routinely in critically ill patients with hypovolemia, burns, or hypoalbuminemia because albumin administration does not *reduce* mortality

Goals of Fluid Therapy

The goals of fluid therapy are:

- To normalize hemodynamic and electrolyte abnormalities
- To maintain daily requirements of fluids and electrolytes
- To replace previous fluid and electrolyte losses
- To replace ongoing fluid and electrolyte losses
- To provide nutrition
- To provide a source for IV drug administration

The choice of fluid therapy depends largely on the clinical situation. Crystalloids are usually preferred to colloids in fluid therapy except in certain situations.

Fluid therapy is not without complications. Some of the complications include fluid overload, resulting in pulmonary edema, electrolyte disturbances such as hyponatremia with hypotonic solutions and hypernatremia with hypertonic solutions, and IV catheter-associated infections and phlebitis. Dangerous hyperkalemia may develop with K^+-containing solutions, particularly in patients with renal failure. Also, hyperchloremic metabolic acidosis (dilutional acidosis) and acute kidney injury may develop with large volumes of normal saline.

How Much Fluid Is Retained in the Intravascular Compartment?

The most frequently asked question in fluid management is: How is the infused fluid either crystalloid or colloid distributed in body compartments? In order to answer this question, recall the percentage of total body water and its distribution in various fluid compartments (see Chap. 1). In a 70 kg man with lean body mass, the total body water accounts for 60% of body weight (42 L), and two-thirds of this water (i.e., 28 L) is in the ICF and one-third (i.e., 14 L) is in the ECF compartment. Of these 14 L of ECF water, 3.5 L (25%) is present in the intravascular and 11.5 L (75%) in the interstitial compartments (Fig. 4.1). Accordingly, if 1 L of D5W is infused, approximately 664 mL will move into the ICF, and 336 mL will remain in the ECF compartment. Of these 336 mL, only 84 mL (25%) will remain in the intravascular compartment (Fig. 4.2) The retention of hypotonic solutions such as 0.45% NaCl is different. 0.45% NaCl is considered to be a 50:50 mixture of normal saline and free water. If 1 L of 0.45% NaCl is infused, the free water (500 mL) is distributed between ICF (333 mL) and ECF (167 mL) compartments (Fig. 4.3). Of 167 mL, only 42 mL (25%) will remain in the intravascular compartment. Considering the other 500 mL, which behaves like 0.9% saline, 375 mL (75%) will move into the interstitial space and 125 mL stays in the intravascular compartment. Thus, the total

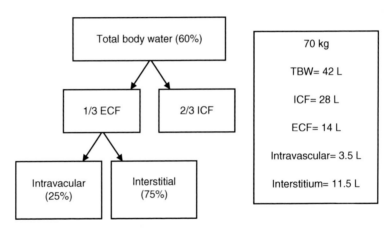

Fig. 4.1 Distribution of total body water (TBW) in a 70 kg man. ECF extracellular fluid volume, ICF intracellular fluid volume

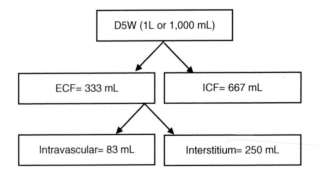

Fig. 4.2 Distribution of 5% decxtrose in water (D5W) in the body. ECF extracellular fluid volume, ICF intracellular fluid volume

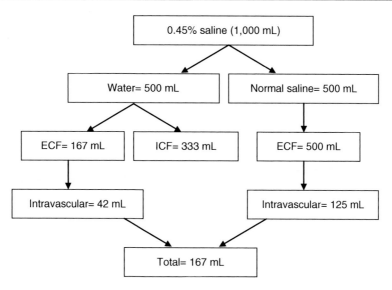

Fig. 4.3 Distribution of half-normal saline in the body. ECF extracellular fluid volume, ICF intracellular fluid volume

Fig. 4.4 Distribution of normal saline in the body. ECF extracellular fluid volume, ICF intracellular fluid volume

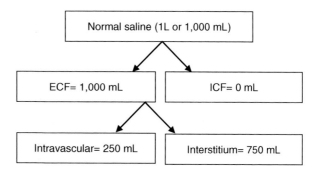

volume remaining intravascularly after 1 L of infusion would be only 167 mL (42 + 125 = 167 mL). On the other hand, more fluid is retained in the intravascular space with isotonic fluids (Fig. 4.4). Infusion of colloids results in even much more retention of fluids in the intravascular compartment. Approximate distribution of various crystalloids and colloids in body compartments in the absence of shock or sepsis is summarized in Table 4.8.

As evident from the Table 4.8, crystalloids are less effective than equivalent volumes of colloids in expanding the intravascular fluid compartment. Despite this benefit of colloids, their use in fluid resuscitation even in hemorrhagic shock is controversial. It should be noted that the percentage distribution of both crystalloids and colloids between compartments may vary in critically ill patients because of altered cell and vascular permeability.

Table 4.8 Approximate distribution of 1 L of IV fluids in body compartments

Fluid	Intracellular (mL)	Interstitial (mL)	Intravascular (mL)
D5W	664	252	84
Normal saline (0.9%)	0	752	248
Ringer's lactate	0	752	248
Albumin (5%)	0	100	900
Albumin (25%)	0	−3,000[a]	4,000
Hetastarch (6%)	0	0	1,000
Dextran-40	0	−1,000[a]	2,000
Packed RBC	0	0	250

[a]Fluid movement from interstitial to intravascular (plasma) compartment

Maintenance Fluid and Electrolyte Therapy

Maintenance fluid therapy is aimed at replacing fluids lost during the course of a day after stabilization of the patient. The daily requirements for water and electrolytes aredetermined by sensible and insensible losses. Insensible losses are from respiration, perspiration, and stools. Although these losses are difficult to estimate, they average about 8–12 mL/kg/day and increase by 10% for each degree of body temperature above 37.2 °C (99 °F). In a 70 kg afebrile man, the insensible loss is 560–840 mL. The sensible loss equals daily urine output, which varies from 500 to 2,000 mL, depending on the solute intake and urine osmolality. Thus, the total daily water requirement for a 70 kg man is about 1,000–2,000 mL. This translates approximately to 30 mL/kg/day. The requirements for Na^+ are variable, because the kidneys regulate Na^+ excretion. It is generally estimated that 1–2 mEq/kg/day of Na^+ is required for maintenance therapy. The requirement for K^+ is half that of Na^+. Thus, a 70 kg man may need at least 2,000 mL of water with 70–140 mEq of Na^+ and 35–70 mEq of K^+ daily. The crystalloid that best fits this patient's daily requirement is either 0.33% (56 mEq of Na^+) or 0.45% (77 mEq of Na^+) saline solution with KCl in the amount of 20–30 mEq/L. The requirements for other electrolytes depend on their serum levels. Remember that 1 g Na^+ diet gives about 44 mEq, whereas 1 g salt (NaCl) diet gives 17 mEq of Na^+. Do not order hypotonic fluids to a patient whose serum [Na^+] is <136 mEq/L. This will worsen hyponatremia.

Note that the above daily requirements for water, Na^+, and $K^+$are rough guidelines only. Fluid and electrolyte therapy should be individualized based upon daily weight (if possible) and serum electrolytes. Be careful with K^+ replacement in patients with renal failure.

In critically ill patients with ongoing losses from drainages and suction, these fluids should be measured and replaced. Profuse loss from diarrhea can be estimated and replaced with isotonic or appropriate saline solutions while correcting simultaneously other electrolyte abnormalities.

Fluid Therapy in Special Conditions

Patients with mild to severe volume contraction and patients with shock due to several causes are frequently admitted to medical service and the intensive care units for management. In addition, patients with pulmonary disease as well as patients with renal failure develop problems with fluid management. Also, patients with burns, traumatic hemorrhage, and stroke are admitted to surgical service with fluid and electrolyte problems. Therefore, a brief discussion of fluid and electrolyte therapy in these conditions is presented below.

Volume Contraction

Elderly patients and patients from nursing homes are admitted with severe dehydration (volume depletion) because of poor oral intake as well as inability to access water. These patients generally present with altered mental status, hypotension, and fever. The choice of fluid therapy is normal (0.9%) saline. Ringer's lactate can also be used, if the patient has multiple electrolyte deficits. The fluids can be continued until the blood pressure and urine output start improving. Fever, in the absence of infection, also improves with adequate volume replacement, and the patient becomes more alert. With adequate volume replacement, all abnormal laboratory findings return to baseline or normal.

Septic Shock

Septic shock is a condition of altered vascular permeability, fluid leakage into the extravascular space, and multiorgan involvement. Large fluid deficits (up to 10 L) are present in the septic patient. Therefore, fluid therapy is essential to improve cardiac output, blood pressure, and tissue perfusion. Isotonic saline is preferred initially to improve volume status. Fluid challenges of 1 L of saline can be given with CVP monitoring. Ringer's lactate, if indicated, can be used. Routine use of colloids is not recommended unless the patient has anemia in which case packed RBCs are infused to raise Hb level to 9–10 g/dL. Occasionally, patients need infusion of 25% albumin to raise serum albumin levels >2 g/dL and minimize peripheral edema. Vasopressor support is required if crystalloids alone do not improve blood pressure. Three hundred to 500 mL of colloids can also be given in 30 min to improve hemodynamics.

As mentioned above, normal saline is widely used as a volume expander in patients with septic shock. However, infusion of balanced solutions has been shown to cause less adverse effects such as hyperchloremic metabolic acidosis and acute kidney injury. It should be noted that the cost of these balanced solutions limits their use worldwide.

Hemorrhagic Shock Due to Gastrointestinal Bleeding

Hemorrhagic shock can result from massive gastrointestinal bleeding. The therapeutic goals are to restore the circulating blood volume and to restore adequate Hb levels. Transfusion of packed RBCs is recommended if Hb level is <7 g/dL. Raising Hb level above 9–10 g/dL is not necessary. Patients with Hb levels between 7 and 10 g/dL should be evaluated for clinical instability and inadequate oxygen delivery. If Hb level is stable, administration of crystalloids (isotonic saline) is preferred. Frequently, patients need both transfusion of packed RBCs and administration of normal saline to prevent vascular collapse.

Hemorrhagic Shock Due to Trauma

The important therapeutic goals are to improve the circulating blood volume and to restore adequate Hb levels. Crystalloid solutions are very effective in restoring intravascular volume. Therefore, crystalloid solutions are an ideal first-line treatment that should be started as soon as possible. The fluid of choice is Ringer's lactate, because it can replace some of the interstitial fluid and electrolyte deficits that may be present during hypovolemic shock. It is recommended that trauma patients should receive blood transfusion, if they are not stabilized after receiving 2 L of Ringer's lactate or if they deteriorated following a brief stabilization. Transfusion of packed RBCs is required if Hb level is <7 g/dL. Maintenance of Hb levels >9–10 g/dL has not been shown to be beneficial. Transfusion of FFP is indicated for coagulopathy and platelet transfusion for a platelet count <100,000/µL.

Hypertonic saline (7.5%) alone or in combination with 6% dextran is also effective for trauma patients, particularly in patients with head trauma. It lowers the volume requirements and also improves survival in these patients requiring surgery.

Cardiogenic Shock

Cardiogenic shock is usually not associated with increased microvascular permeability. Therefore, the fluid requirement is not substantial. A crystalloid solution is probably the choice of initial fluid therapy because the patients in cardiogenic shock are not hypooncotic. The use of colloid can lead to changes in cardiac filling pressure, resulting in pulmonary vascular congestion. Crystalloid therapy is usually guided by the pulmonary capillary wedge pressure and cardiac output.

Adult Respiratory Distress Syndrome (ARDS)

Because of generalized vascular permeability changes, patients with ARDS demonstrate signs of decreased intravascular volume and circulatory shock, as well as pulmonary alveolar edema and hypoxemia. The management, therefore, involves restoration of intravascular volume and preservation of gas exchange. Both crystalloid and colloid therapy was found to be effective and safe; however, crystalloid (saline) infusion may occasionally worsen pulmonary edema without impairing gas exchange. Therefore, colloid rather than crystalloid infusion is suggested. Furthermore, colloids are more potent volume expanders than crystalloids and produce greater increases in cardiac output and systemic oxygen delivery. Despite these beneficial effects, crystalloids are generally recommended in most of the patients with ARDS unless the patients are anemic and hypoalbuminemic in which case colloids are the choice of fluid resuscitation. The major goal of fluid therapy in ARDS is to minimize the increases in pulmonary hydrostatic pressure. For this purpose, frequent measurements of pulmonary capillary wedge pressure or CVP and radiographic as well as clinical evaluation for pulmonary edema are essential.

Phases of Fluid Therapy in Critically Ill Patients

Fluid therapy is an early intervention in the management of acutely ill patients. The selection of resuscitation fluid should be based on the patient's clinical context. The need for fluid therapy in critically ill patients is not static but varies depending on the hemodynamic status. Therefore, a conceptual model for fluid management has been proposed. This model includes four phases: (1) rescue or salvage, (2) optimization, (3) stabilization, and (4) de-escalation.

Rescue phase is characterized by life-threatening shock (hypotension and poor organ perfusion), which requires rapid fluid bolus therapy. Optimization phase is less life threatening and requires fluid boluses of 250–500 mL in 15–20 min to restore cardiac output and organ perfusion. During the stabilization phase, fluid management is aimed at maintaining adequate intravascular volume (maintenance of fluid balance). De-escation phase is characterized by measures of recovery, including weaning from ventilator and vasoactive support and treatment of volume overload by appropriate measures. It should be noted that these phases are not mutually exclusive but interrelated.

Study Questions

Case 1 A 24-year-old woman is admitted for fever with chills and weakness. She is found to be hypotensive and tachycardic. Blood cultures are positive for *Staphylococcus aureus*, and the diagnosis of septic shock is made. There is no peripheral edema. Based upon the sensitivity, the patient is started on vancomycin. Pertinent labs:

Na^+ = 144 mEq/L	Glucose = 80 mg/dL
K^+ = 5.1 mEq/L	Total protein = 5.8 g/dL
Cl^- = 88 mEq/L	Albumin = 2.0 g/dL
HCO_3^- = 20 mEq/L	Hemoglobin = 10 g/dL
BUN = 30 mg/dL	Hematocrit = 30%
Creatinine = 1.7 mg/dL	Urinary Na^+ = 10 mEq/L

Question 1 What is the appropriate initial fluid therapy for this patient?

Answer Relative intravascular volume depletion is usual in septic shock. This patient has evidence of intravascular volume depletion. Therefore, the choice of fluid is normal saline. Rapid infusion of at least 1 L of saline is needed within an hour and then at least 150–200 mL/h until blood pressure, tissue perfusion, and oxygen delivery are acceptable. Note that the patients with septic shock can develop pulmonary edema at pulmonary capillary wedge pressures <18 mmHg.

Question 2 Does the patient need blood transfusion (packed RBCs) to raise Hb levels >9–10 g/dL?

Answer No. The patient needs transfusion of packed RBCs once her Hb drops below 7 g/dL.

Question 3 At what stage does the patient need infusion of 5% albumin?

Answer If the blood pressure does not improve with substantial amount of normal saline and the patient has trace edema, infusion of albumin may help to restore blood pressure and tissue perfusion. In a patient with intravascular volume depletion due to diarrhea or other causes, the presence of peripheral edema may imply adequate volume replacement. However, peripheral edema may be present in patients with septic shock without adequate volume replacement because of extravasation of fluid into the interstitium due to increased vascular permeability. Vasopressors, in addition to albumin, may be required to improve blood pressure, tissue perfusion, and gas exchange.

The above patient received a total of 10 L normal saline. There is trace peripheral edema. Her serum [Cl⁻] is 115 mEq/L.

Question 4 Which one of the following statements about hyperchloremia is correct?

(A) Hyperchloremia causes renal vasoconstriction.
(B) Chloride-restrictive fluids decrease the incidence of AKI and the need for RRT in critically ill patients.
(C) Hyperchloremic acidosis from saline causes systemic hypotension.
(D) Saline infusion is associated with longer time to first micturition compared to Ringer's lactate infusion.
(E) All of the above.

The answer is E All of the above statements are correct (E). Although crystalloid rather than colloids is recommended as initial choices of fluid resuscitation in ICU patients, hyperchloremia resulting from large volume infusion of saline may have several adverse effects on renal function. Initial studies in animals showed renal vasoconstriction, resulting in decreased renal blood flow and GFR (A is correct). Clinically, chloride-rich fluid administration to ICU patients caused higher incidence of AKI and is a requirement for RRT than chloride-restrictive fluids (B is correct). Induction of hyperchloremia in animals led to a dose-dependent systemic hypotension (C is correct). In human volunteers and patients, high-chloride fluids caused longer time to first urination compared to low-chloride fluids. In noncardiac surgery patients, hyperchloremia was associated with poor postoperative outcomes (D is correct).

Case 2 A 30-year-old man is admitted to the trauma service with multiple abdominal wounds that required splenectomy and repair of several organs. He has multiple surgical drainages. His blood pressure is 120/80 mmHg with a pulse rate of 80 beats/min. His labs:

Na^+ = 134 mEq/L	Glucose = 80 mg/dL
K^+ = 3.1 mEq/L	Ca^{2+} = 7.8 mg/dL
Cl^- = 88 mEq/L	Phosphate = 3.5 mg/dL
HCO_3^- = 21 mEq/L	Hemoglobin = 11 g/dL
BUN = 10 mg/dL	Hematocrit = 34%
Creatinine = 1.1 mg/dL	Urinary Na^+ = 12 mEq/L
	Urinary K^+ = 10 mEq/L

Question 1 What is the appropriate fluid therapy for this patient?

Answer This patient has multiple electrolyte problems because of nonrenal losses. Therefore, the appropriate fluid for initial therapy is Ringer's lactate, which contains Na^+, Cl^-, K^+, Ca^{2+}, and lactate. This fluid should be continued until all electrolyte abnormalities are corrected.

Question 2 What would happen if D5W or normal saline is given?

Answer Since the patient has hypokalemia, dextrose would further lower serum $[K^+]$. This may cause weakness and arrhythmia. Normal saline alone may not improve electrolyte abnormalities.

One week later, the serum creatinine and BUN rose to 2.1 and 40 mg/dL, respectively. The patient is found to have acute kidney injury due to acute tubular necrosis. His serum $[K^+]$ is 4.8 mEq/L and he is euvolemic. His blood pressure is 120/80 mmHg.

Question 3 What would happen if Ringer's lactate is continued?

Answer Continuation of Ringer's lactate would cause hyperkalemia because of acute kidney injury. Therefore, either D5W or 0.45% saline should be used as maintenance fluid therapy. Normal saline can be used if the patient develops volume depletion and hypotension.

Case 3 A 50-year-old man is admitted for dizziness, weakness, and blurred vision. His serum glucose is 1,400 mg/dL, and serum $[Na^+]$ is 158 mEq/L. He has orthostatic blood pressure and pulse changes.

Question 1 What is the appropriate fluid for this patient?

Answer This patient lost both water and Na^+ in the urine, causing orthostatic blood pressure and pulse changes. Therefore, hemodynamic instability rather than hypertonicity should be corrected first. Normal saline is the appropriate IV fluid in this patient. Once blood pressure is stabilized, 0.45% NaCl should be given. If the glucose level reaches around 200 mg/dL, D5 0.45% NaCl can be continued.

Question 2 Match the following cases with appropriate IV solutions.

1. A 40-year-old patient with septic shock
2. A nondiabetic subject with chest pain and normal blood pressure
3. A 25-year-old patient with AIDS and diarrhea
4. A postoperative patient with serum $[Na^+]$ of 120 mEq/L and altered mental status
5. A 30-year-old patient with ARDS
6. An elderly patient with positive stool guaic and normal blood pressure
7. A nondiabetic patient with increased pulse rate (90 beats/min) and serum $[K^+]$ of 5.5 mEq/L

(A) Normal (0.9%) saline
(B) 0.45% saline
(C) D5W
(D) 3% NaCl
(E) D5 ½ (0.45%) normal saline

Answers 1 = A; 2 = C; 3 = A; 4 = D; 5 = A; 6 = A; 7 = E

Case 4 A 70-year-old man is admitted for elective surgery of his prostate gland. He weighs 70 kg. His serum electrolytes and glucose are normal. He is kept NPO (nothing per mouth).

Question 1 Write the fluid and electrolyte orders in this patient for 24 h.

Answer Before you write the orders, estimate approximate daily values for (1) urine output, (2) insensible loss, and (3) requirements for Na^+, K^+, and energy. These are:

$$\text{Urine output} = 1{,}400 \text{ mL}$$
$$\text{Insensible loss} = 600 \text{ mL}$$
$$Na^+ = 70 \text{ mEq/L}$$
$$K^+ = 40 \text{ mEq/L}$$

Thus, the daily fluid requirement is 2.0 L. The IV orders should be:

1. Half-normal (0.45%) saline at 83 mL/h for 12 h
2. D5W with KCl 40 mEq at 83 mL/h for 12 h

These orders would deliver approximately 2 L of fluid, 77 mEq of Na^+ and 40 mEq of K^+, and 50 g of glucose to prevent starvation ketosis. For IV medications, either D5W or normal saline (usually 50–100 mL per medication) can be ordered. Your total fluid order should include fluid that is required for medications.

Suggested Reading

1. Agrò FE, editor. Body fluid management. From physiology to therapy. Italia: Springer-Verlag; 2013.
2. Hahn RG, editor. Clinical fluid therapy in the perioperative setting. Cambridge: Cambridge University Press; 2011.
3. McDermid RC, Raghunathan K, Romanovsky A, et al. Controversies in fluid therapy: type, dose and toxicity. World J Crit Care Med. 2014;3:24–33.
4. Moritz MI, Ayus JC. Maintenance intravenous fluids in acute ill patients. N Engl J Med. 2015;373:1350–60.
5. Myburgh JA, Mythen MG. Resuscitation fluids. N Engl J Med. 2013;369:1243–51.
6. Rewa O, Bagshaw SM. Principles of fluid management. Crit Care Clin. 2015;31:785–801.
7. Semler MW, Rice TW. Sepsis resuscitation. Fluid choice and dose. Clin Chest Med. 2016;37:241–50.
8. Varrier M, Ostermann M. Fluid composition and clinical effects. Crit Care Clin. 2015;31:823–37.
9. Vincent J-L, De Backer D. Circulatory shock. N Engl J Med. 2013;369:1726–34.

Diuretics

5

Diuretics promote Na^+ and water excretion. Excretion of Na^+ in the urine is called *natriuresis*, whereas *diuresis* refers to increased urine flow rate. In clinical medicine, two types of diuresis are recognized: solute diuresis and water diuresis. Solute diuresis results from a decrease in the renal tubular reabsorption of solute. Since water reabsorption follows solute reabsorption, inhibition of solute reabsorption generally diminishes water transport. However, water diuresis can be promoted without solute diuresis by drugs, which impair the action of antidiuretic hormone (ADH). Examples include ADH receptor blockers (vaptans) and lithium. This chapter reviews briefly the various groups of diuretics, their physiologic action, clinical use, and complications.

Classification of Diuretics

Diuretics can be classified according to their chemical structure and site of action. Accordingly, they are divided into the following groups: (1) osmotic diuretics, (2) carbonic anhydrase inhibitors, (3) loop diuretics, (4) distal tubule diuretics, and (5) K^+-sparing diuretics (Table 5.1). Each of these diuretic groups differs in its natriuretic potency.

© Springer Science+Business Media LLC 2018
A.S. Reddi, *Fluid, Electrolyte and Acid-Base Disorders*,
DOI 10.1007/978-3-319-60167-0_5

Table 5.1 Classification of diuretics

Group	Chemical nature	Prototype drug(s)	Site of action	Mechanism of action	Relative natriuretic potency
Osmotic diuretics	Polysaccharide	Mannitol	Predominantly proximal tubule and loop of Henle	Inhibition of tubular reabsorption of solute and water	Dose dependent (>10%)
Carbonic anhydrase inhibitors	Sulfonamide	Acetazolamide	Proximal tubule	Inhibits carbonic anhydrase	1–3%
Loop diuretics	Sulfonamide phenoxyacetic acid-derivative	Furosemide Bumetanide Torsemide Ethacrynic acid	Thick ascending Henle's loop	Inhibit Na/K/2Cl cotransporter	20–25%
Distal tubule diuretics	Benzothiadiazine or its derivatives	Chlorothiazide Hydrochlorothiazide Chlorthalidone Metolazone Indapamide	Early distal convoluted tubule	Inhibit Na/Cl cotransporter	5%
K+- sparing diuretics	Steroid pyrazine carboxamides Pteridine derivative	Amiloride Triamterene Spironolactone Eplerenone	Cortical collecting duct	Inhibit ENaC (amiloride and triamterene) Antagonize MR receptors (spironolactone and eplerenone)	1–3%

ENaC epithelial Na channel, *MR* mineralocorticoid receptor

Physiologic Effects of Diuretics

In addition to their actions on Na^+ and water, diuretics exert several other physiologic effects in the kidney. These include changes in renal blood flow (RBF), glomerular filtration rate (GFR), concentration and dilution of urine, and excretion of several other electrolytes. The physiologic effects of diuretics are summarized in Table 5.2.

Clinical Uses of Diuretics

The primary action of diuretics is to increase Na^+ and water excretion in patients with edema of variable causes. Diuretics are also used to treat hypertension and other nonedematous conditions. Table 5.3 summarizes the disease conditions that are treated with diuretics.

Table 5.2 Physiologic effects of diuretics

	Osmotic diuretics	CA inhibitors	Loop diuretics	Thiazide diuretics	K^+-sparing diuretics
Hemodynamics					
RBF	↑↑	↓	↑	↓	NC
GFR	↑	↓	NC	↓	NC
Urinary excretion					
Na^+	↑↑	↑	↑↑	↑↑	↑
K^+	↑	↑	↑↑	↑	↓↓
Cl^-	↑	↓	↑	↑	↑
HCO_3^-	↑	↑↑	NC	NC	↑
Ca^{2+}	↑	NC	↑↑	↓	NC
Phosphate	↑	↑↑	↑	↑	NC
Mg^{2+}	↑	NC	↑↑	↑	NC
Urine volume	↑↑	↑	↑↑	↑↑	↑
T^cH_2O	↑	↑	↓	↓	NC

↑ slight increase, ↑↑ moderate increase, ↓ slight decrease, *NC* no change, ↓↓ moderate decrease, *T^cH_2O* electrolyte-free water clearance

Table 5.3 Clinical uses of diuretics

Disease condition	Diuretics commonly used	Mechanism/effect
Generalized edema states		
Congestive heart failure	Furosemide, metolazone, or both, Spironolactone	↑ Excretion of Na^+ and water to reduce edema
Liver cirrhosis with ascites	Spironolactone, furosemide, or both	↑ Excretion of Na^+ and water prevention of hypokalemia
		↓ Edema
Nephrotic syndrome	Furosemide, amiloride	↑ Excretion of Na^+ and water
		↓ Edema
Idiopathic edema	Hydrochlorothiazide, furosemide	↓ Edema by promoting Na^+ and H_2O excretion

(continued)

Table 5.3 (continued)

Disease condition	Diuretics commonly used	Mechanism/effect
Localized edema		
Pulmonary edema	Furosemide, bumetanide	↓ Pulmonary congestion by removing Na^+ and water
Cerebral edema	Mannitol	↓ Intracranial pressure
Nonedematous states		
Acute kidney injury	Furosemide, mannitol	Improve urine flow and convert oliguric (<400 mL urine) to nonoliguric (>400 mL urine) failure
Chronic kidney disease (GFR < 60 mL/min)	Furosemide, metolazone	↑ Excretion of Na^+ and water Thiazides other than metolazone do not work at GFR < 30 mL/min
Hypertension	Thiazides	↓ Plasma volume and cardiac output
Renal calcium stones	Hydrochlorothiazide	↓ Ca^{2+} excretion
Nephrogenic diabetes insipidus	Hydrochlorothiazide	↓ Plasma volume and polyuria
Acute hypercalcemia	Furosemide	↓ Ca^{2+} absorption in thick ascending limb and promotes calciuria
Glaucoma	Acetazolamide	↓ HCO_3^- and Na^+ transport and ↓ aqueous humor formation

Table 5.4 Complications of diuretic use

Fluid, electrolyte, and acid–base disorders
Extracellular fluid volume depletion
Hyponatremia (mostly thiazide diuretics)
Hypokalemia
Hyperkalemia (K^+-sparing diuretics)
Hypocalcemia and hypercalciuria (loop diuretics)
Hypercalcemia (thiazide diuretics)
Hypomagnesemia (thiazide and loop diuretics)
Hypophosphatemia (all except K^+-sparing diuretics)
Metabolic acidosis (Acetazolamide and K^+-sparing diuretics)
Metabolic alkalosis (thiazide and loop diuretics)
Metabolic disorders
Hyperuricemia (thiazides cause both hyper- and hypouricemia)
Hyperglycemia (thiazides and loop diuretics)
Hyperlipidemia (thiazide and loop diuretics)
Gynecomastia (mostly spironolactone)
Sexual dysfunction (mostly spironolactone)
Toxicities
Hypersensitivity reactions
Deafness
Pancreatitis
Renal calculi

Complications of Diuretics

Chronic use of diuretics causes several complications, which can be considered under three categories (Table 5.4).

Study Questions

Case 1 A 60-year-old woman was brought to the emergency room by her husband for progressive shortness of breath. She has hypertension for 20 years and is on a thiazide diuretic (hydrochlorothiazide). Physical examination reveals a moderately built woman in acute respiratory distress. Her blood pressure is 180/110 mmHg with a pulse rate of 96/min. Lungs have crackles. Heart examination shows an S_3 gallop. She has 2–3 mm pitting edema in lower extremities. Chest X-ray shows pulmonary edema.

Question 1 Based on physical findings and the chest X-ray, what type of diuretic would you use to relieve this patient's pulmonary congestion?

Answer The appropriate diuretic to use is a loop diuretic. The most commonly used loop diuretic is furosemide (40–80 mg IV). It promotes Na^+ and water excretion within 30–60 min, if given intravenously. Furosemide also causes vasodilation of the pulmonary vasculature in patients with congestive heart failure. By decreasing ventricular filling pressure and cardiac oxygen consumption, furosemide improves cardiac output as well. Bumetanide (1–2 mg) can also induce natriuresis and diuresis.

Question 2 What would happen if mannitol was given to this patient?

Answer Although mannitol promotes Na^+ and water diuresis, it increases extracellular fluid volume and would thus worsen her pulmonary congestion.

Question 3 What would you expect the patient's urine osmolality to be after administration of furosemide?

Answer Furosemide acts in the medullary thick ascending limb and inhibits the Na/K/2Cl cotransporter. As a result, the medullary hypertonicity is abolished, thereby preventing the urine concentrating ability of the kidney. Despite sufficient volume depletion, the patient's urine osmolality will not exceed >400 mOsm/kg H_2O and is usually similar to plasma osmolality (isosthenuria).

Case 2 A 30-year-old woman is admitted for nausea, vomiting, headache, and blurred vision for 1 week. Examination of her eyes reveals papilledema, and CT scan of the head shows hydrocephalus (increased intracranial fluid). The patient is started on mannitol to decrease the intracranial pressure.

Question 1 Discuss the effect of mannitol on RBF and GFR.

Answer Mannitol is an osmotic diuretic. It extracts water from the intracellular compartment to the extracellular compartment and expands the extracellular fluid volume. Also, mannitol and other osmotic diuretics dilate the afferent arteriole. As a result of these effects, the RBF is increased. A slight increase in GFR is also observed due to an increase in glomerular capillary pressure (P_{GC}).

Question 2 What would happen to the urinary excretion of electrolytes in this patient?

Answer In general, osmotic diuretics cause an increase in the urinary excretion of all electrolytes, including Na^+, K^+, Cl^-, HCO_3^-, Ca^{2+}, Mg^{2+}, and phosphate.

Case 3 A 50-year-old man with cirrhosis of the liver is admitted for altered mental status (confusion, irritability, etc.). Physical examination shows ascites and pitting edema in both lower extremities. He is started on several medications, including spironolactone.

Question 1 What effect does spironolactone have on serum $[K^+]$ and acid–base balance?

Answer Spironolactone is a competitive antagonist of aldosterone by antagonizing the mineralocorticoid receptor. By counteracting the effect of aldosterone, spironolactone inhibits K^+ secretion in the cortical collecting duct, causing hyperkalemia. Spironolactone also inhibits H^+ secretion at the same site, causing metabolic acidosis in cirrhotic patients.

Suggested Reading

1. Hoorn EJ, Wilcox CJ, Ellison DH. Diuretics. In: Skorecki K, et al., editors. Brenner & Rector's the kidney. 10th ed. Philadelphia: Elsevier; 2016. p. 1702–33.
2. Reddy P, Mooradian AD. Diuretics: an update on the pharmacology and clinical uses. Am J Ther. 2009;16:74–85.
3. Seldin D, Giebisch G, editors. Diuretic agents. Clinical physiology and pharmacology. San Diego: Academic Press; 1997.

Disorders of Extracellular Fluid Volume: Basic Concepts

6

In Chap. 3, we discussed how NaCl and water are handled by various segments of the nephron. Since Na^+ is the major extracellular electrolyte, the total amount of this electrolyte and its accompanying anion (Cl^-) determine the extracellular fluid (ECF) volume. Therefore, retention or excretion of Na^+ by the kidneys is critical for the regulation of ECF volume. This regulation of NaCl is precise in normal individuals. In a steady state, urinary Na^+ approximates dietary Na^+, as the kidneys are major excretory organs of Na^+ besides gastrointestinal tract and skin. Low salt intake results in low excretion of Na^+. Conversely, high salt intake results in high excretion of Na^+. Any disturbance in this regulation activates or inhibits neural and hormonal mechanisms, leading to appropriate change in Na^+ excretion by the kidneys. This chapter discusses the basic concepts that characterize ECF volume depletion and conditions that are associated with the development of volume expansion and edema formation.

Mechanisms of Volume Recognition

How does the kidney respond to changes in Na^+ intake? Several components participate in the regulation of NaCl:

1. Sensors
2. Afferent neural mechanisms (pathways)
3. A coordinating integrative control (vasomotor) center in the medulla
4. Efferent neural mechanisms (pathways)
5. Kidneys

Sensors called baroreceptors perceive changes in volume; they are located in the vascular system and other areas of the body (Table 6.1). Anatomically, signals are sent regarding volume changes from the carotid sinus through the Hering's nerve to the glassopharyngeal nerve (cranial nerve IX) and then to the vasomotor center in the medulla. Signals from the aortic arch are sent through the vagus nerve

© Springer Science+Business Media LLC 2018
A.S. Reddi, *Fluid, Electrolyte and Acid-Base Disorders*,
DOI 10.1007/978-3-319-60167-0_6

Table 6.1 Afferent and efferent mechanisms involved in renal Na⁺ excretion

Afferent mechanisms	Efferent mechanisms
High-pressure (arterial) volume receptors	Glomerular filtration rate
Carotid sinus	Peritubular capillary Starling forces
Aortic arch	Tubular luminal composition
Intrathoracic low-pressure (venous) receptors	Medullary blood flow
Cardiac atria	Humoral factors
Pulmonary veins	Renin–angiotensin–aldosterone system
Hepatic volume receptors	Prostaglandins
Intrarenal volume receptors	Kallikrein–kinin system
Juxtaglomerular apparatus	Atrial natriuretic factor
Arterial perfusion pressure receptors	Antidiuretic hormone
Interstitial pressure receptors	Nitric oxide
Central nervous system receptors	

(cranial nerve X) to the same vasomotor center. High-pressure receptors play an important role in blood pressure regulation; however, they are also important players in volume regulation. Compared to high-pressure receptors, low-pressure receptors located in atria and pulmonary veins play a much more prominent role in volume regulation. Once these afferent mechanisms reach the vasomotor center, they send signals to the kidney via efferent mechanisms for appropriate response. The coordination of these afferent and efferent mechanisms is responsible for maintenance of Na⁺ and fluid balance.

Let us see how the afferent and efferent mechanisms operate when salt intake is low.

First, a decrease in salt intake causes a decrease in ECF volume, which stimulates the baroreceptors (afferent mechanisms); then the CNS integrative control center sends a message via the efferent mechanisms to the kidney to conserve Na⁺ and water to restore volume. The mechanisms involved are:

1. Renin–angiotensin II (AII)–aldosterone
2. Sympathetic nervous system (SNS)
3. Antidiuretic hormone (ADH)
4. Atrial natriuretic peptide (ANP)

Renin causes the formation of AII, which promotes renal vasoconstriction as well as aldosterone release; the latter stimulates renal tubular reabsorption of Na⁺. Second, increase in SNS (norepinephrine) causes renal afferent and efferent arteriolar vasoconstriction, resulting in a decrease in renal blood flow (RBF) and a slight decrease in GFR. This causes an increase in filtration fraction (GFR/RBF), leading to a decrease in peritubular hydrostatic pressure and an increase in plasma oncotic pressure. These changes in Starling forces favor Na⁺ reabsorption by peritubular capillaries. Norepinephrine also stimulates renin secretion and AII formation. Third, ADH secretion increases, which promotes water reabsorption. Finally, the synthesis of ANP, which promotes excretion of Na⁺, is decreased. The net result is a decrease in Na⁺ excretion and maintenance of Na⁺ and water balance.

When Na^+ intake increases, the ECF volume also increases. The afferent mechanisms sense this excess ECF volume, and the vasomotor center conveys a message via the efferent mechanisms to restore volume. This is achieved by the inhibition of salt- and water-retaining mechanisms (renin–angiotensin–aldosterone, SNS, and ADH) and the activation of salt-losing mechanisms (ANP). Alterations in physical factors also inhibit Na^+ reabsorption in peritubular capillaries. As a result of these changes, urinary excretion of Na^+ is promoted to maintain normal volume.

Conditions of Volume Expansion

So far we have discussed how ECF volume is regulated by afferent and efferent mechanisms in a subject with low or high salt intake. However, these mechanisms fail to operate appropriately in volume-expanded states. In clinical practice, three major conditions of excess fluid volume are usually seen. They are:

1. Congestive heart failure
2. Cirrhosis
3. Nephrotic syndrome

The above clinical conditions are associated with salt and water retention despite excess ECF volume. These patients are in a positive Na^+ balance because their Na^+ excretion is less than Na^+ intake. The retention of Na^+ and water occurs in congestive heart failure and cirrhosis in the absence of renal parenchymal disease.

Let us see how patients with ECF volume expansion retain Na^+. To gain insight into the mechanism of Na^+ retention, one should understand the concept of effective arterial blood volume and distinguish it from ECF volume.

Concept of Effective Arterial Blood Volume (EABV)

A fundamental characteristic of expanded ECF volume conditions, as stated above, is avid retention of Na^+ and development of edema. Therefore, it is essential to understand the concept of EABV in these conditions. EABV is not a measurable quantity. It refers to a component of the ECF volume that perfuses tissues. In a healthy individual, both ECF volume and EABV are normal; therefore, the excretion of Na^+ is normal. This relationship is disturbed in conditions such as congestive heart failure (CHF) and cirrhosis. For example, CHF is a condition of ECF volume expansion. The expected increase in Na^+ excretion to this volume expansion does not occur. Instead, the excretion of Na^+ decreases. The kidney thus behaves as if it were responding to a low-volume state. This decrease in Na^+ excretion is explained by the concept of EABV. In CHF and cirrhosis, EABV is decreased. This decrease in EABV is sensed by baroreceptors, with resultant activation of salt-retaining mechanisms, as seen in states of low salt intake. As a result, Na^+ is retained despite an increase in ECF volume. Therefore, the ECF volume and EABV are not identical in these conditions. Although no adequate experimental evidence supports the concept of EABV, it is generally believed that EABV reflects "underfilling" of the arterial system in both CHF and cirrhosis. Thus, EABV is decreased in these conditions. Let us see how EABV is an important trigger in Na$^+$ retention in CHF and cirrhosis.

Formation of Edema

In order to understand the formation of edema, it is essential to learn Starling forces that are operative in transcapillary fluid exchange. In the body, fluid is filtered across all capillaries into the interstitial space, which is then returned to the blood stream via the lymphatic system. Nearly 3–5 L of fluid is filtered at the arteriolar end, and most of it is reabsorbed at the venous end. Any excess fluid and protein that remain in the interstitium will be returned to the blood via the lymphatic system. Thus, the plasma and interstitial fluid volumes and protein concentration are maintained at near-normal levels. This maintenance of volumes is governed by Starling forces, and these forces are:

Hydrostatic pressure of the capillary (P_c)—pressure that pushes the fluid out of capillaries

Hydrostatic pressure of the interstitium (P_i)—pressure that opposes P_c

Colloid oncotic pressure of the capillary (Π_c)—pressure that opposes P_c

Colloid oncotic pressure of the interstitium (Π_i)—pressure that opposes Π_c

These pressures for fluid movement can be arranged in the Starling equation as follows:

$$J_v = K_f \left[\left(P_c - P_i \right) - \sigma \left(\Pi_c - \Pi_i \right) \right]$$

where J_v is the rate of fluid flow across the capillary, K_f is the filtration coefficient of the capillary, σ is the reflection coefficient of the capillary to plasma proteins, and others represent Starling forces. K_f represents the surface area and the number of pores of the capillary for fluid transfer. When σ is 1, the passage of plasma proteins across the capillary is restricted, whereas 0 represents free passage of plasma proteins. The σ for plasma proteins is approximately 0.95. The values for both K_f and σ differ considerably from tissue to tissue. Figure 6.1 explains how these pressures operate at the arterial and venous ends of the capillary.

Recently, the Starling equation has been revised in view of the demonstration of endothelial glycocalyx and a small protein-free zone called subglycocalyx space (sg), which participate in filtration. According to the revised theory of filtration, there is no reabsorption of fluid at the venous end, as shown in Fig. 6.1. Also, the oncotic pressure differences are set up between the plasma side of the endothelial surface layer (glycocalyx) (Πp) and subglycocalyx space (Πeg), thus eliminating the role of interstitial colloid oncotic pressure. Since there is no reabsorption at the venous end, the filtered fluid is returned to circulation via lymph. This results in an increase in lymphatic flow. Thus, the revised concept of filtration differs from Starling principles in three ways: (1) no reabsorption at the venous end, (2) no role for interstitial oncotic pressure, and (3) the lymphatic drainage is much higher than originally proposed by Starling. In view of these changes, the revised equation can be written as follows:

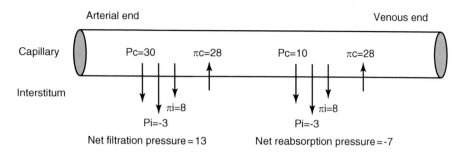

Fig. 6.1 Starling forces that operate at the arterial end and venous end of the capillary for filtration and reabsorption of fluid. The numbers reflect approximate pressures in mmHg. *Arrows* point toward the direction of flow

$$J_v = K_f \left[\left(P_c - P_i \right) - \sigma \left(\Pi_p - \Pi_{sg} \right) \right]$$

Although, the revised equation is appropriate for fluid exchange in the capillary, the exact oncotic pressure differences in various capillaries are not clearly known. Until these pressures are known, this author prefers to use the original Starling principles of fluid exchange in capillaries.

In general, edema is formed when Starling forces are altered. In addition, the inefficiency of lymphatics to drain fluid from the interstitium into the blood aids in the accumulation of fluid, causing edema. In CHF, due to backward failure, edema is formed because of accumulation of fluid in the venous end, which raises the hydrostatic pressure (P_c) to such an extent that it overcomes the net reabsorption pressure, resulting in the filtration of fluid from the capillary into the interstitium. Because of edema, decreased EABV persists. With low cardiac output (forward failure), Na$^+$ and water reabsorption continues, leading to altered Starling forces and edema formation. Formation of edema in cirrhosis and nephrotic syndrome is due to the persistent activation of salt- and water-retaining mechanisms and alterations in Starling forces. In nephrotic syndrome, an increase in the K_f of the capillary endothelium, permitting protein leakage, and activation of ENaC by serine protease are primarily responsible for edema formation (see Chap. 7–9).

Suggested Reading

1. Doucet A, Favre G, Deschênes G. Molecular mechanism of edema formation in nephrotic syndrome: therapeutic implications. Pediatr Nephrol. 2007;22:1983–90.
2. Rondon-Berrios H. New insights into the pathophysiology of oedema in nephrotic syndrome. Nefrologia. 2011;31:148–54.
3. Schrier RW. Decreased effective blood volume in edematous disorders: what does this mean? J Am Soc Nephrol. 2007;18:2028–31.
4. Slotki IN, Skorecki KL. Disorders of sodium balance. In: Skorecki K, et al., editors. Brenner & Rector's the kidney. 10th ed. Philadelphia: Elsevier; 2016. p. 390–459.

Disorders of ECF Volume: Congestive Heart Failure

7

Congestive heart failure (CHF) is a condition in which the cardiac output is decreased due to heart disease. However, the kidney is intrinsically normal. Despite normal kidney function, CHF is characterized by Na^+ retention and extracellular fluid (ECF) volume expansion. Decreased cardiac output in CHF is due to both "backward" and "forward" failure. In backward failure, accumulation of blood in the venous system causes increased hydrostatic pressure and filtration of fluid into the interstitium. This eventually leads to a decrease in plasma volume. In forward failure due to a decrease in cardiac contraction, enough blood is not supplied to the tissues due to which the kidneys cannot excrete Na^+ and water normally. In high-output CHF conditions such as AV shunts and beriberi, there is a decrease in peripheral vascular resistance due to shunting of the blood from arterial to venous side creating a situation similar to that of backward or forward failure. In both low-output and high-output cardiac failure, decreased effective arterial blood volume (EABV) persists, and this "underfilling" then activates salt-retaining mechanisms and nonosmotic release of antidiuretic hormone (ADH). The effect of atrial natriuretic peptide (ANP) on Na^+ excretion is attenuated. The major site for Na^+ reabsorption in CHF is the proximal tubule. Plasma volume increases and cardiac output improves. If these mechanisms persist despite excess plasma volume, edema is formed due to altered Starling forces. Figure 7.1 shows mechanisms that promote Na^+ reabsorption in CHF.

© Springer Science+Business Media LLC 2018
A.S. Reddi, *Fluid, Electrolyte and Acid-Base Disorders*,
DOI 10.1007/978-3-319-60167-0_7

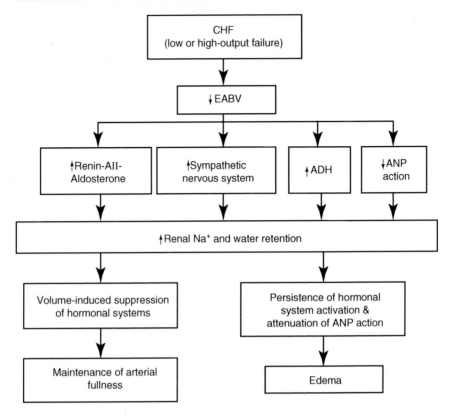

Fig. 7.1 Mechanisms of renal Na⁺ and water retention and edema formation in CHF

Clinical Evaluation

A brief discussion of clinical evaluation of CHF is presented here. The most common presentation of patients with heart failure (acute or chronic) is dyspnea due to pulmonary congestion and volume overload. Foot and leg discomfort due to edema and abdominal discomfort due to ascites are also frequently presented complaints. Taking history of prescribed medications, dietary salt intake, over-the-counter medications such as nonsteroidal anti-inflammatory drugs (NSAIDs), dizziness, syncope, palpitations, and alcohol use is an integral part of clinical evaluation.

Physical examination starts with taking the blood pressure and pulse rate, and orthostatic changes, if indicated. Neck, lung, heart, and abdominal examination for jugular–venous distention (JVD), crackles and pleural effusion, marked S_3 and P_2, murmurs, and ascites should be performed. Examination of lower extremities for pulses, edema, skin discoloration, and touch to coolness is extremely important. Mental status such as depression, confusion, forgetfulness, and difficulty in concentration also needs to be evaluated.

Pertinent labs include complete blood count (CBC), Na^+, K^+, Cl^-, HCO_3^-, BUN, creatinine, and glucose. Other tests include Ca^{2+}, Mg^{2+}, and phosphate. If Ca^{2+} is low, albumin is obtained. Liver function tests and lipid panel are needed, as indicated. Echocardiography (ECHO) and other tests are ordered as per the suggestion of a cardiologist.

Pertinent electrolyte abnormalities in patients with heart failure are hyponatremia and hyper- or hypokalemia. BUN is more important in patients with acute heart failure, as a level >43 mg/dL has a prognostic significance. Liver function tests are abnormal in many patients with right heart failure or biventricular failure. Anemia (< 10 g/dL) is also common in many patients with heart failure.

Treatment of CHF

Only management of edema is discussed. Effective medical therapy of CHF depends on understanding the abnormal physiologic processes that cause salt and water retention as well as venous congestion. Generalized edema affects all organ functions, including the myocardium with resultant decrease in left ventricle (LV) contractility, coronary blood flow, and ventricular compliance. Therefore, reduction in edema formation is an essential component of the overall management of CHF. The following therapeutic measures apply to most of the patients with mild to severe chronic CHF. Educating the patients about their condition and providing information about salt restriction and daily weight as a measure of salt and fluid intake are extremely helpful in long-term management of CHF.

Management of Edema

Ambulatory Patient

1. Restrict Na^+ to 2 g (88 mEq) or 5 g (85 mEq) salt diet. Avoid salt substitutes because they contain K^+, and hyperkalemia is possible in patients with renal dysfunction. Salt restriction improves diuretic and angiotensin-converting-enzyme inhibitor (ACE-I)'s effectiveness.
2. Restrict water to avoid hyponatremia, if patients are on thiazide diuretics.
3. Use diuretics, preferably loop diuretics, if salt and water restriction fails. Start furosemide at 20 mg orally twice daily, and follow natriuresis and diuresis. Increase the dose, if necessary. Bumetanide or torsemide can be substituted for furosemide, if patient is noncompliant to a twice-daily dose or long-acting loop diuretic is needed.
4. Addition of a thiazide diuretic (metolazone) to loop diuretic may be helpful in some patients. Like furosemide, metolazone works in patients with low GFR.
5. Suspect diuretic resistance in a compliant patient when the patient is gaining weight and signs and symptoms of edema are not improving on adequate regimen of diuretics. Patients develop diuretic resistance with acute or chronic use of

loop diuretics. This happens immediately following the first dose of furosemide, which induces more Na^+ and water loss than intake. A new steady state is reached in < 1 week, and additional doses of diuretic do not increase any electrolyte loss than intake. This is called the breaking phenomenon. The mechanism for this lack of response is not clearly understood; however, diuretic-induced renin secretion by macula densa independent of volume status and also volume depletion which activates sympathetic nervous system seem to stimulate postdiuretic Na^+ reabsorption. Were it not for the breaking phenomenon, the patient would lose all the fluid and salt and become extremely volume depleted.

Diuretic resistance due to chronic use is related to several factors. First, general volume depletion promotes Na^+ reabsorption in the proximal tubule with less delivery to other segments of the nephron. Second, loop diuretics are protein bound and are not filtered but secreted in the proximal tubule. Hypoalbuminemic conditions impair this secretion, causing less delivery of the diuretic to their site of action (thick ascending limb of Henle's loop). Third, the duration of action of furosemide is short so that postdiuretic Na^+ reabsorption is enhanced, and finally, loop diuretics deliver more Na^+ to the distal tubule. As a result, hyperplasia and hypertrophy of thiazide-sensitive epithelial cells occur, and these cells increase their Na^+ reabsorption. Low urinary Na^+ levels may indicate diuretic resistance.

6. Do not stop diuretic abruptly without restricting salt intake to avoid avid Na^+ reabsorption.
7. Diuretics promote excretion of water-soluble vitamins, and long-term therapy in CHF patients reduces folate and thiamine levels. Supplementation is, therefore, recommended.
8. Weight and orthostatic blood pressure and pulse rate changes are mandatory during each visit in patients on diuretics.

In-Hospital Patient with Acute Decompensated Heart Failure (ADHF)

1. Acute decompensated heart failure (ADHF) is the most common cause of hospital admission in elderly patients. For these patients, IV furosemide (5–10 mg/h) should be started until an optimal volume status is achieved. Continuous IV is superior to IV boluses, as the former infusion method was associated with good urine output, reduced hospital stay, and reduced mortality. Follow serum albumin concentration. A combination of albumin (25–50 g of 5% albumin) and 40–60 mg of furosemide can be tried for hypoalbuminemic patients. Note that this combination may not cause natriuresis and diuresis in all patients.
2. In addition to loop diuretics, nesiritide (brain natriuretic factor, BNP) can be given intravenously with or without furosemide to improve pulmonary capillary wedge pressure. Note that excessive diuresis by BNP can raise serum creatinine levels and precipitate acute cardiorenal syndrome.
3. If edema does not improve and patient has hyponatremia, oral vasopressin receptor (V_2) antagonist such as tolvaptan (15 mg) can be given. This results in water excretion (aquaresis) with improvement in serum sodium and weight.

4. When diuretic resistance is evident and nesiritide treatment no longer helps the patient and renal function worsens, ultrafiltration using continuous venovenous hemofiltration for fluid removal should be considered. Several advantages of hemofiltration over diuretic therapy have been reported, as shown below.

   (a) Removal of fluid and Na^+.
   (b) Hypokalemia less common.
   (c) Removal of proinflammatory cytokines.
   (d) Inhibition of renin–AII–aldosterone system.
   (e) Reduced length of hospital stay.
   (f) Decreased rehospitalization rate for heart failure.
   (g) Improved quality of life.
   (h) If the procedure is done carefully, prerenal azotemia can be prevented.

Note that ultrafiltration is expensive and is not devoid of complications, such as bleeding from anticoagulation and infection from catheter placement.

Inhibition of Renin–AII–Aldosterone, Sympathetic Nervous System, and ADH

Pharmacologic inhibition of the above salt- and water-retaining hormones helps not only contractility but also edema. ACE-Is, angiotensin receptor blockers (ARBs), or direct renin inhibitors reduce afterload and improve contractility. These drugs also cause vasodilation of the efferent arteriole by removing vasoconstrictive effect of AII. As a result of this vasodilation, more plasma flows into the peritubular capillaries, causing an increase in hydrostatic pressure and a decrease in oncotic pressure. The net effect is reduced Na^+ reabsorption. Aldosterone antagonist such as low-dose spironolactone or aldosterone receptor antagonist, eplerenone, improves contractility in CHF patients with reduced cardiac output. As stated above, tolvaptan or other approved ADH receptor antagonists promote water excretion. β-blockade with carvedilol or nevibolol suppresses sympathetic tone and improves contractility. African-American patients with CHF may benefit from a combination of nitrate and hydralazine. Thus, removal of fluid overload with a loop diuretic and improvement in contractility by vasodilators may improve CHF. In hospitalized patients, nesiritide is helpful in the inhibition of renin–AII–aldosterone system. Inotropes such as dobutamine and milrinone can improve cardiac function and urine output.

Cardiorenal Syndrome

Cardiorenal syndrome (CRS) is a recently described entity that refers to the interactivity between the heart and the kidney. Both organs have a cross talk between them in health and disease. Renal dysfunction carries poor prognosis in hospitalized patients with ADHF. The Acute Decompensated Heart Failure National Registry (ADHERE) database study reported that of all the variables, only high admission levels of BUN ($\geq$43 mg/dL) followed by a systolic blood pressure <115 mmHg and

Table 7.1 Classification of cardiorenal syndrome

Type	Description	Recommended treatment
Type 1	Acute cardiac decompensation (e.g., cardiogenic shock, ADHF) leading to acute kidney injury (AKI)	Diuretics, inotropes, nesiritide, and pressors, as indicated. Hold ACE-Is in view of acute increase in creatinine
Type 2	Chronic heart failure leading to progressive chronic kidney disease (CKD)	Loop and K^+-sparing diuretics, vasodilators, including ACE-Is
Type 3	AKI leading to acute cardiac disorders (fluid overload, CHF, arrhythmias due to hyperkalemia)	Treat cardiac disorders appropriately
Type 4	CKD leading to chronic heart failure due to fibrosis, anemia, etc.	Loop diuretics, ACE-Is, ARBs, correction of anemia, and other drugs as indicated
Type 5	Systemic diseases (e.g., diabetes, lupus) leading to both cardiac and kidney dysfunction	Treat the underlying disease and institute appropriate management to prevent cardiac and kidney disease

creatinine levels ≥ 2.75 mg/dL predicted high mortality in hospitalized patients with heart failure. Similarly, patients with acute kidney injury or chronic kidney disease may suffer a cardiovascular event, such as flash pulmonary edema, increased pre-load, and arrythmias. Thus, the relationship between the heart and the kidney is intricate and unavoidable.

The mechanisms that lead to CRS are incompletely understood. A classification of CRS has been developed to enhance our understanding of the pathophysiology of this syndrome (Table 7.1).

Study Questions

Case 1 A 60-year-old African-American woman with a past medical history of hypertension is admitted for dyspnea (shortness of breath) and weight gain of 10 lbs in the last 2 months. She denies chest pain, palpitations, dizziness, and syncope. She is on hydrochlorothizide and enalapril (an ACE-I) and noncompliant to diet. Her blood pressure is not well controlled on several clinic visits. Currently, her blood pressure is 160/96 mmHg with a pulse rate of 100 beats/min. She has no orthostatic changes. Pertinent physical examination includes JVD, crackles, an S_3, and pitting edema in her lower extremities. Chest X-ray shows pulmonary congestion. Her eGFR is >60 mL/min.

Question 1 Discuss the reason for her weight gain.

Answer Dietary noncompliance results in high Na^+ intake. Upon questioning, it was known that she was taking ibuprofen (Motrin) for leg pain. Both excess Na^+ intake and ibuprofen lead to fluid retention and eventually leg and pulmonary edema. Ibuprofen, an NSAID, decreases renal blood flow and GFR. Also, NSAIDs promote Na^+ reabsorption in the thick ascending limb and collecting duct. The net result is retention of Na^+ and the development of edema and weight gain.

Question 2 Describe this patient's EABV and urinary Na⁺ excretion.

Answer The EABV in patients with CHF is generally decreased, although the ECF volume is increased. Because of low EABV, the proximal tubule reabsorbs most of the filtered load of Na⁺ with urinary [Na⁺] <10 mEq/L.

Question 3 How would you manage her symptoms?

Answer The patient's shortness of breath will improve with diuresis by administering a loop diuretic such as furosemide. IV 40 mg bolus should be started with recording of urine output. Prompt urine output starts at 30 min and peaks between 1 and 2 h. This diuresis decreases LV filling pressures with improvement in dyspnea. Although no relationship between diuretic dose and the extent of diuresis is established in heart failure patients, doses from 20 to 400 mg daily have been used.

Question 4 Is bolus dosing better than continuous infusion of furosemide?

Answer Both of these approaches have been used in CHF patients. Bolus (BID dose) dosing of furosemide may have a good diuretic effect for 4–6 h, followed by a subtherapeutic effect for 6–8 h; during this period, Na⁺ reabsorption may be enhanced. This rebound effect may not be seen with continuous infusion. According to one meta-analysis, continuous infusion was associated with greater urine output, less renal dysfunction, lower mortality, and shorter length of stay as compared with bolus dosing. However, a few studies showed no difference between bolus and continuous infusion.

Question 5 What was her hospital course?

Answer With bolus furosemide (40 mg), the patient started having good diuresis. She had a urine volume of >3 L in 24 h, and her symptoms improved. IV furosemide (BID) was continued for another 24 h and then switched to oral furosemide 80 mg/day. She lost 12 lbs in 4 days. Her blood pressure decreased to 140/80 mmHg. She was instructed by a dietician regarding salt intake.

Question 6 How would you manage her edema in the outpatient setting?

Answer Restriction of salt to 5 g/day with no added salt or salt substitute is necessary. Medications should include oral furosemide 40 mg BID and ramipril 10 mg QD instead of enalapril. Patient should be seen in the clinic in 2 weeks. Advise her not to take NSAIDs, but acetaminophen as needed.

Two weeks later, she returns to the clinic. She has no shortness of breath. Her blood pressure is 140/82 mmHg with a pulse rate of 78 beats/min. She has trace edema in lower extremities. Serum chemistry is normal, but LDL cholesterol is 148 mg/dL. Atorvastatin 40 mg is prescribed, and a 6-week appointment is given.

After 24 weeks, her blood pressure was 156/90 mmHg, she gained 6 lbs., and developed pitting edema in lower extremities. Her urinary [Na⁺] was 20 mEq/L, despite adherence to salt diet.

Question 7 What would you do next?

Answer Based on her urinary [Na^+] and weight gain, she is reabsorbing Na^+ distal to the thick ascending limb of Henle's loop. Therefore, a thiazide-type diuretic such as metolazone 2.5–5 mg should be started to inhibit Na^+ reabsorption. During follow-up, furosemide dose can be increased to TID. Diuretic resistance should be suspected, if there is no response in edema or weight gain.

Case 2 A 72-year-old man with history of hypertension, type 2 diabetes, coronary artery disease with stent placement, and CHF is admitted for dyspnea at rest. He noticed swelling of his legs for 4 weeks despite salt restriction and diuretics. His LV ejection fraction (EF) is 40%. Meds: humalog (75/25) 20 units QD, furosemide 40 mg BID, metolazone 2.5 mg QD, spironolactone 12.5 mg QD, carvedilol 12.5 mg BID, ramipril 10 mg QD, atorvastatin 40 mg QD, clopidogrel 75 mg QD, and aspirin 81 mg QD. Physical examination: blood pressure 100/60 mmHg, pulse 102 beats/min, marked JVD, crackles, increased S_3, positive hepatojugular reflex, and pitting edema up to knees. Labs: Na^+ 134 mEq/l, K^+ 3.8 mEq/L, Cl^- 90 mEq/L, HCO_3^- 28 mEq/L, BUN 46 mg/dL, creatinine 1.8 mg/dL, eGFR <60 mL/min, and glucose 100 mg/dL. $HbA1_c$ 7%. Urinalysis is significant for 2+ proteinuria. Electrocardiogram shows tachycardia. He weighs 98 kg.

Question 1 How would you treat the patient initially?

Answer The patient needs symptomatic relief immediately from volume overload. Continuous IV furosemide (5 mg/h) is probably better than IV bolus because of established safety profile, greater urine output, and less renal impairment. If diuresis is poor on furosemide, nesiritide should be tried until urine output is improved. The recommended dose of nesiritide is 2 µg/kg bolus followed by 0.01 µg/kg/min. Nesiritide causes vasodilation in the venous and arterial, including coronary vasculature. It also decreases venous and ventricular pressures with slight increase in cardiac output. As a result, dyspnea may improve. With the use of nesiritide, the requirement for furosemide decreases. If urine output is not adequate, nitroglycerine at 20 µg/min should be considered. Since nitroglycerine causes hypotension, monitoring of blood pressure is extremely important, and the drug should be discontinued once systolic blood pressure is <90 mmHg.

The patient improved symptomatically over a 48 h period; however, his urine output and edema did not improve substantially. His weight decreased from 98 to 96 kg. Repeat labs show creatinine of 2.1 mg/dL. His blood pressure is maintained at 100/56 mmHg.

Question 2 What would be the next appropriate step?

Answer Adrenergic agonists such as dobutamine should be considered in view of low EF. Dobutamine improves cardiac output by decreasing afterload and increasing inotropy. Renal perfusion also improves at doses of 1–2 µg/kg/min.

Despite dobutamine, the urine output did not improve significantly in 24 h. Another inotrope, milrinone, which is a phosphodiesterase inhibitor was started with a bolus dose of 25 µg/kg followed by 0.1 µg/kg/min to improve inotropy. Milrinone blocks the degradation of cAMP, leading to Ca^{2+} influx into the myocyte and enhanced contractility. Blood pressure, urine output, and edema did not improve. Serum chemistry shows creatinine level of 3.2 mg/dL.

Question 3 What would you do next?

Answer The patient developed type 2 cardiorenal syndrome. Diuretics, nesiritide, and nitroglycerine should be discontinued. Hemofiltration is the best option for this patient. Continuous venovenous hemofiltration should be started for removal of fluid. Along with fluid removal, creatinine also improves. Continuous venovenous hemodiafiltration is needed in some patients.

Suggested Reading

1. Hadjiphilippou S, Kon SP. Cardiorenal syndrome: review of our current understanding. J Royal Soc Med 2015;o:1–6.
2. House AA, Haapio M, Lassus J, et al. Therapeutic strategies for heart failure in cardiorenal syndromes. Am J Kidney Dis. 2010;56:759–73.
3. Liang KV, Williams AW, Greene EL, et al. Acute decompensated heart failure and the cardiorenal syndrome. Crit Care Med. 2008;36(Suppl 1):S75–88.
4. Schrier RW. Renal sodium excretion, edematous disorders, and diuretic use. In: Schrier RW, editor. Renal and electrolyte disorders. 7th ed. Philadelphia: Kluwer; 2010. p. 45–85.

Disorders of ECF Volume: Cirrhosis of the Liver

8

Na$^+$ and water retention and extracellular fluid (ECF) volume expansion, leading to formation of edema and ascites, are the most common clinical findings in patients with severe liver disease. The initiating process for these clinical manifestations is hepatic cell death. Pathologically, in cirrhosis, the liver is characterized by fibrosis and nodular regeneration. Liver function tests (aminotransferases, bilirubin, alkaline phosphatase) are abnormal.

Similar to congestive heart failure (CHF), retention of Na$^+$ and water occurs in cirrhosis as a result of activation of salt- and water-retaining mechanisms rather than intrinsic abnormalities of the kidney. As in CHF, there is a decrease in effective arterial blood volume (EABV) due to arterial vasodilation in the splanchnic circulation prior to edema formation. This decrease in EABV, in turn, activates the neurohumoral vasoconstrictors and antidiuretic hormone (ADH) release (Fig. 8.1). As a result, Na$^+$ reabsorption is increased in the proximal and distal tubules. Water reabsorption is promoted by ADH. Resistance to atrial natriuretic peptide (ANP) also seems to contribute to Na$^+$ retention. When these mechanisms persist despite adequate plasma volume, alterations in the Starling forces promote edema formation. The mediators of the splanchnic vasodilation seem to be nitric oxide, endotoxin, and prostaglandins.

© Springer Science+Business Media LLC 2018
A.S. Reddi, *Fluid, Electrolyte and Acid-Base Disorders*,
DOI 10.1007/978-3-319-60167-0_8

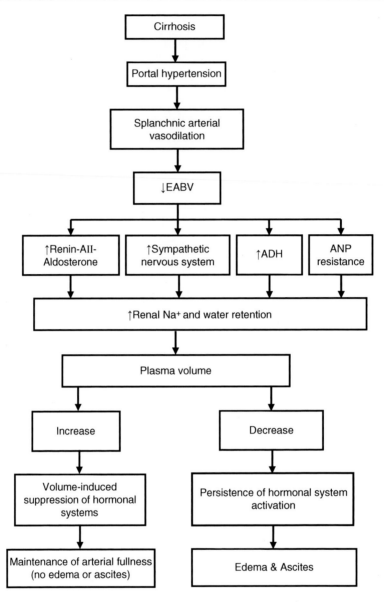

Fig. 8.1 Mechanisms of renal Na⁺ and water retention and edema and ascites formation in cirrhosis. *EABV* effective arterial blood volume, *ADH* antidiuretic hormone, *ANP* atrial natriuretic peptide, *AII* angiotensin II

Clinical Evaluation

A brief discussion of clinical evaluation of cirrhosis is presented here. The most common presentations of patients with cirrhosis (acute or chronic) are dyspnea, abdominal discomfort due to ascites, and lower leg edema. Taking history of pre-scribed medications, dietary salt intake, over-the-counter medications such as non-steroidal anti-inflammatory drugs (NSAIDs), dizziness, and recent alcohol use is an integral part of clinical evaluation.

Physical examination starts with measuring blood pressure and pulse rate and orthostatic changes, if indicated. Neck, lung, heart, and abdominal examination for jugular venous distention (JVD), crackles and pleural effusion, marked S_3 and P_2, murmurs, and ascites should be performed. Examination of lower extremities for pulses, edema, and skin discoloration is extremely important. Mental status, such as depression, confusion, forgetfulness, and difficulty in concentration, needs to be evaluated for encephalopathy.

Pertinent laboratory tests include complete blood count (CBC), Na^+, K^+, Cl^-, HCO_3^-, blood urea nitrogen (BUN), creatinine, and glucose. Other tests include Ca^{2+}, Mg^{2+}, phosphate, and albumin. Liver function tests and lipid panel are needed as indicated.

Pertinent electrolyte abnormalities in patients with cirrhosis are hyponatremia and hyper- or hypokalemia due to diuretics. BUN and creatinine levels will explain the status of the kidney function. Liver function tests are abnormal in many patients with cirrhosis. Anemia (< 10 g/dL) is also common in many patients.

Treatment of Edema

1. Restrict dietary Na^+ to 88 mEq (2 g Na^+ diet). Less than 60 mEq Na^+ diet may be unpalatable. Patients gain weight on unrestricted salt diet. Remember that reten-tion of 135–140 mEq of Na^+ will increase the ECF volume by 1 L or increase the weight by 1 kg.
2. Water restriction may not be necessary until serum Na^+ falls <130 mEq/L.
3. Measure spot urine [Na^+] during routine outpatient visit to document dietary compliance. Determination of weight at home and in the office is extremely helpful. Ideal weight loss in patients without edema is approximately 0.5 kg/day.
4. If salt and water restriction fail, start spironolactone at 100 mg/day, and stepwise increase the dose every 7 days to a maximum of 400 mg/day. If no response is seen in edema or hyperkalemia is present, start furosemide 20–40 mg/day. Evaluate weight, edema, and volume status in 7 days and then every 2 weeks. Titrate furosemide dose to 160 mg/day.

5. At times, measurement of a spot urine (preferably 24 h urine) Na^+/K^+ ratio may be helpful in selecting appropriate diuretic agent in patients with resistant edema. If the ratio is <1, the patient may respond to spironolactone alone, and furosemide may be the right choice in those whose ratio is >1. This avoids the combined use of spironolactone and furosemide and resultant excess volume depletion.

6. Bed rest is sometimes helpful. Na^+ is retained by the kidneys during daytime when the patient is walking, and it is excreted during recumbency. Note that there are no clinical trials to show that bed rest improves edema or promotes the efficacy of medical therapy.

Formation of Ascites

From Fig. 8.1, it is clear that Na^+ and water are retained even in early stages of cirrhosis because of activation of renin–angiotensin II (AII)–aldosterone, sympathetic nervous system (SNS), and nonosmotic release of ADH. However, edema and ascites may not be evident in some patients because of their strict dietary regimen. If the above management of edema fails, patients start developing ascites, which is the most common complication of cirrhosis. About 60% of patients with compensated cirrhosis develop ascites within 10 years during their course of disease. Patients with portal hypertension (portal vein pressure >12 mm Hg) only develop ascites. Noncirrhotic causes also cause ascites, but they are not discussed in this chapter. Tradionally three theories have been proposed in the formation of ascites in cirrhotic patients: (1) underfill, (2) overfill, and (3) peripheral vasodilation theories.

The underfill theory suggests that ascites formation begins when a critical imbalance of the Starling forces (increase in portal hydrostatic pressure and decrease in colloid oncotic pressure) develops in the hepatic sinusoids and splanchnic circulation with resultant transudation of fluid into the peritoneal cavity. This imbalance in the Starling forces is explained as follows. Unlike other capillaries in the body, hepatic sinusoids are highly permeable to proteins (albumin). As a result, the colloid oncotic pressure decreases in hepatic sinusoids. However, the sinusoidal hydrostatic pressure remains unchanged, which pushes the plasma from the vascular space into the lymphatics of the sinusoids. The cirrhotic liver generates high volumes of lymph (>20 L/day), and when lymph production exceeds the rate of removal by the thoracic duct, the excess lymph "spills" over the liver into the peritoneal cavity to form ascites. As ascites increases, a decrease in intravascular volume occurs which is perceived as a reduction in EABV. This reduction in EABV stimulates Na^+ retention and water-retaining mechanisms, resulting in further increase in ascites and edema. Thus, formation of ascites occurs prior to Na^+ retention. Although the underfill theory has been supported by some studies, other studies showed increased plasma volume in cirrhotics. This led to the development of overfill theory.

According to the overfill theory, Na^+ retention by the kidney precedes the development of ascites. It seems that the hepatic venous outflow obstruction signals renal Na^+ retention independent of decreased EABV. This Na^+ retention causes an increase in plasma volume, cardiac output, and splanchnic blood flow with resultant increase in portal pressure. This portal hypertension in association with an increase in hydrostatic pressure pushes fluid into the interstitium. Subsequently, the fluid overflows into the peritoneal cavity to form ascites.

These two theories do not adequately explain the formation of ascites in all cirrhotics. A third theory called peripheral vasodilation theory was proposed, which states that portal hypertension activates vasodilatory mechanisms mostly mediated by nitric oxide (NO) overproduction that eventually leads to splanchnic and peripheral arteriolar vasodilation. This arteriolar vasodilation causes underfilling of the vascular space and EABV. EABV is not due to true hypovolemia as in underfill theory but related to profound enlargement of the arterial tree due to arterial vasodilation. Underfilling of the arterial circulation is sensed by the arterial baroreceptors with resultant stimulation of renin–AII–aldosterone, SNS, and ADH axis. The net effect of this axis is retention of Na^+ and water by the kidneys, leading to increased plasma volume and development of ascites as well as edema (Fig. 8.1). Thus, Na^+ retention occurs following arterial vasodilation. Inhibition of NO synthesis prevents arterial vasodilation and Na^+ as well as water retention.

In mild to moderate stages of cirrhosis, arterial vasodilation is moderate, and the lymph that is generated is easily returned to the circulation by the thoracic duct. During this process, the EABV is preserved due to transient increase in Na^+ and water reabsorption. The resultant increase in plasma volume suppresses the renin–AII–aldosterone, SNS, and ADH action. Therefore, no edema or ascites is formed (Fig. 8.1).

Treatment of Ascites

The European Association for the Study of the Liver guidelines classify ascites into three grades based on the amount of fluid accumulation in the peritoneal cavity. This grading system avoids unnecessary therapeutic measures. Table 8.1 shows the grading system and suggested treatment for ascites.

Table 8.1 Grading of ascites and suggested treatment

Grade	Definition	Suggested treatment
Grade 1 ascites	Small volume (mild) detectable by ultrasound	No treatment. How frequently patients progress to grade 2 ascites is unknown
Grade 2 ascites	Moderate amount of fluid with distention of abdomen	Salt restriction and diuretics
Grade 3 ascites	Large amount of fluid with marked distention of abdomen	Large-volume paracentesis, with salt restriction and diuretics

Salt Restriction

1. Na^+ diet (88 mEq/day) or 5 g salt (1 teaspoon) diet (85 mEq).
2. No restriction of water unless patient has hyponatremia.

Diuretics

1. Spironolactone and furosemide. Patients with first episode of moderate ascites should receive spironolactone 100 mg/day with increasing dose every 7 days to a maximum of 400 mg/day. Monitor serum K^+. If no response to spironolactone or hyperkalemia is evident, start furosemide at 40 mg/day to a maximum of 160 mg/day. Maintain combination therapy ratio at 100 (spironolactone) to 40 (furosemide) mg. With this combination, serum $[K^+]$ is usually maintained at normal levels.
2. Patients with recurrent tense ascites should be started simultaneously with both spironolactone and furosemide, as suggested above. Weight loss during diuretic therapy should be approximately 0.5 kg/day for nonedematous patients and approximately 1 kg/day for edematous patients. The combination therapy reduces length of stay for hospitalized patients.
3. Some patients may gain weight despite on salt restriction and diuretic use. Before they are considered diuretic resistant, it is necessary to measure urine $[Na^+]$ for dietary compliance. A spot urine Na^+/K^+ ratio may be helpful. Diuretic-resistant patients will have a ratio <2.5, whereas those that are sensitive to diuretics will have a ratio >2.5.
4. Lower the dose of diuretics once ascites is minimal or absent. Discontinue diuretics when hyponatremia or hypovolemia is present. Also, discontinuation of diuretics is warranted when the patient develops renal impairment or hepatic encephalopathy.
5. When the patient is admitted for diuretic-induced hypovolemia, colloid (5% albumin) is better than crystalloid (normal saline) therapy to prevent accumulation of ascitic fluid. However, in some patients with less ascites, normal saline can be considered to reduce the need for albumin use.

Large-Volume Paracentesis

1. Large-volume paracentesis (LVP), removal of 5–7 L at one time, is the treatment of choice for patients with grade 3 ascites, followed by administration of 6–8 g/L of albumin to prevent circulatory dysfunction. Albumin is more effective than other plasma expanders.
2. Patients should receive maximum dose of diuretics after LVP to prevent reaccumulation of ascites.
3. Drugs such as NSAIDs and aminoglycosides are contraindicated in patients with ascites. Also, drugs such as angiotensin-converting enzyme (ACE) inhibitors or

angiotensin receptor blockers (ARBs) should be avoided as they lower blood pressure and increase serum creatinine.

4. Contrast study in a patient with normal renal function is not contraindicated. However, the benefit–risk ratio should be evaluated for contrast study in a patient with renal impairment.

Refractory Ascites

Refractory ascites is defined as ascites that does not respond to salt restriction and maximum doses of diuretics and recurs immediately after LVP. These patients retain Na^+. Generally, ascitic fluid $[Na^+]$ is similar to that of plasma $[Na^+]$. If serum $[Na^+]$ is 130 mEq/L, removal of 5 L of ascites is equal to removing approximately 650 mEq of Na^+. Assuming the patient is consuming 5 g salt diet (85 mEq) and excreting 13 mEq in the urine and stool, the patient retains a net of $72 (85 - 13 = 72)$ mEq/day. Thus, removal of 5 L of ascitic fluid is equivalent to removal of 9 days of retained Na^+ (72 mEq $\times 9 = 648$ mEq). For this reason, frequent therapeutic LVPs with albumin are recommended. It should be noted that serial paracenteses predispose patients to infection, protein malnutrition, and other complications. Diuretics should be discontinued in these patients if their urine Na^+ is <30 mEq/L. Use of midodrine (7.5 mg orally 3 times/day) has been shown to improve urine volume, urine Na^+ excretion, mean arterial pressure, and survival in patients with refractory ascites.

Transjugular intrahepatic portosystemic shunt (TIPS) is an alternative to repeated LVPs; however, TIPS is associated with precipitation of hepatic encephalopathy. Also, TIPS did not show any survival benefit over serial LVPs. Liver transplantation is definitely indicated in some of these patients with refractory ascites.

Some studies have shown improvement in ascites following weekly infusion of albumin, and daily use of clonidine (0.075 mg twice daily), or subcutaneous injection of octreotide.

Hepatorenal Syndrome

Hepatorenal syndrome (HRS) is defined as the development of renal failure in a patient with advanced liver disease and ascites. It may also occur in patients with acute liver failure. Renal failure is not related to intrinsic renal disease. In 2015, the criteria for HRS have been revised (Table 8.2).

Thus, HRS is the diagnosis of exclusion. Two types of HRS have been described. Type 1 HRS is characterized by rapidly progressive decline in renal function over a 2-week period. It is usually precipitated by spontaneous bacterial peritonitis. Type 2 HRS is associated with slow decline in renal function, and survival is better than patients with type 1 HRS.

The pathogenesis of HRS involves a decrease in EABV with activation of neurohormonal systems and severe vasoconstriction of the afferent arteriole. As a result,

Table 8.2 Criteria for HRS

1	Diagnosis of cirrhosis and ascites
2	Diagnosis of AKI according to ICA-AKI criteria
3	No response after 2 days of diuretic withdrawal and plasma volume expansion with albumin 1 g per kg of body weight
4	Absence of shock
5	No current or recent use of nephrotoxic drugs (NSAIDs, aminoglycosides, iodinated contrast media, etc.)
6	No macroscopic signs of structural kidney injury*defined as
	Absence of proteinuria (>500 mg/day)
	Absence of microhematuria (>50 RBCs cells per high-power field)
	Normal findings on renal ultrasonography

*Patients who fulfil these criteria may still have structural damage such as tubular damage. Urine biomarkers will become an important element in making a more accurate differential diagnosis between HRS and acute tubular necrosis. *AKI* acute kidney injury, *ICA* International Club of Ascites, *NSAIDs* nonsteroidal anti-inflammatory drugs, *RBCs* red blood cells

renal blood flow decreases. In addition, arterial blood pressure also decreases because of systemic vasodilation, resulting in low cardiac output. There is also a coexistence of systemic inflammation that contributes to low cardiac output. Relative adrenal dysfunction has also been implicated in the pathogenesis of HRS. All of these mechanisms impair cardiac function and renal blood flow, leading to renal dysfunction in HRS.

Treatment

Pharmacologic treatment has been shown to improve the clinical course of type 1 HRS and is the choice of therapy. The most commonly used combination is vasoconstrictors and albumin. Vasoconstrictors that have been tried frequently in clinical trials are vasopressin, terlipressin (an analogue of vasopressin with greater effect on V_1 than V_2 receptor), norepinephrine, midodrine, and dopamine. Vasoconstrictors are used to counteract the splanchnic vasodilation and albumin for expansion of arterial volume. Octreotide, a long-acting somatostatin analogue, reduces portal hypertension and causes splanchnic vasoconstriction. The aim of vasoconstrictor therapy is to improve mean arterial pressure. It has been shown that an increase in mean arterial pressure >5 mmHg improved renal function in patients with type 1 HRS irrespective of the agents used. Midodrine at a dose of 7.5 mg three times a day to a patient with recurrent or refractory ascites improved urine volume, urine Na^+ excretion, mean arterial pressure, and survival. Also, vasoconstrictor therapy alone with or without albumin reduced mortality in both types of HRS. The combinations of agents that have been tried most frequently in clinical trials are shown below.

1. Combination 1 (terlipressin + albumin). Terlipressin (not yet approved in the USA) starting dose is 1 mg IV q4–6 h. Increase the dose to 2 mg q4–8 h, if serum creatinine does not decrease by 25% from baseline by day 3 up to a maximum of

12 mg/day as long as there are no side effects. Simultaneously start 25% albumin at 1 g/kg followed by daily doses of 20–50 g. Continue treatment to a maximum of 14 days. This is the preferred combination.

2. Combination 2 (midodrine + octreotide + albumin). Midodrine (an α1 agonist)— start with 7.5–12.5 mg orally q8 h, as needed, to increase the mean arterial pressure by 10 mmHg from baseline. Also, start octreotide 100–200 μg subcutaneously q8 h. Also, start 25% albumin at 1 g/kg followed by 20–50 g/day. Duration of treatment is 14 days. This is the preferred combination when terlipressin is not available.

3. Combination 3 (norepinephrine + albumin). Start with norepinephrine at 0.5–3.0 mg/h IV until the mean arterial pressure increases by at least 10 mmHg from baseline. Simultaneously start 25% albumin at 1 g/kg followed by 20–50 g/day. The maximum duration of treatment is not well established. However, patients who do not improve their renal function after 4 days of treatment may not reverse their HRS and require other treatment modalities (see below).

The above combination regimens have shown reversal of HRS in 25–83% of patients compared with 8.7–12.5% with albumin alone. If HRS recurs, retreatment with one of the above combinations should be started. It is interesting to note that HRS due to acute liver disease with fulminant hepatic failure may not respond to any of the above combinations. There are several contraindications for vasoconstrictor therapy in HRS: (1) coronary artery disease, (2) cardiac arrhythmias, (3) respiratory or cardiac failure, (4) severe hypertension, (5) cerebrovascular accidents, (6) peripheral vascular disease, and (7) severe bronchospasm.

Other Treatment Modalities

1. TIPS alone or in combination with pharmacologic therapy
2. Hemodialysis or peritoneal dialysis (not preferred treatments)
3. Continuous venovenous hemofiltration (CVVH)
4. Continuous venovenous hemodiafiltration (CVVHDF)
5. Extracorporeal albumin dialysis system (molecular adsorbent recirculating system or MARS)
6. Orthotopic liver transplantation

Study Questions

Case 1 A 50-year-old woman with alcohol abuse presents to the emergency department for the first time with dyspnea, worsening abdominal distention, and swollen legs for the last 4 weeks. Past medical history includes 1 pint of alcohol a day for 20 years. She is not on any medications. She eats regular diet. Blood pressure is 124/68 mmHg with a pulse rate of 80 beats/min. She has crackles, an S_3, tense ascites, and pitting edema up to the knees. Pertinent labs: serum [Na$^+$] 128 mEq/L, [K$^+$] 3.6 mEq/L, and creatinine 0.8 mg/dL. Chest X-ray shows pulmonary congestion.

Question 1 Does this patient have a Na$^+$ or water problem or both?

Answer This patient has both Na$^+$ and water problems. On the basis of physical examination, she has an excess total body [Na$^+$]. In addition to cirrhosis, she has CHF. Both liver disease (cirrhosis) and CHF are characterized by decreased EABV. As a result, the patient will retain both Na$^+$ and water.

Question 2 What would her urinary Na$^+$ excretion be?

Answer Since her EABV is decreased with activation of neurohormonal system, her excretion of Na$^+$ would be < 10 mEq/L.

Question 3 How would you treat this patient?

Answer Since her major problem is Na$^+$ and water retention, restriction of both will help lose weight. Since the patient has crackles with pulmonary congestion, she would benefit from IV infusion of a loop diuretic such as furosemide (40 mg BID). Spironolactone at 100 mg should be started initially with an increase every 2–3 days by 100 mg up to 400 mg/day. If urine output is not adequate, furosemide up to 160 mg (80 mg BID) should be tried. Bed rest is advisable to improve cardiac output and glomerular filtration rate (GFR). Her ascites and CHF should improve. If her ascites does not improve despite the above treatment modality, LVP with 5% albumin (6–8 g/L) replacement is recommended. Daily weight, blood pressure, and intake/output (I/O) should be recorded.

   With the above management, she lost 14 kg in 7 days. Her serum [Na$^+$] is 134 mEq/L, and creatinine remains at 0.8 mg/dL. She received education about restricted Na$^+$ diet and abstinence of alcohol and was discharged on spironolactone 400 mg QD and furosemide 80 mg BID. She was given clinic appointment in 2 weeks. In the clinic, she was found to have severe volume depletion and weight loss of another 4 kg. Her ascites did not increase during this 2-week period.

Question 4 What would you do next?

Answer She should be hospitalized for volume replacement and stabilization. Diuretics should be stopped, and 5% albumin should be given (100 g/day). A liter of normal saline can be considered with 50 g of 5% albumin the next day. Daily weight with blood pressure and I/Os should be followed. On discharge, furosemide dose should be decreased to 40 mg BID with reducing dose of spironolactone, as indicated.

Case 2 A 38-year-old man with cirrhosis due to hepatitis C develops refractory ascites requiring LVP (5–7 L) every 2 weeks with albumin infusion. He is on furosemide and spironolactone at the maximum doses, but not on any prophylactic antibiotics. He has been stable for over 6 months. This time, he comes to the clinic with a complaint of abdominal discomfort and pain. Following a LVP (6 L), he is admitted for possible spontaneous bacterial peritonitis (SBP) and antibiotic therapy. His

Na$^+$ is 130 mEq/L, creatinine 1.3 mg/dL, and bilirubin 8 mg/dL. His urinalysis is benign other than bilirubin. His urine Na$^+$ is < 10 mEq/L. Ascitic fluid white blood cell (WBC) count is 500, and culture result is pending.

Question 1 How would you manage the patient?

Answer Diuretics should be discontinued. A third-generation cephalosporin, either cefotaxime (2 g IV q8 h) or ceftriaxone (1 g q12 h), should be started based on estimated GFR (eGFR). Albumin (5%) at 1.5 g/kg at diagnosis and 1 g/kg on day 3 may substantially decrease the development of HRS. This combination (antibiotic and albumin) therapy should be continued for a minimum of 5 days.

Despite the combination therapy, his bilirubin and creatinine increased to 10 mg/dL and 2.4 mg/dL, respectively. His urine analysis is still benign.

Question 2 What is the diagnosis, and how would you treat the patient?

Answer The patient developed type 1 HRS, since 30% of patients with SBP develop HRS. Vasoconstrictor therapy with albumin should be started. The combination therapy either one or two, as described under HRS, should be started. If no response is seen in 14 days, other options such as CVVH or CVVHDF, TIPS, or liver transplantation should be considered.

Suggested Reading

1. Angeli P, Ginès P, Wong F, et al. Diagnosis and management of acute kidney injury in patients with cirrhosis: revised consensus recommendations of the International Club of Ascites. J Hepatol. 2015;62:968–74.
2. Durand F, Graupera I, Ginès P, et al. Pathogenesis of hepatorenal syndrome: implications for therapy. Am J Kidney Dis. 2016;67:318–28.
3. Ginès P, Cardenas A, Sola E, et al. Liver disease and the kidney. In: Coffman TM, et al., editors. Schrier's diseases of the kidney. 9th ed. Philadelphia: Lippincott Williams & Wilkins; 2013. p. 1965–96.
4. Runyon BA. Introduction to the revised American Association for the study of liver disease practice guideline management of adult patients with ascites due to cirrhosis 2012. Hepatology. 2013;57:1651–3.

Disorders of ECF Volume: Nephrotic Syndrome

9

Unlike patients with congestive heart failure (CHF) and cirrhosis, patients with nephrotic syndrome have some underlying renal disease. Also, effective arterial blood volume (EABV) is not decreased in all patients with nephrotic syndrome. This syndrome is characterized by proteinuria in excess of 3.5 g/day, hypoalbuminemia, hyperlipidemia, edema, and lipiduria. The mechanism for salt and water retention is not clear. The traditional ("underfill") theory implies that loss of protein in the urine causes hypoalbuminemia and decreased plasma oncotic pressure. These factors favor fluid movement into the interstitium, resulting in intravascular hypovolemia and activation of salt-retaining mechanisms (Fig. 9.1). Two lines of evidence, however, argue against this traditional theory. First, not all patients with congenital deficiency of albumin (analbuminemia) develop edema. Second, some patients with nephrotic syndrome have either normal or increased intravascular volume despite hypoalbuminemia. This evidence suggests that mechanisms other than hypoalbuminemia and decreased intravascular volume play a role in renal retention of Na^+ in nephrotic syndrome.

Experimental evidence also suggests that Na^+ and water retention occurs in the kidney due to an intrarenal cause independent of salt-retaining mechanisms. As a result, the plasma volume is expanded, and this overfilled plasma volume leaks into the interstitium to cause edema. This is called the "overfill" theory (Fig. 9.1). The major site for Na^+ reabsorption in patients with nephrotic syndrome is the collecting duct. This formed the basis of molecular theory.

According to this theory, Na^+ retention in patients with nephrotic syndrome occurs by the overactivity of the epithelial Na^+ channel (ENaC) in principal cells of the collecting duct. ENaC is inhibited by amiloride. Studies also have shown that the activity of Na/K-ATPase located in the basolateral membrane of the principal cell is enhanced. The net effect is avid Na^+ reabsorption. It seems that ENaC activity is increased by locally generated plasmin from plasminogen. Plasminogen is filtered at the glomerulus in nephrotic syndrome. When it reaches the cortical

© Springer Science+Business Media LLC 2018
A.S. Reddi, *Fluid, Electrolyte and Acid-Base Disorders*,
DOI 10.1007/978-3-319-60167-0_9

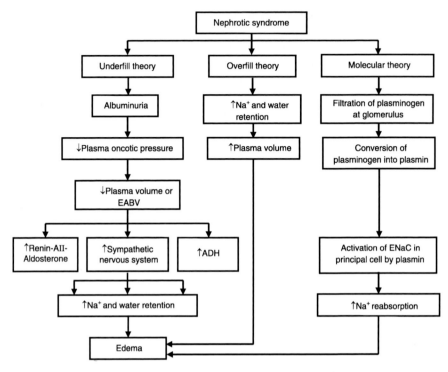

Fig. 9.1 Mechanisms of renal Na$^+$ and water retention and edema formation in nephrotic syndrome

collecting duct, it is split into plasmin by urokinase, and plasmin activates the ENaC to reabsorb Na$^+$, resulting in low excretion of Na$^+$. Thus, edema is formed in nephrotic syndrome.

Finally, the roles of atrial natriuretic peptide (ANP) and brain natriuretic peptide (BNP) have been implicated in the formation of edema in nephrotic syndrome. The levels of both of these hormones are elevated in nephrotic syndrome; however, their diuretic and natriuretic effects are blunted, resulting in retention of Na$^+$ and water and edema formation.

Clinical Evaluation

A brief discussion of clinical evaluation of nephrotic syndrome is presented here. The most common presentation of patients with nephrotic syndrome is leg edema. Taking history of prescribed medications, dietary salt intake, over-the-counter medications such as nonsteroidal anti-inflammatory drugs (NSAIDs), dyspnea, and dizziness is an integral part of clinical evaluation.

Physical examination starts with taking blood pressure and pulse rate, and orthostatic changes, if indicated. Neck, lung, heart, and abdominal examination for

Table 9.1 Pertinent serology in nephrotic syndrome

Test	Comment
VDRL	Patients with positive VDRL test with nephrotic syndrome may have underlying minimal change disease or membranous nephropathy
ASO (antistreptolysin) titers	To rule out postinfectious glomerulonephritis (GN)
Complement (C3 and C4)	Low complements in postinfectious GN, lupus nephritis, membranoproliferative GN, and cryoglobulinemia
HIV, hepatitis B and C, as indicated	To recognize the respective diseases
cANCA and pANCA	To recognize Wegener's granulomatosis (granulomatosis with polyangitis) and microscopic polyarteritis

VDRL venereal disease research laboratory, *cANCA* cytoplasmic antineutrophil cytoplasmic antibodies, *pANCA* perinuclear antineutrophil cytoplasmic antibodies

JVD, crackles and pleural effusion, marked S_3 and P_2, murmurs, and ascites should be performed. Examination of lower extremities for pulses, edema, and skin discoloration is extremely important.

Pertinent laboratory tests include complete blood count (CBC), Na^+, K^+, Cl^-, HCO_3^-, blood urea nitrogen (BUN), creatinine, and glucose. Other tests include Ca^{2+}, Mg^{2+}, phosphate, and lipid panel. Urine analysis, protein-to-creatinine ratio, and if possible 24 h urine for protein and creatinine need to be ordered routinely. Serum protein electrophoresis should be ordered for protein excretion other than albumin. Routine serology (Table 9.1) is necessary.

Pertinent electrolyte abnormalities in patients with nephrotic syndrome are hyponatremia and hyper- or hypokalemia due to diuretic use. Anemia (< 10 g/dL) is also common in many patients with nephrotic syndrome.

Treatment

1. Treat the underlying cause of nephrotic syndrome. Use immunosuppressive agents (steroids, cyclophosphamide, cyclosporine, mycophenolate mofetil, and other agents, as indicated).
2. Restrict dietary Na^+, as suggested for CHF and cirrhosis.
3. Use combination of loop diuretic and amiloride to improve edema. Also, spironolactone can be used in place of amiloride.
4. Restrict dietary protein intake to < 1 g/kg/day, if serum albumin is < 2 g/dL.
5. Use angiotensin-converting enzyme inhibitors (ACE-Is) or angiotensin receptor blockers (ARBs) to improve proteinuria and prevent progression of renal disease.
6. Addition of small doses (12.5–50 mg) of spironolactone in combination with ACE-I or ARB to improve proteinuria and prevent progression of renal disease.
7. Follow serum K^+, as hyperkalemia is rather common.
8. The use of statin is important to improve lipids and proteinuria.
9. Avoid NSAIDs.

10. Avoid excess diuresis, as volume depletion precipitates acute kidney injury.
11. Consider ultrafiltration, if diuretic resistance develops.
12. Note that edema resolves once proteinuria is improved.
13. Do not use the combination of furosemide and triamterene, as the latter inhibits the secretion of the former in the proximal tubule.

Study Questions

Case 1 A 46-year-old man is referred to you by a primary care physician for evaluation of proteinuria and leg edema for 3 months. The patient is healthy otherwise. He is not on any medications; however, he has a long history of smoking. The patient noticed edema of lower extremities 2 months ago. Blood pressure is 132/80 mmHg with a pulse rate of 74 beats/min. Physical examination is normal other than pitting edema in lower extremities. Serum chemistry and CBC are normal. Serum albumin is 3.2 g/dL. Urinalysis reveals 4+ proteinuria and fatty casts. Urine protein-to-creatinine ratio is 7.2, and 24 h protein is 7.1 g. His urinary Na^+ is 142 mEq/L. He weighs 94 kg. The patient agrees to renal biopsy, which shows membranous nephropathy. Work-up for secondary causes of membranous nephropathy is negative. He has no insurance.

Question 1 What is your initial management of edema?

Answer Restriction of Na^+ (88 mEq) in the diet is the first step in the management. Furosemide 40 mg QD and lisinopril (an ACE-I) 20 mg QD should be started to improve edema and proteinuria.

Patient returns to your office in 2 weeks with worsening edema. There is no change in blood pressure. His weight is now 95 kg. The urinary Na^+ is 132 mEq/L, and total protein excretion is 6.9 g.

Question 2 Does his urinary Na^+ reflect dietary intake or the effect of furosemide?

Answer Although furosemide increases both diuresis and natriuresis initially, a few days later new equilibrium is established, and daily excretion of Na^+ no longer exceeds daily intake. Therefore, the urinary Na^+ of 132 mEq/L reflects his daily intake and not the effect of furosemide. ACE-I does not have its full effect in a patient with noncompliance to low Na^+ intake.

Question 3 How would you manage the edema?

Answer The patient should adhere to low-salt diet, and with furosemide he will have a negative Na^+ balance. Also, lisinopril promotes Na^+ excretion by alteration in Starling forces in the peritubular capillaries.

Two weeks later, he returns to your office with slight improvement in edema. His urinary Na^+ is 79 mEq/L, and his weight is 93 kg. Serum chemistry is normal except for K^+ of 3.4 mEq/L.

Question 4 What would you do next?

Answer Adding amiloride 5 mg QD seems appropriate in this patient. This avoids hypokalemia and also improves edema.

Question 5 Does reduction in proteinuria improve edema?

Answer Yes. In any patient with nephrotic syndrome due to a glomerular lesion, either immunosuppression induced or spontaneous resolution of nephrotic syndrome improves edema. In this patient, his glomerular disease may respond to immunosuppressive therapy and should be tried.

Four weeks later, his edema has improved with proteinuria of 6.1 g. He weighs 89 kg. Hypokalemia resolved. His albumin is 3.5 g/dL, but LDL cholesterol is 124 mg/dL.

Question 6 What would you do next?

Answer Adding atorvastatin 20 mg QD is appropriate to improve both LDL cholesterol and proteinuria.

Question 7 What are your final therapeutic strategies in this patient?

Answer The therapeutic strategies in this patient are:

1. Restrict Na^+ in the diet to 85–88 mEq/day.
2. Continue the combination of furosemide and amiloride.
3. Use other loop diuretics (bumetanide or torsemide), if necessary.
4. Reduce proteinuria with an ACE-I or ARB and immunosuppressive drugs with tapering.
5. Restrict protein intake to < 1 g/kg/day.
6. Continue atorvastatin, and follow liver function tests and creatine kinase.
7. Avoid NSAIDs, and, if needed, suggest acetaminophen for pain.
8. Avoid excess diuresis and hypovolemia.

Case 2 A 54-year-old obese woman with type 2 diabetes, hypertension, and coronary artery disease is admitted for refractory edema associated with weakness and difficulty in walking. She is on maximum doses of furosemide, spironolactone, indapamide, and an ACE-I. She follows diet as per her physician. Her urine output is 600 ml/day. Her blood pressure is 120/76 mmHg. Pulse rate is 82 beats/min. Serum chemistry is normal except for creatinine of 1.6 mg/dL. Hemoglobin A1c is 7%. Other medications include insulin, atorvastatin, vitamin D, and aspirin. Her 24 h proteinuria is 8.2 g.

Question 1 How does diuretic resistance develop?

Answer Diuretic resistance in a compliant patient is defined as gaining of weight and edema despite adequate regimen of diuretics. Diuretic resistance is related to several factors. First, relative volume depletion promotes Na^+ in the proximal tubule with less delivery to other segments of the nephron. This is related to activation of sympathetic nervous system and renin–AII–aldosterone system. Second, loop diuretics are protein bound and are not filtered but secreted in the proximal tubule. Hypoalbuminemic conditions impair this secretion, causing less delivery of the diuretic to its site of action (thick ascending limb of Henle's loop). Third, the duration of action of furosemide is short so that postdiuretic Na^+ reabsorption is enhanced, and finally, loop diuretics deliver more Na^+ to the distal tubule. As a result, hyperplasia and hypertrophy of thiazide-sensitive epithelial cells occur, and these cells increase their Na^+ reabsorption. Low urinary Na^+ levels may indicate diuretic resistance.

Question 2 How does hypoalbuminemia cause diuretic resistance in nephrotic syndrome?

Answer Diuretic resistance due to hypoalbuminemia is a well-recognized phenomenon. First, furosemide is >95% protein bound, and this complex is delivered to the proximal tubule for secretion. In hypoalbuminemia, less protein binding results in more free drug availability (increase in volume of distribution) and less secretion. Second, the metabolic clearance of furosemide is increased in hypoalbuminemia, and third, even the small amount of furosemide that is secreted into the tubular lumen binds to the filtered albumin with resultant decrease in delivery to the site of action.

Question 3 Does the combination of furosemide and albumin increase natriuresis and diuresis?

Answer As previously stated, hypoalbuminemia blunts the natriuretic effect of furosemide. Initially, it was shown that premixing of furosemide with albumin enhanced natriuresis in adult and pediatric patients with nephrotic syndrome. Other studies have failed to confirm this observation. A few case reports in patients with CHF and hypoalbuminemia have shown beneficial effects of the combination of furosemide and albumin. Thus, this combination therapy should be individualized.

Suggested Reading

1. Doucet A, Favre G, Deschènes G. Molecular mechanism of edema formation in nephrotic syndrome: therapeutic implications. Ped Nephrol. 2007;22:1983–90.
2. Duffy M, Jain S, Harrell N, et al. Albumin and furosemide combination for management of edema in nephrotic syndrome: a review of clinical studies. Cell. 2015;4:622–30.
3. Elhassan EA, Scrier RW. Disorders of extracellular volume. In: Johnson RJ, Feehally J, Floege J, editors. Comprehensive clinical nephrology. 5th ed. Philadelphia: Elsevier Saunders; 2015. p. 80–93.
4. Rondon-Berrios H. New insights into the pathophysiology of oedema in nephrotc syndrome. Nefrologia. 2011;31:148–54.
5. Siddall EC, Radhakrishnan J. The pathophysiology of edema formation in the nephrotic syndrome. Kidney Int. 2012;82:635–42.

Disorders of ECF Volume: Volume Contraction

10

As stated in Chap. 6, the maintenance of extracellular fluid (ECF) volume is dependent on the extracellular concentration of Na^+ ($[Na^+]$). An increase in total body Na^+ causes an expansion in ECF volume, and a decrease in total body Na^+ reduces ECF volume. Most of the critically ill patients and patients with less availability of salt and water develop volume contraction, because it is rather difficult to induce volume contraction in humans with normal renal function. The signs and symptoms of volume contraction depend on the rapidity of Na^+ loss. Sudden loss of Na^+ causes a marked reduction in blood pressure and cardiac output, whereas slow and sustained loss results in a slight decrease in blood pressure. Pure water loss results in hypertonicity with high serum $[Na^+]$, whereas loss of both Na^+ and water leads to low blood pressure.

Causes of Volume Contraction

Volume depletion can be caused by many conditions. Generally, loss of Na^+ occurs through renal as well as extrarenal routes, as shown in Table 10.1.

© Springer Science+Business Media LLC 2018
A.S. Reddi, *Fluid, Electrolyte and Acid-Base Disorders*,
DOI 10.1007/978-3-319-60167-0_10

Table 10.1 Extrarenal and renal causes of Na⁺ loss

Extrarenal loss	Renal loss
Gastrointestinal losses	*Na⁺ loss by the normal kidney*
Vomiting	Diuretics
Diarrhea	Adrenal insufficiency
Nasogastric suction	Decreased renin production
Fistulas	*Na⁺ loss by the abnormal kidney*
Bleeding	Chronic kidney disease
Transcellular losses	Diuretic phase of acute kidney injury
Acute pancreatitis	Postobstructive diuresis
Ileus	Renal transplantation
Peritonitis	Salt-losing nephropathy
Small bowel obstruction	Tubulointerstitial diseases
Pleural effusions	
Skin losses	
Excessive sweating	
Burns	
Inflammatory skin diseases	
Cystic fibrosis	

Dehydration vs Volume Depletion

Generally, dehydration and volume depletion are used interchangeably in clinical practice. Although both of them are bedside diagnoses, they differ in certain aspects. Dehydration results from pure water loss with high serum [Na⁺]. Most of this water loss (two-thirds) is from the intracellular fluid (ICF) compartment and very little from the intravascular compartment. Blood pressure is, therefore, either slightly low or normal. Patients with volume depletion lose Na⁺ and water mostly from the ECF (intravascular) compartment. As a result, they have orthostatic blood pressure and pulse changes. Thus, the pathophysiology of these two conditions is different with some differences in signs and symptoms (Table 10.2). Treatment of these conditions is also different.

Types of Fluid Loss

It is customary to classify fluid losses into *hypotonic*, *isotonic*, or *hypertonic* volume contraction. The term contraction is used here to denote both dehydration and volume depletion. *Hypotonic* volume contraction occurs as a result of electrolyte (salt) in excess of water loss. This excess electrolyte loss causes a decrease in plasma osmolality, which shifts water from the ECF to the ICF compartment to maintain osmotic equilibrium (see Chap. 1). Thus, the ICF compartment is expanded. Diuretic use is an example. *Isotonic* volume contraction is due to the loss of salt and water in proportionate amounts, i.e., 154 mEq of Na⁺ and 154 mEq of Cl⁻ for each liter of water. As a result, the plasma osmolality does not change, and therefore, no shift in water between

Table 10.2 Pertinent clinical and laboratory features of volume contraction

Clinical evaluation	Dehydration	Volume depletion
History		
Dietary history of Na$^+$ and water intake	Yes	Yes
History of renal disease	Yes	Yes
History of medications (diuretics)	Yes	Yes
History of travel, diarrhea, vomiting, bleeding	Yes	Yes
History of symptoms: thirst, weakness, dizziness, lethargy	Yes (more thirst)	Yes (less thirst)
Physical examination		
Low blood pressure	Yes	Yes
Orthostatic blood pressure and pulse changes	No	Yes
Poor skin turgor	+	+++
Dry mucous membranes	+++	+
↓ Urine output	+++	++
Laboratory data		
Serum [Na$^+$]	High	Normal to slightly low
Serum osmolality	High	Normal
Serum creatinine	+	++
Serum BUN	+	++
Hematocrit	+	++
Urine osmolality	+++	+
Urine [Na$^+$]	<10 mEq/L	>10 mEq/L
Fractional excretion of Na$^+$	<1%	>2%

+ mild, ++ moderate, +++ severe, ↓ decreased, *BUN* blood urea nitrogen

ECF and ICF compartments occurs. However, the loss of isotonic fluid is entirely from the ECF compartment, resulting in its contraction. Thus, isotonic fluid loss is more likely to produce circulatory collapse. Diarrhea is a cause of isotonic contraction. In *hypertonic* contraction, water loss exceeds salt loss. As a result, the plasma [Na$^+$] and osmolality increase, which causes a shift of water from ICF to ECF compartment. Decreased intake of water, excess sweating, or urinary loss of water and salt due to an increase in serum glucose levels generally cause hypertonic contraction.

Clinical Evaluation

Diagnosis of ECF volume contraction can be made by obtaining appropriate medical history, physical signs and symptoms, and laboratory findings (Table 10.2). At times, it is difficult to distinguish between dehydration and volume depletion at bedside. Studies on water deprivation suggested that at least 10% of water (3–4 L) loss is needed before volume contraction is evident on physical examination. At least 15% of water (>6 L) loss is needed to demonstrate orthostatic changes. Mild deficit (2–4%) in total body water may have a slight increase in pulse rate that is above the expected increase on standing, which is usually not recognized on physical examination.

Treatment

The goals of therapy in a volume-contracted patient are twofold: (1) to improve perfusion pressure to vital organs such as the brain, kidney, and liver and (2) to improve physical symptoms of the patient.

Dehydration

As stated earlier, the patient with dehydration who presents with increased thirst and neurological changes due to hypertonicity should receive water (pure water, if patient can take by mouth, or 5% dextrose in water) slowly to replace the water deficit. If serum [Na$^+$] is >160 mEq/L, it should be lowered by no more than 6–8 mEq/day. In order to achieve this, one needs to calculate water deficit. The patient starts to urinate once fluid is replaced because of improvement in glomerular filtration rate (GFR). Thirst and mental changes will improve once hypertonicity is slowly corrected.

Volume Depletion

Patient with volume depletion should receive intravascular volume expansion with normal (0.9%) saline. This fluid can be given rapidly to restore intravascular volume to improve blood pressure and GFR. Physical signs and symptoms will improve within 24 h.

Study Questions

Case 1   A 70-year-old man is brought to the emergency room for lethargy and dizziness. He has a history of hypertension and atrial arrhythmias. He is on a diuretic (hydrochlorothiazide) and not on any antiarrhythmic drug. His blood pressure is 120/80 mmHg with a pulse rate of 110 (lying) and 100/60 mmHg with a pulse rate of 120 (sitting). He is afebrile. His laboratory values are as follows:

Na$^+$	=	134 mEq/L	Creatinine	=	1.5 mg/dL
K$^+$	=	3.1 mEq/L	Glucose	=	140 mg/dL
Cl$^-$	=	88 mEq/L	Hemoglobin	=	14%
HCO$_3^-$	=	28 mEq/L	Hematocrit	=	50%
BUN	=	40 mg/dL	Urinary Na$^+$	=	20 mEq/L

Question 1   Does this patient have dehydration or volume depletion?

Answer   This patient has volume depletion because of orthostatic blood pressure and pulse changes.

Question 2 Discuss the reason for this patient's dizziness and lethargy.

Answer The patient has orthostatic blood pressure and pulse changes, which are due to intravascular volume depletion probably caused by the diuretic. Increases in blood urea nitrogen (BUN), creatinine, hematocrit, and urinary [Na^+] of 20 mEq/L also indicate volume depletion caused by the loss of both Na^+ and water from the intravascular compartment. When the blood pressure in an elderly hypertensive patient decreases to these levels, the blood flow to the brain and other vital organs is decreased. Both dizziness and lethargy are related to relative hypotension.

Question 3 How would you treat this patient?

Answer As this patient is symptomatic, rapid correction of volume depletion is essential. The initial choice of fluid is normal (0.9%) saline. During the first hour, the patient should receive at least 1 L of normal saline intravenously. Since normal saline remains in the extracellular compartment, it increases blood pressure and also improves perfusion to the kidney and brain. As a result, the GFR increases and the patient's lethargy should improve. Since K^+ is excreted with improvement in GFR, K^+ supplementation is necessary. Subsequent administration of intravenous fluids depends on the serum chemistry.

Question 4 What happens if the patient receives D5W?

Answer D5W is an incorrect fluid for this patient. It does not improve either volume status or blood pressure. Also, serum K^+ level falls because of transcellular shift due to glucose-induced insulin release. This relative hypokalemia may precipitate arrhythmia.

Case 2 A 36-year-old woman is admitted for dizziness, weakness, poor appetite, fatigue, and salt craving for 4 weeks. She has history of asthma and is not on any medications. She has a family history of type 1 diabetes and hypothyroidism. On admission, her blood pressure is 100/60 mmHg with a pulse rate of 100 (sitting) and 80/48 mmHg with a pulse rate of 120 (standing). Her temperature is 99.6 °F. The laboratory test values are as follows:

Na^+	=	124 mEq/L	Creatinine	=	1.8 mg/dL
K^+	=	6.1 mEq/L	Glucose	=	50 mg/dL
Cl^-	=	114 mEq/L	Hemoglobin	=	13%
HCO_3^-	=	20 mEq/L	Hematocrit	=	40%
BUN	=	42 mg/dL	Urinary Na^+	=	60 mEq/L

Question 1 What would be her effective arterial blood volume (EABV)?

Answer The EABV is decreased, as she has hypovolemia (volume depletion).

Question 2 What would be the most likely diagnosis in this patient?

Answer On the basis of orthostatic blood pressure and pulse changes, hyponatremia, hyperkalemia, acute kidney injury, hypoglycemia, and high urine Na^+ excretion, the most likely diagnosis is Addison's disease (glucocorticoid and mineralocorticoid deficiency), which is an autoimmune disorder. Her signs and symptoms are related to volume depletion and electrolyte abnormalities. Hypotension is related to loss of both Na^+ and water caused by deficiency of the above hormones.

Question 3 How would you treat her?

Answer First, replacement of glucocorticoid with hydrocortisone (100 mg IV) with continuation every 6 h is necessary. The patient also requires volume replacement. The ideal fluid is normal saline. The patient may require several liters. Some physicians choose D5W and normal saline. However, with D5W, serum Na^+ may drop initially. Normal saline should be continued until the blood pressure and urine output improve. There is no need to treat the patient with mineralocorticoid preparation.

Suggested Reading

1. Bhave G, Neilson EG. Volume depletion versus dehydration: how understanding the difference can guide therapy. Am J Kidney Dis. 2011;58:302–9.
2. Elhassan EA, Scrier RW. Disorders of extracellular volume. In: Johnson RJ, Feehally J, Floege J, editors. Comprehensive clinical nephrology. 5th ed. Philadelphia: Elsevier Saunders; 2015. p. 80–93.
3. Mange K, Matsura D, Cizman B, et al. Language guiding therapy: the case of dehydration versus volume depletion. Ann Intern Med. 1997;127:848–53.
4. Spital A. Dehydration versus volume depletion and the importance of getting it right. Am J Kidney Dis. 2007;49:721–2.

Disorders of Water Balance: Physiology

11

In this chapter, we will discuss how plasma osmolality and water balance are maintained. Like Na^+ balance, water balance is determined by the amount of water that is ingested and excreted. Therefore, water intake equals water loss. In a normal individual, the major source of water intake is oral fluids. Water is also derived from other sources such as solid foods and intermediary metabolism. Intravenous fluids form the principal source of water intake in hospitalized patients. Dialysis patients may also gain water during treatments.

If water intake and water loss are not equal, the plasma osmolality is altered. However, in a healthy individual, plasma osmolality is controlled within fairly narrow limits (± 1–2%) by the hypothalamic–pituitary–antidiuretic hormone (ADH) axis. Normal plasma osmolality varies from 280 to 295 mOsm/kg H_2O. If plasma osmolality increases by 1–2%, the subject feels thirsty, the circulating ADH levels increase, and the subject drinks fluids. This fluid is retained in the body by the action of ADH in the collecting duct, and the osmolality returns to normal. Opposite changes occur if plasma osmolality is decreased. Although the major influencing factor in maintaining normal plasma osmolality is the sensation of thirst, it is the combined effect of thirst, ADH, and the renal response to ADH that regulates plasma osmolality and water balance. Osmoregulation is the term generally used to refer to the regulation of body fluid osmolality.

Control of Thirst

Thirst is essential to the maintenance of normal body fluid osmolality. It is defined as a desire for water. Abnormal thirst may be physiological or pathological. The main regulator of thirst is the effective osmolality of body fluids (osmotic thirst). For example, an increase in plasma osmolality (hypertonicity) stimulates thirst by causing thirst osmoreceptor cells to shrink. These cells are located in the anterolateral hypothalamus near the third ventricle. Hypovolemia also stimulates thirst (hypovolemic thirst). The mechanism appears to be an increase in angiotensin II.

© Springer Science+Business Media LLC 2018
A.S. Reddi, *Fluid, Electrolyte and Acid-Base Disorders*,
DOI 10.1007/978-3-319-60167-0_11

In contrast, an increase in plasma osmolality due to urea or alcohol does not stimulate thirst because the thirst osmoreceptors do not shrink. These substances, called ineffective osmolytes, penetrate the cell plasma membrane easily and thus are unable to maintain any osmotic gradient. Therefore, the thirst osmoreceptors do not shrink.

Structure and Synthesis of ADH

ADH is a nonapeptide, that is, it contains nine amino acids. Because arginine is located at position 8, ADH is also called arginine vasopressin (AVP). In clinical practice, the terms AVP and ADH are used synonymously. Cysteine is located at both the first and sixth positions; these two amino acids form a disulfide bridge. Removal of this disulfide bridge destroys the biologic activity of ADH. Substitution of lysine for arginine at position 8 yields lysine vasopressin, which is found in pigs.

ADH is synthesized by the supraoptic and paraventricular nuclei of the hypothalamus. It is initially synthesized as a precursor protein called preprohormone. This preprohormone contains a signal peptide, vasopressin, neurophysin II, and copeptin. Subsequently, it is converted into prohormone by removing signaling peptide. This prohormone is composed of three components: vasopressin, neurophysin II, and copeptin. The prohormone is packaged in secretory vesicles within the cell bodies of the hypothalamic nuclei. The secretory vesicles containing the prohormone are transported to the posterior pituitary gland through the hypothalamic neurohypophyseal tract. During this transport, the prohormone is cleaved to form ADH, neurophysin II, and copeptin. Neurophysin II acts as a carrier protein of vasopressin from the hypothalamus to the posterior pituitary gland.

ADH is released from the posterior pituitary gland in response to a stimulus by calcium-dependent exocytosis. The half-life of ADH is 10–25 min, and it is degraded by the liver and kidney. In plasma, it is cleared by a specific enzyme called vasopressinase.

Control of ADH Release

The major physiologic stimulus for ADH release is plasma osmolality. An increase in plasma osmolality stimulates ADH release, while a decrease inhibits ADH release. It has been shown that when plasma osmolality is less than 280 mOsm/kg H_2O, the plasma levels of ADH are undetectable. Conversely, when plasma osmolality is greater than 295 mOsm/kg H_2O, the plasma levels of ADH are greatly increased. An increase in plasma osmolality of 1–2% causes shrinkage of osmoreceptor cells, which in turn causes ADH to be synthesized and released into the circulation. A decrease in osmolality causes swelling of osmoreceptor cells and eventual inhibition of ADH release. Besides osmotic

Table 11.1 Factors (partial list) that influence ADH release

Stimuli	Response
Osmotic	
Increase in plasma osmolality	↑
Decrease in plasma osmolality	↓
Nonosmotic	
Decrease in volume or blood pressure	↑
Increase in volume or blood pressure	↓
Nausea	↑
Pain	↑
Physical stress	↑
Hypoglycemia	↑
Low PO_2 and high PCO_2	↑
α-Adrenergic agents	↓
β-Adrenergic agents	↑
Cholinergic and dopaminergic agents	↑
Angiotensin II	↑
Narcotics	↑
Antimetabolites	↑
Oral hypoglycemics (chlorpropamide)	↑
Ethanol	↓
Phenytoin	↓
Prostaglandins (PGE_2)	↓
Atrial natriuretic peptide	↓

↑ increase, ↓ decrease

stimulus, several other nonosmotic factors have been shown to influence ADH release (Table 11.1).

Copeptin

Copeptin is released with ADH. It is a glycopeptide with 39 amino acids (molecular wt 5 kDa). It is largely neglected until 2006 when it was characterized as a surrogate biomarker of ADH. A linear relationship between ADH and copeptin levels has been demonstrated. Generally it is difficult to measure ADH levels because of low serum concentrations, instability at room temperature, and other technical problems. Therefore, serum ADH levels are not routinely available. Although the assay of copeptin is not commercially available, its measurements seem to be less cumbersome. Similar to ADH, copeptin levels are suppressed by hypoosmolality and elevated in hyperosmolality conditions in healthy individuals. Also, a close relationship between copeptin levels and osmolality has been demonstrated with an osmolality threshold of 282 mOsm/kg H_2O. Stress increases copeptin levels. A few studies have shown that serum levels of copeptin are helpful in the evaluation of hyponatremia and polyuric syndromes (see Chaps. 12 and 13).

Distribution of Aquaporins in the Kidney

Before we discuss the mechanism of action of ADH, it is essential to understand the distribution of water channels (called aquaporins) because of their involvement in water transport across the epithelia. AQPs are membrane water channels that are responsible for water transport in the nephron and other organs. There are 13 mammalian AQPs. In the kidney, AQPs 1–4 are involved in water transport. AQP-1 is expressed in the proximal tubule and the descending limb of Henle's loop at both the apical and basolateral membranes. It is also present in the descending vasa recta. AQP-1 is absent in the thin and thick ascending limbs of Henle's loop where the water permeability is low. AQP-2 is present in the apical membrane of the principal cells of the cortical, outer medullary, and inner medullary collecting duct and in the cells of the inner medullary collecting duct. AQP-3 is expressed predominantly in the basolateral membrane of the principal cells of the collecting duct from cortex to the tip of the papilla, whereas AQP-4 is present in the basolateral membrane of the principal cells of the inner medullary collecting duct. Of the four AQPs, only AQP-2 is regulated by ADH. This hormone stimulates the synthesis and insertion of AQP-2 into the apical membrane of the principal cell to promote water permeability.

Mechanism and Actions of ADH

Mechanism

The main actions of ADH are on the kidney. However, as the name vasopressin implies, ADH has pressor effects on the blood vessels. ADH exerts its effects through membrane receptors. To date, four different ADH receptors have been identified. Vasopressin V_1 receptors are present on the vascular smooth muscle, liver, and glomerular mesangial cells. Binding of ADH to these receptors increases the concentration of cytosolic Ca^{2+} through the inositol triphosphate pathway. Vasopressin V_2 receptors are present on the epithelial cells of the medullary thick ascending limb and the collecting duct. Vasopressin V_3 receptors are present in the kidney, pituitary, heart, and spleen in rats, whereas in humans they are restricted to the pituitary. The vasopressin V_4 receptor (called vasopressin-activated calcium-mobilizing receptor) is present in the kidney, heart, brain, and skeletal muscle.

The vasopressin V_2 receptor is the major receptor responsible for water reabsorption in the collecting duct. Briefly, the binding of ADH to this V_2 receptor in the collecting duct promotes water reabsorption from the tubular lumen by the following mechanism (Fig. 11.1). ADH binds to the V_2 receptor located in the basolateral membrane. The V_2 receptor is coupled with a stimulatory G protein. Activation of G protein stimulates adenylate cyclase, which converts ATP (adenosine triphosphate) into cAMP (cyclic adenosine monophosphate). This cAMP activates protein kinase A, which in turn stimulates intracellular vesicle-containing AQP-2 water channels. These AQP-2 water channels are subsequently translocated to the apical membrane

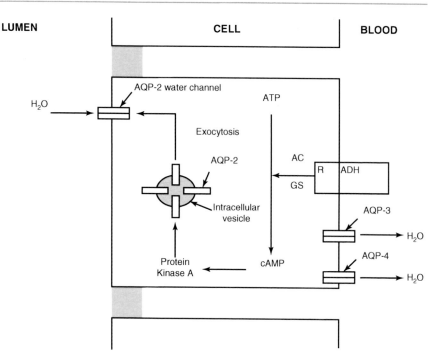

Fig. 11.1 Simplified mechanism of action of ADH on the epithelial cell of the collecting duct. *R* vasopressin V_2 receptor, *AC* adenylate cyclase, *Gs* stimulatory G protein, *AQP-2, AQP-3, and AQP-4* aquaporin-2, aquaporin-3, and aquaporin-4 water channels

by exocytosis of intracellular vesicles for transport of water. This process of translocation is called shuttle hypothesis. Once ADH levels are low, water permeability is decreased with a shift of AQP-2 water channels back into the intracellular vesicles. Water exit at the basolateral membrane is facilitated by AQP-3 and AQP-4 water channels (Fig. 11.1).

Actions

ADH has the following actions in the kidney:

1. In principal cells, it increases water permeability in the cortical and medullary collecting ducts and plays an important role in urinary concentration and dilution.
2. It increases the urea transport in the terminal inner medullary collecting duct, and thus participates in urea recycling in the process of urinary concentration.
3. It activates Na/K/Cl cotransporter and increases NaCl reabsorption in the medullary thick limb of Henle's loop.
4. It stimulates NaCl transport and Na transport via ENaC in the cortical collecting duct.

Urinary Concentration and Dilution

The processes that maintain urinary concentration and dilution are briefly summarized as follows:

1. The kidneys prevent life-threatening deviations in body fluid volume and osmolality by regulating water excretion. During periods of water deprivation, the
   kidneys reabsorb water and excrete a concentrated (hypertonic) urine with an
   osmolality of 1,200 mOsm/kg H_2O. When water intake is excessive, the kidneys
   generate a dilute (hypotonic) urine with an osmolality of 50 mOsm/kg H_2O. Thus,
   the kidney can concentrate or dilute urine depending on water availability.
2. Urine is concentrated because of the combined function of the loop of Henle,
   which progressively generates a high osmolality (hypertonicity) in the medulla
   by a process called *countercurrent multiplication* and the action of ADH on the
   collecting duct to augment water permeability by regulating AQP-2 water channel. Also, NaCl reabsorption in the thick ascending limb of Henle's loop is
   essential to maintain medullary hypertonicity.
3. The medullary hypertonicity created by countercurrent multiplication is maintained by the vasa recta, the blood vessels that supply the medulla, by a process
   called *countercurrent exchange*. Urea, which constitutes about 50% of the solute
   in the medullary interstitium, also plays an important role in the maintenance of
   hypertonicity by a process of urea recycling. ADH plays an important role in
   urea recycling.
4. Dilute urine is formed when ADH levels are low or absent. Dilute urine can also
   result from tubular resistance to ADH action.
5. Several conditions can impair urinary concentration and dilution. For example,
   excessive water intake and low-protein intake causing low urea production or
   inhibition of NaCl reabsorption in the thick ascending limb of Henle's loop-by-
   loop diuretics impair concentrating ability of the kidney. On the other hand, thiazide diuretics impair the diluting ability of the kidney. Patients with a syndrome
   of inappropriate ADH secretion cannot dilute their urine that is proportionate to
   their serum $[Na^+]$.
6. The kidneys' ability to dilute or concentrate the urine is quantitated by measuring the amount of solute-free water (C_{H_2O}) that is excreted or reabsorbed ($T^c_{H_2O}$)
   by the collecting duct.

Measurement of Urinary Concentration and Dilution

The ability of the kidney either to concentrate or dilute the urine can be quantitated
by measuring the urinary osmolality. Under appropriate conditions, the kidney can
dilute urine to as low as 50 mOsm/kg H_2O or can concentrate it up to 1,200 mOsm/
kg H_2O, as described earlier. In dilute urine, more water is excreted than solutes, i.e.,
the renal tubules reabsorbed less and excreted more water. Conversely, in concentrated urine, more solute-free water is reabsorbed. To quantitate the amount of water

excretion or reabsorption, the concepts of free water and osmolar clearance were introduced. According to these concepts, the urine (V) consists of two portions: one portion contains all the solute that is isosmotic to plasma and is called the osmolar clearance (C_{osm}), and the other portion contains solute-free water and is called the free water clearance (C_{H_2O}). C_{H_2O} is clinically used to evaluate plasma [Na^+]. The following equation has been developed to show the relationship among V, C_{osm}, and C_{H_2O}:

$$V = C_{osm} + C_{H_2O}, \qquad (11.1)$$

where V is the total urine volume and C_{osm} is defined by the standard clearance formula as:

$$C_{osm} = (U_{osm} \times V)/P_{osm}, \qquad (11.2)$$

where V is the urine volume in mL/min and U_{osm} and P_{osm} refer to urinary and plasma osmolalities, respectively.

C_{H_2O} is not defined by the clearance formula. Instead, it is defined as the difference between the urine volume and the osmolar clearance. Therefore,

$$C_{H_2O} = V - C_{osm}. \qquad (11.3)$$

How are C_{H_2O} and C_{osm} calculated?

The following example illustrates the significance of C_{H_2O} and C_{osm} in diluted urine.

A volunteer is infused via a central vein with 10 L of D5W (5% dextrose in water), and the following values are obtained:

$$P_{osm} = 280 \ mOsm/kg \ H_2O,$$
$$U_{osm} = 50 \ mOsm/kg \ H_2O.$$

Urine flow rate is 6 mL/min:

$$C_{H_2O} = V - C_{osm}$$
$$= 6 - (50 \times 6/280 \ ) \ or \ 300/280 = 1.07 \qquad (11.4)$$
$$= 6 - 1.07 = 4.93.$$

Of the 6 mL of dilute urine, 4.93 mL accounts for free water (C_{H_2O}), and 1.07 mL represents isosmotic solution containing the entire solute (C_{osm}).

In the above example, the urine was diluted maximally because of excess water or the tubules reabsorbed less water. The opposite phenomenon occurs in an individual with concentrated urine, which is due to water reabsorption. This solute-free reabsorption of water is called *negative free water clearance* (abbreviated as $T^c_{H_2O}$). The abbreviation $T^c_{H_2O}$ stands for the difference between the osmolar clearance and the urine flow rate. Thus,

$$T^c_{H_2O} = C_{osm} - V$$

How is $T^c_{H_2O}$ calculated?

A volunteer is asked not to drink fluids for 12 h; he lost 2% of his body weight. The following values are obtained:

$$P_{osm} = 290 \text{ mOsm/kg H}_2\text{O},$$
$$U_{osm} = 870 \text{ mOsm/kg H}_2\text{O}.$$

Urine flow rate is equal to 0.5 mL/min:

$$C_{osm} = \frac{870 \times 0.5}{290} = 1.5, \tag{11.5}$$

$$T^c_{H_2O} = C_{osm} - V \text{ or } 1.5 - 0.5 = 1 \text{ mL}.$$

This result indicates that 1.0 mL of water was reabsorbed per minute. Another way of stating this is that $T^c_{H_2O}$ is equal to 1 mL/min.

Calculation of Electrolyte–Free Water Clearance

It is clear from the above calculations that plasma and urine osmolalities are needed to calculate $T^c_{H_2O}$. It should be noted that urea is included in the measurement of osmolality and urea is an ineffective osmolyte. Therefore, it does not establish an osmotic gradient for movement of water between two compartments; thus, plasma [Na+] does not change. Changes in serum [Na+] are better predicted by calculating electrolyte–free water clearance ($T^e_{C_{H_2O}}$), which uses serum [Na+] instead of serum osmolality and urine [Na+] and [K+] instead of urine osmolality:

$$T^e_{C_{H_2O}} = V\left(1 - \frac{U_{Na} + U_K}{P_{Na}}\right),$$

where V is 24 h urine volume.

Thus, the concept of $T^e_{C_{H_2O}}$ is used to calculate the kidneys' ability to conserve or excrete the daily intake of fluids to maintain normal serum [Na]. Whenever water balance is disturbed, either hypo- or hypernatremia develops. In such a situation, $T^e_{C_{H_2O}}$ is used. When more water is reabsorbed by nephron segments, less water is excreted in the urine, and $T^e_{C_{H_2O}}$ is negative. As a result, hyponatremia develops. When $T^e_{C_{H_2O}}$ is positive, more water is excreted with a resultant increase in serum [Na+].

When 24 h urine collection is not possible, determination of urine [Na+] and [K+] as well as serum [Na+] in a spot urine sample can be used to predict changes in serum [Na+]. For example, if the sum of urine [Na+] and [K+] exceeds serum [Na+], $T^e_{H_2O}$ is negative. This means that the patient is in a state of free water retention with resultant hyponatremia. Conversely, if the sum of urine [Na+] and [K+] is less than serum [Na+], $T^e_{C_{H_2O}}$ is positive, meaning that the patient has lost free water in the urine. As a result, hypernatremia ensues. The sum of urine [Na+] and [K+] divided by serum [Na+] could also be used in the evaluation of changes in serum [Na+]. In hyponatremia, the ratio is >1, and in hypernatremia it is ≤0.5. A ratio of 1 indicates no change in serum [Na^+].

Disorders of Water Balance

Clinically, disorders of water balance can be divided into those with hypoosmolality and those with hyperosmolality. Since plasma osmolality is largely determined by plasma [Na^+] (Chap. 1), a true decrease in plasma [Na^+] due to water excess results in hypoosmolality (<280 mOsm/kg H_2O). This condition is called hyponatremia. Conversely, an increase in plasma [Na^+] due to water loss causes hyperosmolality (>295 mOsm/kg H_2O), and this clinical condition is called hypernatremia. It is, therefore, evident that water content relative to [Na^+] can alter the plasma osmolality. Hypo- and hypernatremia are discussed in the next two chapters.

Study Questions

Case 1 A 48-year-old woman with small cell lung cancer is brought to the emergency department with altered mental status since 4 days and questionable seizure disorder. Her husband says that the patient is sipping water frequently because of dry mouth. Her BP (blood pressure) is 130/80 mmHg with a pulse rate of 74/min. Following administration of 2 L of 0.45% saline in 24 h, the following laboratory data are obtained:

Serum Na^+ = 114 mEq/L
Serum osmolality = 238 mOsm/kg H_2O
Urine osmolality = 540 mOsm/kg H_2O
Urine Na^+ = 140 mEq/L
Urine K^+ = 34 mEq/L
Urine osmolality = 284 mOsm/kg H_2O
24 h urine volume = 1 L

Question 1 Regarding electrolyte–free water clearance ($T^e_{C_{H_2O}}$), which one of the following is CORRECT?

(a) -0.75 L
(b) -0.52 L
(c) $+0.52$ L
(d) $+0.75$ L
(e) -0.82 L

The answer is B The concept of $T^e_{C_{H_2O}}$ is used to calculate the kidneys' ability to conserve or excrete the daily intake of fluids to maintain normal serum [Na^+]. Whenever water balance is disturbed, either hypo- or hypernatremia develops. In such a situation, calculation of $T^e_{C_{H_2O}}$ is helpful in evaluating serum [Na$^+$] by using the following formula:

$$T^e_{C_{H_2O}} = V\left(1 - U_{Na} + U_K / P_{Na}\right)$$

where V is urine volume/24 h and U_{Na}^+, U_K^+, and P_{Na}^+ are urine Na$^+$, K$^+$, and plasma Na$^+$ concentrations in mEq/L. Substituting the values of the data acquired from the patient, we obtain:

$$T^e_{C_{H_2O}} = 1\left(1 - 140 + 34/114\right) = -0.52 \text{ L}.$$

Whenever the value is negative, the kidney is adding water to the body, resulting in hyponatremia. On the other hand, when $T^e_{C_{H_2O}}$ is positive, the kidney is removing water from the body with resultant hypernatremia. The patient received hypotonic solution with further reduction in serum [Na$^+$]. Thus, option B is correct.

Suggested Reading

1. Brown D, Fenton RA. The cell biology of vasopressin action. In: Skorecki K, et al., editors. Brenner & Rector's the kidney. 10th ed. Philadelphia: Elsevier; 2016. p. 281–302.
2. Christ-Crain M, Morgenthaler NG, Fenske W. Copeptin as a biomarker and a diagnostic tool in the evaluation of patients with polyuria-polydipsia and hyponatremia. Best Pract Res Clin Endocrinol Metab. 2016;30:235–47.
3. Verkman AS. Aquaporins in clinical medicine. Annu Rev Med. 2012;63:306–16.

Disorders of Water Balance: Hyponatremia

12

Hyponatremia is defined as serum or plasma [Na$^+$] <135 mEq/L.

Serum [Na$^+$] is kept between 138 and 142 mEq/L despite wide variations in water intake and is determined by total body Na$^+$, K$^+$, and water content:

$$\text{Serum}\left[\text{Na}^+\right] = \text{Na}^+ + \text{K}^+ / \text{TBW}$$

where Na$^+$ and K$^+$ are total quantities of these cations and TBW is total body water. Therefore, hyponatremia can develop by an increase in total body water, a decrease in Na$^+$ and K$^+$, or a combination of both.

Development of Hyponatremia

Hyponatremia is a condition of water excess relative to Na$^+$. In a normal individual, hyponatremia does not develop unless water intake is greater than renal excretion. A defect in renal water excretion in the presence of normal water intake is a prerequisite for the development of hyponatremia. This defect in water excretion is due to high circulating levels of antidiuretic hormone (ADH). With retention of water, hyponatremic patients are unable to lower their urine osmolality <100 mOsm/kg H$_2$O with the exception of those with psychogenic polydipsia and reset osmostat.

Approach to the Patient with Hyponatremia

Step 1. Measure Serum Osmolality

- Hypoosmolality rules out pseudo (factitious) and hypertonic hyponatremia. Hypotonic hyponatremia is called true hyponatremia (Fig. 12.1).

© Springer Science+Business Media LLC 2018
A.S. Reddi, *Fluid, Electrolyte and Acid-Base Disorders*,
DOI 10.1007/978-3-319-60167-0_12

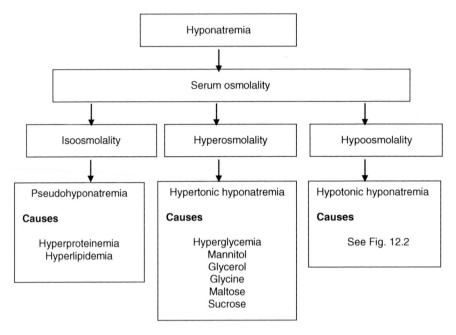

Fig. 12.1 Osmolality in a hyponatremia patient

Step 2. Measure Urine Osmolality and Na⁺ Concentration

Urine osmolality differentiates low osmolality (<100 mOsm/kg H_2O) from high osmolality (>100 mOsm/kg H_2O) conditions. Also urine Na^+ concentration is useful in the differentiation of various causes of hypovolemic, hypervolemic, and euvolemic hyponatremia (Fig. 12.2).

Step 3. Estimate Volume Status

History
- Assess fluid loss (diarrhea, vomiting).
- Review medications such as oral hypoglycemics, antihypertensives, antidepressants, opiates, etc.
- Review medical conditions such as psychiatric illness, cancer, and cardiovascular, thyroid, renal, and liver, including adrenal, disease.
- Check intravenous (IV) fluids for maintenance and medication use.

Physical Examination
- Vital signs with orthostatic changes (very important and mandatory).
- Examination of the neck, lungs, heart, and lower extremities for fluid status.
- Evaluation of mental status is extremely important.
- Based on volume status, classify hypotonic hyponatremia into (Fig. 12.2):

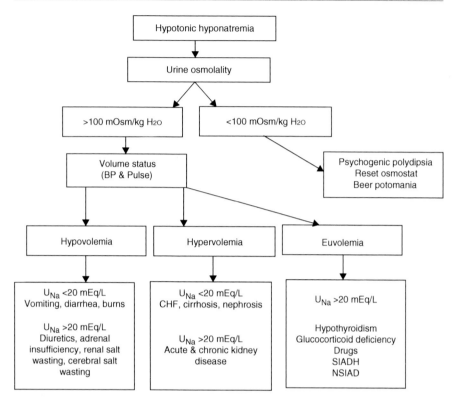

Fig. 12.2 Classification, causes, and diagnosis of hypotonic hyponatremia. *AKI* acute kidney injury, *CKD* chronic kidney disease, *NSIAD* nephrogenic syndrome of inappropriate antidiuresis, *SIADH* syndrome of inappropriate ADH secretion

1. Hypovolemic hyponatremia (relatively more Na^+ than water loss)
2. Hypervolemic hyponatremia (relatively more water than Na^+ gain)
3. Normovolemic hyponatremia (relatively more water relative to Na^+)

Step 4. Obtain Pertinent Laboratory Tests

- Serum chemistry, uric acid, and lipid panel.
- Complete blood count.
- Fractional excretion of Na^+, uric acid, and phosphate is needed occasionally.
- Check liver, thyroid, and adrenal function tests.

Step 5. Know More About Pseudo or Factitious Hyponatremia

- Occasionally serum $[Na^+]$ is artifactually low in patients with severe hyperlipidemia or hyperproteinemia.
- Reduction in $[Na^+]$ is due to displacement of serum water by excess lipid or protein, but the serum osmolality is normal.

- This condition is called *pseudohyponatremia.*
- These patients are asymptomatic because their serum osmolality is normal. Therefore, pseudohyponatremia is called *isotonic hyponatremia.*
- Correction of underlying causes for increased lipids or protein corrects hyponatremia. Therefore, no treatment for isotonic hyponatremia is required.
- In this context, it is important to know how serum Na^+ is determined. Serum Na^+ is determined by ion-selective electrode (potentiometric) method. The determination is done in two ways: indirect and direct. The indirect method involves dilution of serum, whereas the direct method does not require dilution of serum.
- Note that pseudohyponatremia is observed only if serum Na^+ is determined by the indirect ion-selective electrode method, and not by the direct method.
- The following formula can be used to calculated the corrected $[Na^+]$ in the presence of high concentrations of protein and triglycerides:

$$\frac{\text{Measured plasma } Na^+ \times \text{Normal plasma water content} (93\%)}{\text{Calculated water fraction in the presence of high protein or triglyceride levels}}$$

- Table 12.1 provides corrected serum $[Na^+]$ for a fixed $[Na^+]$ measured by indirect method.

Step 6. Know More About Hypertonic (Translocational) Hyponatremia

- Severe hyperglycemia also lowers serum $[Na^+]$ due to water movement from intracellular to extracellular compartment (translocation).
- Serum $[Na^+]$ decreases by 1.6 mEq/L for each 100 mg/dL glucose above normal glucose level (i.e., 100 mg/dL). This correction factor applies to glucose levels up to 400 mg/dL. If serum glucose level is >400 mg/dL, serum $[Na^+]$ decreases by 2.4 mEq/L. However, the correction factor of 1.6 mEq/L should be used until more studies are available to confirm the correction factor of 2.4 mEq/L. Because of hyperglycemia, the serum osmolality is high, and the condition is called *hypertonic hyponatremia.*

Table 12.1 Measured and corrected serum $[Na^+]$ in the presence of high protein or triglyceride concentrations

Total protein (g/dL)	Triglycerides (mg/dL)	Measured Na^+ (mEq/L)	Corrected Na^+ (mEq/L)	Plasma water content (%)
7 (normal)		140	140	93
10		140	142	92
15		140	147	88.5
	3,000	140	143	91.2

- Correction of hyperglycemia corrects hyponatremia.
- Mannitol, sucrose, glycerol, glycine, and maltose also cause hypertonic hyponatremia. These solutes also increase osmolal gap. Osmolal gap is defined as the difference between the measured and calculated serum osmolality. Generally, the measured osmolality is 10 mOsm higher than the calculated osmolality. Values >15 mOsm represent the presence of an osmolal gap.
- Elevated osmolal gap suggests the presence of osmotically active substances that are not included in the calculation of osmolality but are measured in the assay.

Step 7. Rule Out Causes Other than Glucose That Increase Plasma Osmolality

- Urea, methanol, ethanol, and ethylene glycol can also increase plasma osmolality. Calculation of osmolal gap is helpful. These solutes are ineffective osmolytes and are cell permeable. Therefore, they do not cause translocation of water.

Pathophysiology of Hyponatremia

Table 12.2 summarizes the possible mechanisms underlying the generation of hyponatremia. As evident, hyponatremia develops due to an increase in ADH secretion and activity and the kidneys' inability to dilute urine maximally due to impaired water excretion.

Specific Causes of Hyponatremia

It is not possible to discuss all causes of hypotonic hyponatremia. However, it is important to focus on some conditions that are frequently associated with hyponatremia.

Syndrome of Inappropriate Antidiuretic Hormone Secretion

- Syndrome of inappropriate antidiuretic hormone (SIADH) secretion is a common cause of hyponatremia in hospitalized children.
- Usually caused by central nervous system (CNS) disorders, pulmonary disorders, malignancies, and drugs. Some drugs may stimulate the secretion, whereas other drugs may potentiate the action of ADH.
- The diagnostic criteria of SIADH are:
  1. Hypotonic hyponatremia (plasma osmolality <270 mOsm/kg H_2O)
  2. Inappropriate urinary concentration (>100 mOsm/kg H_2O) or inability to dilute urine osmolality below 100 mOsm/kg H_2O
  3. Urinary Na^+ >30 mEq/L on regular diet

Table 12.2 Possible mechanisms of hyponatremia

Cause	Mechanism
Diarrhea and vomiting	Volume depletion→ ↑ADH→ decreased water excretion
Diuretics	Volume depletion→ ↑ADH→ decreased water excretion. Hypokalemia. K⁺ moves out of cells into ECF causing Na⁺ movement into cells to maintain electroneutrality. Thiazides have some other effects
Mineralocorticoid deficiency	Volume depletion→ ↑ADH→ decreased water excretion, ↑Na⁺ excretion
Salt-losing nephropathies	↑ Na⁺ excretion, ↑ADH→ decreased water excretion
Cerebral salt wasting	Volume depletion→ ↑ADH→ decreased water excretion, ↑Na⁺ excretion
Decompensated CHF	↓ EABV→ increased AII-SNS→ ↑Na⁺ and water reabsorption→ decreased delivery to diluting segments and ↑ADH→ decreased water excretion, ↑AQP2 expression
Cirrhosis	The same as earlier
Nephrotic syndrome (hypovolemic)	↓ Water excretion (children)
Nephrotic syndrome (hypervolemic)	Intrarenal mechanisms, leading to Na⁺ and water reabsorption, ↓AQP2 expression
Renal failure	↓ RBF→ ↓GFR→ decreased Na⁺ and water filtration→ decreased water excretion
Psychogenic polydipsia	Water intake exceeds its excretion. ↓ADH and AQP2 expression
Hypothyroidism	↑ADH→ decreased water excretion
Glucocorticoid deficiency	↑ADH→ decreased water excretion, ↑Na/K/2Cl, and ENaC activity→ increased Na⁺ and water reabsorption, ↑AQP2 expression
Drugs	↑ADH secretion and/or potentiation of ADH activity→ decreased water excretion
SIADH	↑ADH→ decreased water excretion
Nephrogenic syndrome of antidiuresis	Mutation in ADH receptor 2→ increased ADH receptor activity→ decreased water excretion, ADH undetectable

EABV effective arterial blood volume, *ENaC* epithelial sodium channel, *RBF* renal blood flow, *SIADH* syndrome of antidiuretic hormone secretion, *CHF* congestive heart failure, *ECF* extracellular fluid, ↑ increased, ↓ decreased

    4. Euvolemia
    5. The absence of thyroid, adrenal, liver, cardiac, and renal disease
- Thus, SIADH is a disease of exclusion.
- Serum ADH levels are usually elevated in many patients due to a defect in osmoregulation.
- Based on serum ADH level response to hypertonic saline, four types of SIADH have been described (Robertson; see Suggested Reading). Normally hypertonic saline increases plasma osmolality and serum [Na⁺], resulting in high ADH levels. Type A patients demonstrate elevated serum ADH levels with erratic fluctuations in response to hypertonic saline, suggesting the lack of relationship between plasma osmolality and ADH levels. These patients usually have small cell lung tumor, and their urine osmolality is fixed at high level (>100 mOsm/kg H₂O). In type B patients, baseline ADH levels are slightly elevated but not that

high as compared with type A patients, and they respond normal to hypertonic saline only when their plasma Na+ or osmolality reaches normal. This type of response is due to "leak" of AVP from damaged neurohypophysis. Some of these patients have malignancy. In type C, the basal ADH levels are low, and the threshold for ADH release is set at lower than normal (usually 284 mOsm/kg H_2O) plasma osmolality. However, the ADH levels increase appropriately at lower plasma Na+ level in response to hypertonic saline. Patients with reset osmostat have this type of SIADH. In type D patients, ADH levels are undetectable and their urine is concentrated. Probably, these patients have mutations in V_2 receptor, similar to those with nephrogenic syndrome of inappropriate antidiuresis (see below).

- Similar to ADH levels, baseline copeptin levels were high compared to controls, suggesting nonsuppressibility in patients with SIADH. Based on plasma copeptin response to hypertonic saline, five types of SIADH have been described (Fenske et al.; see Suggested Reading). Type A patients had high copeptin levels (>38 pmol/L; normal 1–13.8 with a median of 4.2 pmol/L) with no relationship to plasma osmolality. Type B is reset osmostat. These patients showed linear increase in copeptin levels with an increase in plasma osmolality and with low osmotic threshold. Type C patients had copeptin levels in the normal range (2–38 pmol/L) and nonsuppressable by hypoosmolality. There was no copeptin response to hypertonic saline. Type D patients had low copeptin (<2 pmol/L), and DNA sequence of V_2 receptor showed no mutations. Type E patients showed a negative response to increasing plasma osmolality.
- Some major differences exist between Robertson and Fenske et al.'s results with regard to the types (categories) of SIADH. First, only four types of SIADH groups were described by Robertson compared to five groups by Fenske et al. Second, the prevalence of type A patients was 33% in Robertson's study compared to 10% in Fenske et al. study, and, finally, the demonstration of type E patients is an important finding in the study of Fenske et al.
- Besides hyponatremia, patients with SIADH have low uric acid, low blood urea nitrogen (BUN), and low renin and aldosterone levels. Urine [Na+] and FE_{Na} as well as $FE_{uric\ acid}$ are elevated.
- Edema is absent and blood pressure is normal.
- Table 12.3 shows drugs that affect ADH levels and activity.

Cerebral Salt Wasting or Renal Salt Wasting Syndrome

- Cerebral salt wasting (CSW) is similar to SIADH in many aspects except for hemodynamic status and treatment.
- Like SIADH, CSW is associated with CNS diseases.
- CSW was originally described in patients with subarachnoid hemorrhage, although one recent study did not document this association. Subsequently, it was described in patients with tuberculosis and other infections.
- Table 12.4 summarizes similarities and differences between CSW and SIADH.

Table 12.3 Some common drugs that cause hyponatremia by affecting ADH secretion or activity

Drugs that increase ADH release
Antidepressants (e.g., amitriptyline, SSRIs, monoamine oxidase inhibitors)
Antiepileptic drugs (e.g., carbamazepine)
Antipsychotic drugs (e.g., phenothiazine)
Anticancer drugs (e.g., vincristine, cisplatin, cyclophosphamide)
Others: opiates[a], NSAIDs, acetaminophen, ecstasy
Drugs that potentiate ADH action
Chlorpropamide
Carbamazepine
Vincristine
Clofibrate
Nicotine
Narcotics
Ifosfamide
SSRIs
Ecstasy
Drugs that lower or inhibit ADH activity
Alcohol
Phenytoin
Opioids
Vaptans
Drugs that have an unclear effect on ADH
ACE-Is (No ACE-I in the brain. Conversion of AI to AII, which stimulates thirst and ADH release in the brain. Peripherally, ACE-I inhibits degradation of bradykinin, which stimulates ADH)
IVIG
Theophylline
Amiodarone
Amlodipine
Proton pump inhibitors
Reset osmostat
Carbamazepine

[a]Opioids may increase, may decrease, or have no effect on ADH

Nephrogenic Syndrome of Inappropriate Antidiuresis

- Nephrogenic syndrome of inappropriate antidiuresis (NSIAD) is similar to SIADH, but rare.
- First described in 2005 in infants with hyponatremia and high urine osmolality.
- Unlike SIADH, patients with NSIAD have undetectable or extremely low ADH levels.
- NSIAD is a gain-of-function mutation in vasopressin V_2 receptor.
- Treatment is fluid restriction, urea, and vaptans.

Table 12.4 Similarities and differences between CSW and SIADH

Parameter	CSW	SIADH
Hypotonic hyponatremia	Yes	Yes
Volume status	Low	Normal to high
CVP/PCWP	Low	Normal
Orthostatic BP/pulse changes	Yes	No
Hematocrit	High	Normal
Serum uric acid	Low	Low
BUN	High	Low
$FE_{uric\ acid}$	High	High
$FE_{uric\ acid}$ after disease correction	High (persists)	Normal
$FE_{phosphate}$	High	Normal
Urine [Na^+]	High	High
FE_{Na}	High	High
Urine osmolality	High	High
Urine volume	High	Low
Plasma ADH	Normal to high	High
Atrial natriuretic peptide	Normal to high	Normal
Brain natriuretic peptide	Normal to high	Normal
Treatment	Salt, fludrocortisone	Water restriction, 3% saline, loop diuretics, demeclocycline, urea, vaptans

PCWP pulmonary capillary wedge pressure, *CSW* cerebral salt wasting, *SIADH* syndrome of inappropriate antidiuretic hormone secretion

Reset Osmostat

- As described above, reset osmostat is a variant of SIADH because of euvolemia and hyponatremia.
- Usually serum Na^+ levels remain between 125 and 130 mEq/L despite variable salt and water intake.
- Patients with reset osmostat are asymptomatic, and their kidneys demonstrate normal function.
- For example, when patients are challenged with water load (10–15 mL/kg), they can lower urine osmolality to <100 mOsm/kg H_2O, and 80% of water load is excreted in 4 h. Free water excretion is impaired in SIADH.
- Fluid restriction raises urine osmolality above 600 mOsm/kg H_2O.
- Pathogenesis is unclear; however, ADH secretion occurs at low plasma osmolality (<280 mOsm/kg H_2O).
- Patients with alcoholism, malnutrition, spinal cord injury, tuberculosis, and cerebral palsy are prone to develop reset osmostat. Also, reset osmostat is seen in normal pregnancy. Long-term use of DDAVP has been implicated in reset osmostat.
- Distinguishing features from classic SIADH are (1) preservation of both diluting and concentrating capabilities, (2) normal $FE_{uric\ acid,}$ and (3) failure of fluid restriction to improve hyponatremia.

Thiazide Diuretics

- Hyponatremia is a well-documented complication of thiazide diuretics. Thirst and excess water intake may precipitate hyponatremia.
- The major reason for hyponatremia is inability to dilute urine osmolality below 100 mOsm/kg H_2O because of impaired water excretion.
- Urine concentrating ability is preserved.
- Other mechanisms of hyponatremia include (1) volume contraction, (2) early diuretic-induced inactivation of tubuloglomerular feedback system, (3) decreased glomerular filtration rate (GFR) due to earlier two mechanisms, (4) increased release of ADH and increased water reabsorption, and (5) relative decrease in vasodilatory prostaglandin synthesis in elderly subjects with unopposed ADH action.
- Diuretic-induced hypokalemia may further exacerbate hyponatremia by trans-cellular cation exchange, in which K^+ moves out of the cell to improve hypokalemia and Na^+ moves into the cell to maintain electroneutrality.

Ecstasy

- Ecstasy is a popular name for a ring-substituted form of methamphetamine.
- It gained the popularity of a "club drug" among adolescents, young adults, and subjects attending "rave" parties.
- Other side effects include rhabdomyolysis, arrhythmias, and renal failure. It causes symptomatic hyponatremia and sudden death.
- Ecstasy induces ADH secretion and retention of water in the stomach and intestine by decreasing gastrointestinal (GI) motility. Hyponatremia develops as a result of excess water intake and slow reabsorption from the GI tract in the presence of high ADH levels.
- Rapid correction of $[Na^+]$ is indicated in ecstasy-induced hyponatremia.

Selective Serotonin Reuptake Inhibitors

- Selective serotonin reuptake inhibitors (SSRIs) are the most widely prescribed drugs for depression.
- Drugs such as sertraline, paroxetine, and duloxetine inhibit the reuptake of serotonin and improve depression.
- SSRIs have few side effects compared to other antidepressants.
- Hyponatremia is due to drug-induced SIADH.
- Mechanisms include (1) stimulation of ADH secretion, (2) augmentation of ADH action in the renal medulla, (3) resetting the osmostat that lowers the threshold for ADH secretion, and (4) interaction of SSRIs with other medications via p450 enzymes, resulting in enhanced action of ADH.

Exercise-Induced Hyponatremia

- Exercise-induced hyponatremia (EIH) is a serious condition in marathon runners.
- ADH levels are increased despite hyponatremia.
- Water consumption >3 L, body mass index <20 kg/m², excess loss of sweat, nonsteroidal drugs, running time >4 h, and postmarathon weight gain may precipitate hyponatremia.
- Oral supplements or sports drinks rarely cause EIH.
- Rapid correction of [Na⁺] is indicated in EIH.

Beer Potomania

- A syndrome characterized by a history of alcohol abuse, hyponatremia, signs and symptoms of water intoxication, protein malnutrition (chronic alcoholics), low solute intake, and no evidence of diuretic or steroid use.
- Urine osmolality is variable, but may be <100 mOsm/kg H_2O or higher depending on beer intake. Generally urine osmolality is lower than plasma osmolality but can approach 300 mOsm/kg H_2O.
- ADH levels may be suppressed or high at initial presentation.
- Development of hyponatremia depends on solute (e.g., protein, salt) intake.
- An example: If solute intake per day is 250 mOsm and urine osmolality is 100 mOsm/kg H_2O, beer intake >2.5 L can induce hyponatremia.
- Alcoholics with or without hypokalemia are at high risk for osmotic demyelination syndrome (ODS) with rapid correction of hyponatremia.
- Alcoholics with malnutrition and cirrhosis are also at higher risk for ODS.

Poor Oral Intake

- Poor oral intake of protein and salt over days occurs usually in elderly subjects with a slight decrease in glomerular filtration rate (GFR). This type of dietary pattern is called tea and toast diet. It can induce hyponatremia with high water intake similar to that of beer or crash diet potomania with low solute intake.
- Urine osmolality may be <100 mOsm/kg H_2O or higher depending on water intake.
- Protein and salt intake improve both hyponatremia and urine osmolality.
- Certain differences exist between subjects with beer potomania and tea and toast intake. Supply of adequate calories from beer, relatively severe hyponatremia (98 mEq/L), hypokalemia, neurologic manifestations, and excretion of free water with relatively normal GFR are common in subjects with beer potomania compared to those on poor oral intake.

Postoperative Hyponatremia

- Common in hospitalized patients.
- Hypotonic fluids, drugs for pain, and nonosmotic release of ADH are frequent causes.
- Hyponatremia may also occur with normal saline due to retention of water in the presence of ADH. This process is called desalination. When normal saline is infused and intravascular volume is expanded, the kidneys excrete administered NaCl with retention of water, resulting in hyponatremia.
- Patients undergoing hysterectomy or prostate surgery may develop hyponatremia due to irrigation fluids such as glycine.
- Young menstruating women are at risk postoperatively for ODS.

Hypokalemia and Hyponatremia

- Hypokalemia is a rare cause of hyponatremia.
- The reason for hyponatremia is movement of Na^+ from ECF to ICF compartment. At the same time, K^+ moves out of the cell into ECF compartment. This exchange maintains electroneutrality.
- Both hyponatremia and hypokalemia may occur occasionally. Repletion of K^+ alone in the form of KCl may correct serum Na^+ to the desired level without concomitant use of saline.
- Correction of serum $[Na^+]$ is explained by the following way. When KCl is administered, K^+ and Cl^- move into the cell, causing hyperosmolality in the cell. This draws water into the cell with resultant raise in serum $[Na^+]$. Also, when K^+ moves into the cell, H^+ moves out of the cell. This H^+ is buffered by bicarbonate and plasma protein, and the bicarbonate is converted into CO_2 and water. As a result, the plasma osmolality is decreased and water moves into the cell. This raises serum $[Na^+]$.
- When saline is needed, the amount of Na^+ required to achieve the desired level in a patient with both hyponatremia and hypokalemia should include both Na^+ and K^+ concentrations of the solution that should not exceed the total required amount.
- When severe hypokalemia (<2.5 mEq/L) is present with hyponatremia, only KCl may be needed to correct serum Na^+ to the desired level (see question 12).

Diagnosis of Hypotonic Hyponatremia

Figure 12.2 shows the two most important urinary tests in the evaluation of hypotonic hyponatremia:

1. Urine osmolality
2. Urine Na^+ (U_{Na})

As shown in Fig. 12.2, urine osmolality is always >100 mOsm/kg H_2O in all conditions that cause hypotonic hyponatremia except in those conditions of psychogenic polydipsia, beer potomania, and reset osmostat. It is emphasized that U_{Na} is <10 mEq/L only in vomiting, diarrhea, and decompensated congestive heart failure (CHF), cirrhosis, and nephrotic syndrome. Acute kidney injury due to volume depletion also causes low urinary Na^+. Fractional excretion of Na^+ follows that of U_{Na}.

Signs and Symptoms of Hyponatremia

Patients with plasma [Na^+] >125 mEq/L are generally asymptomatic. Symptoms are primarily neurologic, which are related to the severity and rapidity of development of hyponatremia. Gastrointestinal symptoms such as nausea may be the earliest clinical manifestation, followed by headache, yawning, lethargy, restlessness, disorientation, ataxia, and depressed reflexes with [Na^+] <125 mEq/L. In patients with rapidly evolving hyponatremia, seizures, coma, respiratory arrest, permanent brain damage, and death may occur.

Brain Adaptation to Hyponatremia

Cell volume is maintained during extreme conditions of either hypo- or hypertonicity by adjusting its intracellular solute contents. When plasma osmolality is low, water moves into the brain, causing brain swelling and edema. Astrocytes rather than neurons play a role in brain swelling. Blood flow to the brain decreases, leading to brain herniation. Because brain expansion is limited due to the rigid skull, intracranial hypertension develops, and neurologic symptoms occur in a hyponatremic patient. However, the symptoms slowly disappear as the brain begins to adapt to hyponatremia. The major adaptive mechanism is the extrusion of Na^+, Cl^-, K^+, and organic osmolytes (myoinositol, taurine, glycine, etc.) from the brain cell. This results in the reduction of intracellular osmolality, and further water movement into the cell is prevented. Subsequently, the brain volume returns to baseline even in the presence of severe hyponatremia (Fig. 12.3). This adaptation is nearly complete within 48 h. The clinician should keep this simple physiologic mechanism in mind while correcting hyponatremia because slow correction will allow the extruded electrolytes and organic osmolytes to move back into the cell or time to synthesize the organic osmolytes to maintain normal cell volume. For this reason, the guidelines have suggested limits of correction (increase in Na^+) for 24 and 48 h periods (see treatment). There are some factors that may impair brain adaptation to hyponatremia. Table 12.5 shows these factors and their possible mechanisms for impairment of brain adaptation.

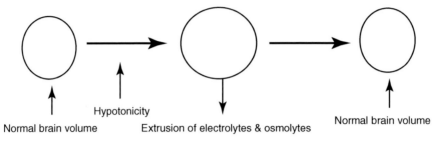

Fig. 12.3   Adaptation of brain volume to hyponatremia

Table 12.5   Factors and their mechanisms that impair brain adaptation

Factor	Mechanism
Children	High brain-to-skull ratio, as brain development is complete before skull development
Young menstruating females	Estrogen inhibition of Na/K-ATPase causing decreased extrusion of Na$^+$
Hypoxia	↓ Cerebral blood flow in the presence of hyponatremia, ↓ATP production, ↑lactate production →low intracellular pH
Increased ADH levels	Cerebral vasoconstriction, hypoperfusion

ATP adenosine triphosphate, *ADH* antidiuretic hormone, ↑ increased, ↓ decreased

Complications of Untreated Chronic Hyponatremia

Even mild chronic hyponatremia is not without complications. Studies have shown cognitive impairment, falls, fractures, and osteoporosis in individuals with serum [Na$^+$] between 126 and 134 mEq/L.

Treatment of Hyponatremia

Hyponatremia is classically defined as acute (<48 h duration) or chronic (>48 h duration) and further characterized as asymptomatic or symptomatic. This classification is important in terms of treatment. Thus, the treatment of hyponatremia depends on four factors:

1. Severity of hyponatremia
2. Duration of hyponatremia
3. Signs and symptoms of hyponatremia
4. Volume status

Treatment of Acute Symptomatic Hyponatremia

1. Acute symptomatic hyponatremia (seizures, respiratory distress, etc.) is a medical emergency.

2. Provide adequate oxygenation. Treat hypoxemia to prevent exacerbation of hyponatremic encephalopathy.
3. Patients at risk for acute symptomatic hyponatremia:
   (1) Postoperative patients receiving hypotonic fluids
   (2) Psychogenic polydipsic patients
   (3) Patients taking ecstasy
   (4) Marathon runners
4. For the above patients, 3% NaCl is the fluid of choice, because its infusion raises serum [Na^+] to a desired level and prevents cerebral edema. Rarely, 5% saline is required. Raise serum Na^+ 6–8 mEq in 3–4 h. Rapid correction to higher than 8 mEq in 24 h may not be that harmful, particularly, in patients with psychogenic polydipsia, patients taking ecstasy, and marathon runners (see Table 12.6). Water restriction should NEVER be used to treat symptomatic hyponatremia, because it takes 24–72 h to increase Na^+ by 5–6 mEq.
5. In all other symptomatic patients, 3% NaCl should also be used. Raise serum Na^+ 1–2 mEq/h for 3 h up to 6 mEq from baseline. Then hold 3% NaCl. If symptoms persist, give another bolus of 100 mL of 3% NaCl. The rate of increase in serum Na^+ is 6–8 mEq in a 24 h period in patients with no risk factors. In high-risk patients, the rate of correction should not exceed 6 mEq in a 24 h period.
6. The above rates of correction can be achieved by giving 1–2 mL/kg/h or 100 mL boluses of 3% NaCl. Repeat these boluses two to three times as needed. Assuming no urine excretion of Na^+, a bolus of 100 mL raises serum [Na^+] by 1 mEq.
7. To avoid overcorrection, it is useful to calculate the amount of Na^+ required to achieve the desired level. If the patient weighs 70 kg and serum [Na^+] is 110 mEq/L, and you wish to increase it to 116 mEq/L, use the following simple formula:

$$\text{Amount of } Na^+ \text{ needed} = \text{Total body water} \times \text{desired } Na^+ - \text{actual } Na^+$$
$$= 70 \times 0.6 \times 116 - 110 \text{ or } 42 \times 6$$
$$= 252 \text{ mEq}$$

1 L of 3% NaCl contains 513 mEq of Na^+.

252 mEq = 494 mL of 3% NaCl. If the patient receives 100–200 mL during the first 3 h to a total of 400–500 mL, and serum [Na^+] reaches 115 mEq, you can stop 3% NaCl.

If the above patient has mild hypokalemia, and you wish to give 40 mEq KCl, you should give 112 mEq of Na^+ and 40 mEq of K^+ separately to a total of 252 mEq.

On the other hand, if you give 40 mEq of KCl and 252 mEq of Na^+ separately, you may overcorrect serum Na^+ level.

8. Note that these calculations are based on the assumption that the patient is not losing any Na^+ in the urine. This is not possible in clinical medicine unless the patient is anuric.
9. Therefore, measure urine volume and urine Na^+ simultaneously with serum Na^+ every 2 h until the symptoms improve. Replace urinary loss of Na^+ with either 3% or 0.9% saline, as needed, to achieve the target Na^+.

10. NEVER correct serum Na⁺ levels above 6–8 mEq in a 24 h period from baseline irrespective of the risk factor.
11. If symptoms persist after serum Na⁺ has risen by 6 mEq/L, look for another cause for the neurologic symptoms.
12. If the patient develops pulmonary congestion, administer furosemide 20–40 mg. With furosemide, the patient loses both electrolytes and water. However, the urine output generally exceeds input, resulting in gradual increase in serum Na⁺ level.
13. If serum Na⁺ levels increase by $> 10\text{–}12$ mEq/L, administer DDAVP 1–2 µg IV with boluses of 5% dextrose in water (D5W) or 4–5 µg subcutaneously, and follow serum Na⁺ level. Repeat every 6–8 h until serum [Na⁺] decreases to a desired level (i.e., 6 mEq/L above baseline).
14. Do not raise serum [Na⁺] >18 mEq/L in a 48-h period.

Treatment of Chronic Symptomatic Hyponatremia

1. Note that overcorrection of serum [Na⁺] predisposes chronic hyponatremic patients to ODS.
2. In chronic hyponatremic patients, cerebral water content increases by only 10%. Therefore, the correction should not exceed 10%.
3. Use 3% NaCl. Do not exceed 1 mEq/h.
4. The maximum rate of correction in a 24 h period should not exceed 6–8 mEq.
5. Once symptoms and signs improve, either water restriction or normal saline should be started with measurements of urine output, urine Na⁺ and K⁺ with replacement of these cations, as needed.
6. In case of overcorrection, relowering of serum [Na⁺] by DDAVP and D5W is necessary to prevent ODS.
7. For fluid overload, furosemide can be given with 3% NaCl or normal saline.
8. Vaptan use also has been advocated prior to discharge. Table 12.6 summarizes the treatment of symptomatic hyponatremia.

Complication of Rapid Correction of Hyponatremia

ODS, previously called central pontine myelinolysis, is a complication of treatment of both acute and chronic hyponatremia (with certain exceptions; see Table 12.6). It occurs due to a rapid increase in serum [Na⁺] of 8–12 mEq in patients with no risk factors or >6 mEq in patients with risk factors above baseline in a 24-h period. The possible mechanism is slow recovery of brain osmolytes during rapid correction of hyponatremia compared to the loss of these osmolytes during the adaptation of brain volume. When serum [Na⁺] is rapidly raised, the plasma osmolality becomes hypertonic to the brain with resultant water movement from the brain. This cerebral dehydration probably causes myelinolysis and ODS.

Table 12.6 Treatment of symptomatic hyponatremia

Onset	Condition(s)	Signs and symptoms	Fluid and rate of correction	Comment
<24 h	Psychogenic polydipsia	Nausea, vomiting, headache, delirium, seizures, coma	3% saline	Overcorrection by >6–8 mEq/L in 24 h may not be harmful
	Marathon runners		100 mL boluses 3–4 times to reach 4–6 mEq/L in first 4–6 h. Hold 3% saline	
	Ecstasy			
24–48 h	Postoperative patients, in particular women and children	As above	As above	Do not exceed 6–8 mEq/L in 24 h
>48 h	*High-risk patients*: alcoholism, cirrhosis, hypokalemia, malnutrition, Na⁺ <105 mEq/L	Nausea Vomiting Fatigue Weakness Seizures	Hypokalemia: KCl Seizures, cirrhosis, Na⁺ <105 mEq/L: 3% saline Alcoholism, malnutrition: normal saline (at times) Do not exceed 4–6 mEq/L in 24 h	DDAVP and D5W for overcorrection

Adapted from Sterns RH. Disorders of plasma sodium- Causes, consequences, and correction. *N Engl J Med* 2015;372:55–65

Risk Factors

Several risk factors for precipitation of ODS have been identified. These are:

1. Chronic hyponatremia
2. Serum [Na⁺] <105 mEq/L
3. Chronic alcoholism
4. Malnutrition
5. Hypokalemia
6. Severe liver disease
7. Elderly women on thiazide diuretics
8. Children
9. Menstruating women
10. Hypoxia
11. Seizures on presentation and overcorrection (>20 mEq/L in 24 h)

Clinical Manifestations

ODS is a biphasic condition Following rapid correction of serum [Na⁺] by >6 mEq/L from baseline in 24 h in hyponatremic patients with above risk factors, the mental status improves and the patients become alert. This condition is followed in 2–3 days by the following manifestations:

1. Short-term memory impairment
2. Paraparesis or quadriparesis
3. Pseudobulbar symptoms (dysarthria or dysphagia)
4. Locked-in syndrome (preserved intellectual capacity without expression)
5. Ataxia
6. Oculomotor abnormalities
7. Mutism
8. Coma

Diagnostic Test

Magnetic resonance imaging (MRI) of the brain. Initially the MRI findings are
normal but may be found 3–4 weeks later after repeat MRI.

Management and Prognosis

The condition is generally irreversible once patients develop paraparesis or pseudobulbar symptoms or locked-in syndrome. Therefore, prevention of ODS is recommended by appropriate treatment of hyponatremia. Four treatment modalities have
been reported with variable success: (1) thyrotropin-releasing hormone, (2) methyl-
prednisolone, (3) plasmapheresis, and (4) IV immunoglobulins. Early reports
showed 100% mortality. Current reports document milder clinical course with substantial improvement in neurologic symptoms in ODS patients. For example, relowering of overtly corrected serum [Na$^+$] by desmopressin and 5% dextrose in water
improved neurologic symptoms in symptomatic hyponatremic patients.

Treatment of Asymptomatic Hyponatremia in Hospitalized Patients

1. Nephrologists are frequently consulted for evaluation of hyponatremia, because
   serum [Na$^+$] fell from 140 to 135 mEq/L due to hypotonic fluids.
2. In such patients, check volume status. For hypovolemic patients, administration
   of normal saline will improve both hemodynamics and serum [Na$^+$]. Avoid hypotonic fluids.
3. If volume is adequate and pseudohyponatremia is excluded, calculate water
   excess. Use the following simple formulas:

Formula 1

$$\text{Water excess} = \text{Total body water}\,(\text{TBW}) \times \text{actual}\left[\text{Na}^+\right]$$
$$= \text{Desired}\left[\text{Na}^+\right] \times \text{New TBW}$$

Example: Weight = 70 kg

Actual [Na⁺] = 110 mEq/L

Desired [Na⁺] = 120 mEq/L

New TBW = 70×0.6 = 42×110/120 = 38.5 L

Water excess = Previous TBW−New TBW

or 42−38.5 = 3.5 L

Formula 2

$$\text{Water excess} = \text{TBW}\left(1 - \frac{\text{Actual}\left[\text{Na}^+\right]}{\text{Desired}\left[\text{Na}^+\right]}\right)$$
$$= 42\times1-110/120$$
$$= 3.5\text{L}$$

4. How to restrict fluids? Generally fluid is restricted to 1 L/day. Although this restriction is adequate, serum [Na⁺] may not improve because of improper electrolyte–free water excretion. As discussed in Chap. 11, the sum of urine [Na⁺] and [K⁺] divided by serum [Na⁺] can be used in the restriction of fluids/day, as follows:

Ratio	Daily fluid intake (mL)
>1	<500
~1	500–700
<1	1,000

5. The simplest way to restrict fluids in hospitalized patients is to measure 24 h urine output. For example, if the total urine volume is 1,000 mL, restrict the total intake (water plus other fluids) to 1,000 mL/day so that the patient will lose daily insensible loss of 500 mL. This loss of 500 mL would raise serum [Na⁺] by 1 mEq/L. We generally do not include metabolic water production from food (about 300 mL) as an intake because many patients may be only on IV fluids.

Treatment of Asymptomatic Chronic Hyponatremia Due to Syndrome of Inappropriate Antidiuretic Hormone Secretion in Ambulatory Patients

1. Treat the underlying cause of SIADH.
2. Restrict fluid, as mentioned earlier.
3. If the patient is noncompliant to fluid restriction, enhance Na⁺ and protein intake to increase solute and water excretion. Furosemide (40 mg) can be tried with high Na⁺ intake.
4. Pharmacologic therapy can be started in some patients. Demeclocycline at 300–600 mg twice daily induces nephrogenic diabetes insipidus. The drug takes 3–4 days to have an effect. The major problem with demeclocycline is nephrotoxicity, and in particular cirrhotic patients develop acute kidney injury.

5. Osmotic diuresis (more water than Na^+ excretion) can be induced in some patients with noncompliance to water restriction. Urea at doses 30–60 g can be effective. Polyuria, GI discomfort, and unpalatability are some of the adverse effects of urea. Urea is usually mixed with orange juice to make it palatable.

6. Drugs such as lithium and V_2 receptor antagonists (vaptans) can be used to suppress ADH action. Lithium (900–1,200 mg/day) can be used. However, it has a narrow therapeutic and toxic range. Polyuria and neurotoxicity are major adverse effects of lithium. Close monitoring of serum $[Na^+]$ is necessary as hypernatremia due to polyuria is rather common, if fluid intake is not adequate.

7. Among vaptans, conivaptan (IV) and tolvaptan (oral) are available in the USA. Although clinical experience is limited, tolvaptan has been used with encouraging results. Vaptans cause water diuresis and, therefore, are called aquaretics. Na^+ loss is negligible. It is better to start the first dose in the hospital to follow the pattern of hyponatremia. Diuresis starts 2–4 h following 15 mg of tolvaptan intake. Serum $[Na^+]$ should be checked in 2–4 h, as Na^+ response is unpredictable. Dose can be increased to 30 or 60 mg at 24 h intervals. Allow free water intake, which may counteract abrupt increase in serum $[Na^+]$. Use tolvaptan only when serum $[Na^+]$ is <125 mEq/L. Avoid vaptans in patients with cirrhosis.

8. Conivaptan can be used to treat hyponatremia in neurosurgical patients with or without other therapies. Case reports and case series suggest that a single or multiple doses of conivaptan (10–40 mg IV over a 30 min period or boluses) improved serum $[Na^+]$ by 4–6 mEq/L in 24 h. No significant adverse effects, including ODS, were observed. In one case report, the 22-year-old woman had motor vehicle accident and subsequently developed hyponatremia (128 mEq/L) due to SIADH. Due to suspicion of cerebral edema and decreased cerebral perfusion, the patient received a bolus of conivaptan (20 mg), and serum Na^+ level increased from 128 to 148 mEq/L in 8 h and intracranial pressure dropped from 11–15 to 2 mmHg. Fortunately no adverse events were noted with rapid increase in serum Na^+ level. Thus, conivaptan can be used to treat hyponatremia in neurosurgical ICUs.

Treatment of General Causes of Hyponatremia

Table 12.7 summarizes optimal treatment of hyponatremia due to various causes.

Table 12.7 Treatment of hyponatremia

Cause	Treatment	Comment
Pseudohyponatremia	None	Treat underlying cause
Hypertonic hyponatremia due to hyperglycemia	Correct glucose with insulin. Normal saline for hypotension, followed by 0.45% saline to improve volume and hypernatremia	In a hypotensive and hypernatremic patient, normal saline is hypotonic to plasma osmolality
Diarrhea	Normal saline. KCl, if hypokalemic	Replace electrolyte loss in secretory diarrhea
Vomiting	Normal saline. KCl, if hypokalemia present	Treat the cause

Table 12.7 (continued)

Cause	Treatment	Comment
Salt-losing syndromes	Normal saline	Follow other electrolytes
Cerebral salt wasting	Normal saline, fludrocortisone	NaCl tablets in outpatient setting
CHF and cirrhosis	Salt restriction, loop diuretics, water restriction for hyponatremia. Vaptans (in CHF only), if water restriction fails and diuretic resistance develops	Edema and hyponatremia improve. Monitor serum [Na$^+$] frequently when tolvaptan is used
Acute and chronic kidney injury	Water restriction	Follow serum creatinine
Primary polydipsia	Water restriction	Treat underlying cause
Hypothyroidism	Thyroxine	Follow thyroid function tests
Glucocorticoid deficiency	Hydrocortisone	Follow serum [Na$^+$] and blood pressure
SSRIs	Water restriction	Do not use hydrochlorothiazide (HCTZ) concomitantly
HCTZ	Discontinue HCTZ. KCl alone is sufficient to raise serum [Na$^+$] in mild hyponatremia. Use NaCl tablets	Do not overcorrect K$^+$ deficit. Careful in using both normal saline and KCl
Exercise-induced hyponatremia (symptomatic)	3% NaCl until serum [Na$^+$] reaches 125 mEq/L or symptoms improve	Avoid pure water intake >3 L and nonsteroidal drug use
Low solute intake (tea and toast diet)	Increase dietary salt and protein intake. Water restriction is helpful	Follow urine osmolality. Seen commonly in elderly subjects
Beer potomania	Dietary salt and protein. Normal saline, as indicated. Water restriction may help in some patients	Follow urine osmolality
Postoperative hyponatremia (asymptomatic)	Normal saline	Follow urine electrolytes and osmolality. Avoid hypotonic solutions when serum [Na$^+$] <138 mEq/L. Hold normal saline once euvolemia is achieved

SSRIs selective serotonin reuptake inhibitors, *CHF* congestive heart failure

Study Questions

Case 1 A 47-year-old man comes to the emergency department with complaints of weakness, dizziness on standing, and poor appetite. Past medical history includes hypertension and CHF with ejection fraction of 30%. The patient says that he developed these symptoms following an increase in furosemide from 80 to 120 mg BID 1 week ago by his cardiologist. He was thirsty and drinking fluids, mostly water.

On physical examination, blood pressure (BP) is 110/70 mmHg, pulse rate is 88/min in sitting position, and 90/60 mmHg with a pulse rate of 104/min upon standing. The lungs are clear to auscultation. Also, cardiac examination is normal. There is no peripheral edema.

Serum	Urine
Na^+ = 128 mEq/L	Na^+ = 40 mEq/L
K^+ = 3.1 mEq/L	K^+ = 30 mEq/L
Cl^- = 88 mEq/L	Osmolality = 400 mOsm/kg H_2O
HCO_3^- = 30 mEq/L	
Glucose = 90 mg/dL	
BUN = 30 mg/dL	
Creatinine = 2.1 mg/dL	
Total protein = 7.1 g/dL	
Osmolality = 274 mOsm/kg H_2O	

Question 1 Is pseudohyponatremia present?

Answer No. Serum glucose and total protein are normal.

Question 2 Are other solutes such as mannitol or glycine present?

Answer No, because the osmolal gap is normal, excluding the presence of mannitol and glycine.

Question 3 How would you treat the patient?

Answer This patient has hypotonic hyponatremia with extracellular fluid volume (ECV) depletion due to a deficit in total body Na^+ and water (Na^+ deficit > water deficit). As a result, the patient has orthostatic BP and pulse changes (hypovolemic hyponatremia). Hypovolemia stimulates ADH release, and water is retained despite hypoosmolality. This type of hypotonic hyponatremia responds to replacement of Na^+ and water. The appropriate IV fluid is normal (0.9%) saline, which not only raises BP but also improves Cl^-. However, severe hypokalemia may develop due to saline-induced diuresis. Therefore, addition of 20–40 mEq of KCl to normal saline initially is sufficient to maintain serum $[K^+]$ at baseline. Oral KCl is usually preferred, if the patient can take it by mouth. Correction of hypokalemia also corrects hyponatremia.

Question 4 Is 3% saline or Ringer's lactate indicated?

Answer 3% NaCl is not indicated as the patient has no severe CNS symptoms. Ringer's lactate is an alternative to normal saline to improve Na^+ and water status, but it will raise serum $[HCO_3^-]$ even further.

Question 5 Is 0.45% saline or D5W indicated?

Answer 0.45% saline is a hypotonic solution that does not have enough Na^+ to compensate for the lost Na^+, even though it may provide more water than normal saline. D5W is inappropriate because it lowers serum [K⁺] even further by translocation into the cell.

Case 2 A 72-year-old woman, who lives alone, was admitted for weakness, inability to walk, and forgetfulness over a 2-week period of time. She cooks her own meals. She is slightly lethargic. Physical examination shows BP 124/74 mmHg, pulse 78/min, and no orthostatic hypotension. Lung and heart examination are normal. The laboratory results are:

Serum	Urine
Na⁺ = 120 mEq/L	Volume = 1 L/day
K⁺ = 3.6 mEq/L	Na⁺ = 20 mEq/L
Cl⁻ = 88 mEq/L	K⁺ = 12 mEq/day
BUN = 6 mg/dL	Urea nitrogen = 246 mg
Creatinine = 0.5 mg/dL	Osmolality = 110 mOsm/kg H₂O
Glucose = 90 mg/dL	

Question 1 How did she develop hyponatremia?

Answer Based on physical examination, the patient has euvolemic hyponatremia. Generally, the typical American diet generates a minimum of 600 mOsm per day (assuming 60 g protein intake). All of these mOsm are excreted in either 12 L of urine, if urine osmolality is 50 mOsm/kg H₂O, or 0.5 L of urine if urine osmolality is 1,200 mOsm/kg H₂O (total mOsm/urine osmolality or 600/50 = 12 L or 600/1,200 = 0.5 L). Thus, a normal individual with intact diluting and concentrating ability can excrete urine from 0.5 to 12 L without any change in water balance (or plasma osmolality).

The patient has urine osmolality of 110 mOsm/kg H₂O; therefore, she can excrete all her mOsm in 2.2 L of urine (110/50 = 2.2 L). However, her total mOsm were only 110, suggesting poor solute intake. If this patient drinks >2.7 L (2.2+0.5 L insensible loss) of fluids daily and her solute excretion is only 110 mOsm, she will be in a positive water balance with subsequent development of hyponatremia.

Question 2 Why is she unable to dilute her urine maximally?

Answer The lack of solute intake impairs the kidney's ability to dilute the urine to 50 mOsm/kg H₂O, as reduced solute excretion limits water excretion.

Question 3 What is the appropriate treatment of her hyponatremia?

Answer Encourage oral intake of food with 60 g protein, salt (100 mEq Na⁺), and 40–60 mEq K⁺.

Case 3 A 44-year-old menstruating woman had abdominal surgery lasting for 4 h. Perioperatively, she received normal saline to maintain BP and urine output. Postoperatively, she received 0.45% saline at 120 mL/h and morphine for pain. Her urine output was 110 mL/h; 24 h later, she was awake and complained of nausea and headache. The following laboratory results were available at the time of consultation:

Serum [Na⁺] = 130 mEq/L
Urine [Na⁺] = 100 mEq/L
Urine [K⁺] = 30 mEq/L
Urine osmolality = 440 mOsm/kg H_2O
Urine output = 100 mL/h
Preop [Na⁺] = 139 mEq/L
Weight = 64 kg

Question 1 Why did she develop hyponatremia?

Answer The reasons for the development of hyponatremia are (1) hypotonic fluid relative to urine osmolality and (2) nonosmotic release of ADH due to morphine and pain.

Question 2 Are nausea and headache significant?

Answer Yes. These symptoms are related to acute decrease in serum [Na⁺] and are probably early manifestations of impending encephalopathy in this menstruating woman.

Question 3 Calculate water excess in this patient.

Answer   Water excess = Total body water $(TBW) \times$ actual $\left[Na^+ \right]$
$$= Preop \left[Na^+ \right] \times New\ TBW$$

Weight = 64 kg
TBW = $64 \times 0.5 = 32$ L
Actual [Na⁺] = 130 mEq/L
Preop [Na⁺] = 139 mEq/L
New TBW = $32 \times 130/139 = 29.92$ L
Water excess = Previous TBW−New TBW
or $32 - 29.92 = 2.1$ L
Alternative calculation:

Preop total body Na^+ = $TBW \times Serum \left[Na^+ \right]$ or $32 \times 139 = 4,448$

Current water balance = Total body Na^+ / Actual $\left[Na^+ \right]$ or $4,448 / 130 = 34.2$ L

Water excess = Current TBW − Preop TBW or $34.2 - 32 = 2.2$ L

Question 4 Which one of the following IV fluids is appropriate for this patient?

(A) 0.9% NaCl
(B) Ringer's lactate
(C) 3% NaCl

The answer is C The patient has acute symptomatic (<48 h) hyponatremia. Therefore, 3% NaCl is appropriate. The rate of increase is 1–2 mEq/h to the maximum of 6 mEq in 3 h or until symptoms improve. Note that the rate of increase should not exceed by 8 mEq in a 24-h period.

Question 5 Write an order for 3% NaCl.

Answer 2 mL/kg (130 mL) to run in 30 min. One liter of 3% NaCl contains 513 mEq of Na$^+$; therefore, 130 mL contains 67 mEq.

Question 5 Assuming no change in her urine output, urine [Na$^+$], [K$^+$], and osmolality, calculate the expected increase in serum [Na$^+$].

Answer Calculate her total body Na$^+$:

$$\text{Total body Na}^+ = \text{New TBW} \times \text{Actual} \left[\text{Na}^+ \right]$$
$$34.2 \times 130 = 4,446 \text{ mEq}$$

Calculate her new total body Na$^+$ and new TBW:

$$\text{New total body Na}^+ = \text{Total body Na}^+ + \text{Infused Na}^+ \text{or}$$
$$4,446 + 67 = 4,513 \text{ mEq}$$
$$\text{New TBW} = 34.2 + 0.13(3\%\text{saline}) = 34.33 \text{ L}$$
$$\text{Expected serum} \left[\text{Na}^+ \right] = 4,513 / 34.33 = 131.45$$
$$\text{or } 1.45(131.45 - 130 = 1.45) \text{mEq} / \text{L increase}$$

Question 6 What is the next appropriate step?

Answer Repeat 100 mL boluses of 3% NaCl twice with close monitoring of serum [Na$^+$] and urine [Na$^+$], [K$^+$], and osmolality.

Question 7 Why are 0.9% NaCl and Ringer's lactate NOT appropriate for this patient?

Answer Both are hypotonic fluids compared to her urine osmolality (440 mOsm/kg H$_2$O). Therefore, her serum [Na$^+$] decreases further.

Case 4 A 60-year-old woman with history of lung cancer is admitted for weakness and lethargy for 4 weeks. Her serum [Na$^+$] is 120 mEq/L. She weighs 60 kg. Her serum osmolality is 250 mOsm/kg H$_2$O. Urine osmolality is 616 mOsm/kg H$_2$O. The diagnosis of SIADH has been made.

Question 1 What would be her serum [Na$^+$], if she receives 1 L of isotonic (normal) saline?

Answer The selection of fluids in the treatment of SIADH depends on a clear-cut understanding of the fluid, serum, and urine osmolalities. In addition, the physician should evaluate the TBW as well as the total body Na$^+$ (TB$_{Na}$) content. I would like to use TB$_{Na}$ content rather than total plasma osmolality, because both calculations would yield similar results. A systematic approach would yield the correct answer.

First, calculate TBW and TB$_{Na}$ of the patient as follows:

$$TBW = Wt(kg) \times \% \text{ of water} / kg$$
$$60 \times 0.5 = 30 \text{ L}$$
$$TB_{Na} = TBW \times Serum\left[Na^+\right]$$
$$30 \times 120 = 3,600 \text{ mEq}$$

Second, calculate the amount of urine volume that is required to excrete the mOsm of normal saline. This can be calculated by dividing urine mOsm into mOsm of normal saline.

The new serum [Na$^+$] can be obtained as follows:

$$\text{mOsm in normal saline} = 308\left(Na^+ = 154 \text{ and } Cl^- = 154\right)$$
$$\text{mOsm in urine} = 616\left(\text{osmolality}\right)$$
$$\text{Amount of urine required to excrete } 308 \text{ mOsm} = 308 / 616 = 0.5 \text{ L}$$

The patient received 1 L of normal saline; however, she excreted all these mOsm in 0.5 L of urine. Therefore, the patient retained 0.5 L of free water, which causes the TBW to increase from 30 to 30.5 L. Assuming the TB$_{Na}$ remains at 3,600 mEq, the new serum [Na$^+$] would be

$$3,600 / 30.5 = 118 \text{ mEq} / L$$

Thus, in a patient with the diagnosis of SIADH, administration of normal saline would result in a decrease rather than an increase in serum [Na$^+$].

Question 2 What would be her serum [Na$^+$], if she receives 1 L of 3% NaCl?

Answer The new serum [Na$^+$] can be calculated in a similar fashion, as described earlier.

$$\text{mOsm in } 3\% NaCl = 1,026\left(Na^+ = 513, Cl^- = 513\right)$$
$$\text{mOsm in urine} = 616$$
$$\text{Urine volume needed to excrete } 1,026 \text{ mOsm} = 1,026 / 616 = 1.67 \text{ L}$$

Thus, the patient excreted more urine than intake (1 L), and the new TBW = 30–0.67 = 29.3 L and new serum [Na$^+$] = 3,600/29.3 = 123 mEq/L.

Question 3 What would be her serum [Na$^+$], if she receives 1 L of 3% saline and furosemide 60 mg and her urine osmolality is reduced to 308 mOsm/kg H$_2$O?

Answer The new serum [Na⁺] can be calculated in a similar fashion, as shown above.

$$\text{mOsm in } 3\%NaCl = 1,026$$

$$\text{mOsm in urine} = 616$$

Urine volume needed to excrete 1,026 mOsm = 1,026/308 = 3.3 L.
Thus, the patient excreted more urine than intake (1 L), and the new TBW is

$$\text{New TBW} = \text{TBW} + \text{Infused saline}(1\,L) - \text{Urine volume}$$

$$30 + 1 - 3.3 = 27.7$$

$$\text{New seum}\left[Na^+\right] = 3,600 / 27.7 = 130\,\text{mEq} / L$$

It should be noted that these are approximate calculations and vary from patient to patient. Therefore, frequent determinations of serum and urine electrolytes as well as urine osmolality are required in the management of symptomatic hyponatremia in a patient with SIADH.

Case 5 An 80-year-old woman was admitted for nausea, headache, and psychosis for 2 days. Past medical history includes hypertension, and her physician increased hydrochlorothiazide (HCTZ), from 12.5 to 25 mg daily. The patient was drinking water more than usual. Her BP was 120/70 mmHg with a pulse rate of 80. There were no orthostatic BP and pulse changes. She weighs 70 kg. EKG showed slight prolongation of QT interval. Pertinent labs:
Serum [Na⁺] = 112 mEq/L
Serum [K⁺] = 3.2 mEq/L
Serum [Cl⁻] = 90 mEq/L
Serum glucose = 90 mg/dL
Serum uric acid = 3.2 mg/dL
Urine osmolality = 220 mOsm/kg H_2O

Question 1 How frequent is diuretic-induced hyponatremia?

Answer Hyponatremia is a well-documented complication of diuretic use. About 73% of cases of hyponatremia were related to thiazide diuretic use. Twenty percent of cases were attributed to a combination of thiazides and K⁺-sparing diuretics, and 8% were related to furosemide use. Thus, HCTZ rather than furosemide is the most common cause of hyponatremia.

Question 2 How does HCTZ rather than furosemide cause hyponatremia?

Answer HCTZ or other thiazide diuretics impair maximum urinary dilution without affecting concentrating ability. Urine osmolality is usually >100 mOsm/kg H_2O among thiazide users. The expected urine osmolality for this degree of hyponatremia (112 mEq/L) with normal diluting capacity should be about 50 mOsm/kg

H_2O. However, this patient is unable to lower urine osmolality <100 mOsm/kg H_2O because of the effect of HCTZ on renal water handling. HCTZ decreases free H_2O clearance (i.e., more water reabsorption), resulting in urine osmolality >100 mOsm/kg H_2O.

Furosemide impairs both diluting and concentrating ability of the kidney. Because of its inability to concentrate urine, furosemide causes more water excretion with urine osmolality similar to that of serum (isosthenuria). Therefore, furosemide alone does not cause hyponatremia, but a combination of HCTZ and furosemide can result in hyponatremia. However, some patients may develop hypotonic hyponatremia with orthostatic BP and pulse changes with chronic use of furosemide due to total body Na^+ and water loss (case 1).

Question 3 How would you treat her hyponatremia?

Answer This patient has acute symptomatic hyponatremia, which requires immediate treatment. Although controversial, treatment should be prompt in view of preventing progression of cerebral edema and hypoxia, which far exceed the risk of osmotic demyelination. Initially, serum $[Na^+]$ should be corrected at the rate of 1–2 mEq/L/h from 112 to 118 mEq/L in 3–4 h or until symptoms resolve. The maximum rate of correction in a 24-h period should not exceed by 6 to 118 mEq/L. Limit the correction to 126 mEq/L in a 48-h period. Administration of hypertonic saline should be adjusted to the target serum $[Na^+]$ by frequent determinations of serum and urine Na^+ and K^+ levels.

Question 4 How much Na^+ is needed to raise serum $[Na^+]$ from 112 to 118 mEq/L?

Answer She weighs 70 kg, and her total body water is 35 L (70×0.5). The amount of serum Na^+ that needs to be increased is 6 mEq. Therefore, the amount of Na^+ that is required is 210 mEq (35 L×6=210). In clinical practice, more than 210 mEq are required, as the patient needs replacement of excreted Na^+ and K^+ in the urine.

Question 5 Is restriction of fluids and 0.9% NaCl appropriate for this patient?

Answer No. Restriction of fluids and administration of normal saline are not appropriate for acute symptomatic hyponatremia, although adequate after relief of symptoms.

It has been shown that slow correction of thiazide-induced symptomatic hyponatremia in 18–56 h may be associated with a high rate of permanent neurologic damage. Thus, prompt correction to relieve symptoms is required.

Question 6 Is correction of hypokalemia with KCl sufficient to relieve her symptoms?

Answer Although administration of KCl alone raises serum $[Na^+]$ by transcellular distribution and can improve her symptoms, the increase in serum $[Na^+]$ is unpredictable. Sometimes overcorrection of serum $[Na^+]$ is possible.

This patient received a total of 60 mEq of KCl IV separately in 3 h, and her serum [K⁺] was 3.8 mEq/L. Repeat EKG was normal. Serum [Na⁺] was 117 mEq/L in 3 h after receiving a total of 190 mEq of Na⁺ and 60 mEq of K⁺. Her symptoms improved. HCTZ was discontinued, and no residual symptoms or neurologic deterioration was observed in 2 and 6 weeks follow-up.

Case 6 A 28-year-old woman was admitted for nausea, vomiting, blurred vision, and questionable seizures. She was electively intubated for airway protection. Further history was obtained from her mother, who stated that the patient had non-bloody diarrhea for 2 days and drank several liters of water. The patient is a strict vegan, and in good health, and does not take any medications. Physical examination revealed a thin female with a BP of 116/72 mmHg with a pulse rate of 98 beats/min. Lung and heart examination were normal. There was no peripheral edema. Her weight was 64 kg. Six weeks ago, she delivered a healthy baby and her serum [Na⁺] was 140 mEq/L. The laboratory results showed:

Serum	Urine
Na⁺ = 114 mEq/L	Na⁺ = <20 mEq/L
K⁺ = 2.7 mEq/L	K⁺ = 6 mEq/L
Cl⁻ = 78 mEq/L	Osmolality = 40 mOsm/kg H₂O
HCO₃⁻ = 17 mEq/L	
Creatinine = 0.5 mg/dL	
BUN = 4 mg/dL	
Glucose = 100 mg/dL	
Uric acid = 2.9 mg/dL	
Osmolality = 240 mOsm/kg H₂O	

Question 1 Assuming her total output (diarrheal fluid, urine output, and insensible loss) is 2 L/day, how much water she may have consumed that lowered her serum [Na⁺] from 140 to 114 mEq/L?

(A) 8 L
(B) 9 L
(C) 11 L
(D) 13 L
(E) 15 L

The answer is C First, calculate her TBW and total body Na⁺ prior to admission, and then calculate water excess.

$$\text{TBW} = 64 \times 0.5 = 32\,\text{L}$$

Previous total body $Na^+ = \text{TBW} \times \text{Serum}\left[Na^+\right]$ or $32 \times 140 = 4,480$ mEq

New TBW = 4,480 / 114 = 39.3 L

Water excess = 39.3 − 32 = 7.3 L

Second, add total output for 2 days (4 L) to water excess of 7.3 L. Therefore, the patient may have consumed approximately 11 L of water. Thus, answer C is correct.

In the emergency department, she received 100 mL of 3% NaCl, and her urine output was noted to be 200 mL/h. She also received 40 mEq of KCl. Repeat serum [Na⁺] in 4 h was 119 mEq/L. She was extubated. The patient did not receive any IV fluids or other interventions for the next 20 h. After 24 h, her serum [Na⁺] was 131 mEq/L.

Question 2 Which one of the following is the MOST appropriate next step in the management of her hyponatremia?

(A) D5W at 100 mL/h
(B) Free water boluses at 200 mL Q6H via N/G tube
(C) 0.45% saline at 100 mL/h
(D) Restrict fluid to 1 L/day
(E) DDAVP 1–2 μg IV or 4 μg subcutaneously with boluses (250 mL) of D5W

The answer is E The patient had an increase of 17 mEq of serum [Na⁺] in 24 h because of increased urine output. This is an expected overcorrection. The appropriate management at this time to prevent further increase in serum [Na⁺], and demyelination, if any, is by administration of DDAVP and D5W. Studies in animals and humans suggest that this type of management is appropriate to prevent further increase in serum [Na⁺]. Thus, option E is correct. Infusion of hypotonic solutions alone is not sufficient to reverse demyelination.

Although she had excess water intake and her correction >8 mEq/L may not be that harmful, she may be at risk for osmotic demyelination because of relative hypokalemia and poor solute intake. Therefore, relowering of serum [Na⁺] to 124–126 mEq/L is justified.

Question 3 Was DDAVP started late?

Answer Yes. DDAVP 1–2 μg IV should have been started when her urine output was 200 mL/h so that her serum [Na⁺] would have been maintained around 124–126 mEq/L.

Case 7 A 49-year-old man is brought to the emergency department for evaluation of nausea, fatigue, and weakness for 24 h. His wife says that he had been having binge drinking without any food intake. He is not taking any medications. On physical examination, he is euvolemic. His weight is 70 kg. BP is 100/60 mmHg with a pulse rate of 82. Serum and urine chemistries are:

Serum [Na⁺] = 122 mEq/L
Serum [K⁺] = 3.8 mEq/L

Serum BUN = 8 mg/dL
Serum creatinine = 0.6 mg/dL
Serum osmolality = 230 mOsm/kg H_2O
Urine osmolality = 75 mOsm/kg H_2O
Urine Na^+ = 10 mEq/L
Urine K^+ = 20 mEq/L

Question 1 In this patient, the most likely diagnosis is beer potomania. Assuming no urine output in 2–3 h, which one of the following is the MOST appropriate therapy for this patient?

(A) D5W
(B) 0.9% NaCl
(C) 3% NaCl
(D) 0.45% NaCl
(E) Fluid restriction and NaCl tablets

The answer is B Treatment of acute symptomatic hyponatremia due to binge drinking is a therapeutic challenge to physicians because of waning and waxing symptoms. A review of the literature on treatment of hyponatremia due to beer ingestion shows the following treatment modalities: 0.9% NaCl, 0.45% NaCl with KCl supplementation, 3% NaCl, fluid restriction, and no treatment. Thus, treatment of hyponatremia seems to depend on the severity and duration of onset of symptoms.

This patient has mild to moderate symptoms of hyponatremia. The appropriate treatment appears 0.9% saline rather than 3% saline. Rapid correction of serum $[Na^+]$ to 128 mEq/L by 3% saline is not necessary in this patient. Furthermore, rapid correction of serum $[Na^+]$ to >130 mEq/L in an alcoholic may precipitate ODS. Frequent determination of serum electrolytes is needed to continue 0.9% saline and KCl replacement, as hypokalemia is a risk factor for ODS, in addition to rapid correction of serum $[Na^+]$. Initiation of diet will improve serum $[Na^+]$.

D5W is not the fluid of initial choice in this patient, because it is converted into free water, and may lower serum $[Na^+]$ even further. Also, it may precipitate hypokalemia as well. D5W can be started, if caloric intake is needed after serum $[Na^+]$ reaches approximately 128 mEq/L. Also, fluid restriction with supplementation of NaCl tablets is not the appropriate choice.

Case 8 A 27-year-old man with subarachnoid hemorrhage developed persistent hyponatremia. He complains of weakness, mild dizziness, and vomiting. Physical examination reveals a BP of 114/70 mmHg, pulse of 106 beats/min, respiratory rate of 16/min, and a temperature of 99.1 F. Cardiac exam is normal. Lungs are clear to auscultation. There is no peripheral edema. He receives 2.5 L of normal saline daily without much improvement in serum $[Na^+]$.

Laboratory studies:

Serum	Urine
Na^+ = 122 mEq/L	Osmolality = 700 mOsm/kg H_2O
K^+ = 4.2 mEq/L	Na^+ = 100 mEq/L
Cl^- = 96 mEq/L	K^+ = 24 mEq/L
HCO_3^- = 27 mEq/L	Volume = 4 L/24 h
BUN = 22 mg/dL	
Glucose = 80 mg/dL	
Total protein = 7.69 g/dL	
Uric acid = 3.5 mg/dL	
$FE_{uric\ acid}$ = 18% (normal <10%)	
$FE_{phosphate}$ = 26% (normal <20%)	

Question 1 Which one of the following is the MOST likely cause of this patient's hyponatremia?

(A) Pseudohyponatremia
(B) Late vomiting
(C) Adrenal insufficiency
(D) Cerebral salt wasting (CSW)
(E) SIADH

The answer is D Pseudohyponatremia is related to extremely high levels of proteins and triglycerides. Although triglycerides were not measured, his total protein concentration was normal. Also, the plasma osmolality is low. Therefore, this patient does not have pseudohyponatremia.

Vomiting is a consideration; however, serum [Cl^-] and urinary K^+ levels are not consistent with vomiting. In general, patients with late vomiting conserve Na^+ and excrete low Na^+ because of volume depletion. Also, K^+ excretion is enhanced in both early and late vomiting. Therefore, option B is incorrect.

Adrenal insufficiency is also a consideration in view of normal to low BP and increased pulse rate as well as increased urinary Na^+ excretion. However, normal Cl^-, HCO_3^-, and glucose levels exclude the diagnosis of adrenal insufficiency.

Hypotonic hyponatremia, low serum uric acid level, relatively normal BP, high urine Na^+, and osmolality suggest the diagnosis of SIADH. However, high pulse rate, slightly elevated HCO_3^-, and BUN levels are unusual in patients with SIADH. Also, high urine volume is unusual in SIADH. Patients with SIADH are euvolemic and lower their serum Na^+ levels with normal saline. Although $FE_{uric\ acid}$ is high, increased $FE_{phosphate}$ is not high in SIADH. The clinical presentation of this patient is suggestive of volume depletion, rather than euvolemia. Therefore, SIADH is unlikely in this patient.

CSW is the most likely cause of this patient's hyponatremia. Hypovolemia and serum as well as urine studies are consistent with CSW. Thus, option D is correct.

Case 9 A 40-year-old woman is admitted for hysteroscopic myomectomy for menorrhagia. Past medical history is unremarkable. Preoperative serum [Na⁺] was 139 mEq/L. The operating time was 2 h. During this time, she received 20 L of 1.5% glycine as an irrigating solution. She also received 2 L of Ringer's lactate. Serum chemistry obtained within 2 h showed the following values:

Na⁺ = 120 mEq/L
K⁺ = 3.9 mEq/L
BUN = 14 mg/dL
Glucose = 90 mg/dL
Osmolality = 290 mOsm/kg H_2O.

Question 1 Why did she develop hyponatremia within 2 h?

Answer Hysteroscopic myomectomy is a surgical procedure for the treatment of menorrhagia and fibroids requiring several liters of hypotonic glycine or sorbitol as an irrigating solution. These solutions are also used in transurethral resection of the prostate. During this irrigation procedure, substantial amount of glycine enters the circulation and expands the extracellular fluid (ECF) volume. Like glucose, glycine is also an osmotic agent and promotes translocation of water from intracellular fluid (ICF) to ECF compartment. Thus, hyponatremia develops by dilution and translocation of water within 2 h after irrigation with glycine. After 2 h, glycine enters the cell for metabolism.

Question 2 Does serum osmolal gap help in the analysis of dilutional and translocational causes of hyponatremia?

Answer Yes. In this patient, the calculated serum osmolality is 250 mOsm/kg H_2O, whereas the measured osmolality is 290 mOsm/kg H_2O. The osmolal gap, therefore, is 40, which accounts for the decrease in serum [Na⁺] from 139 to 126 mEq/L. This calculation is based on the assumption that serum [Na⁺] decreases by 1.6 mmol/L per 5 mmol/L of solute (glycine) confined to the ECF. Accordingly, 40 mOsm (or mmol/L) of glycine would lower serum [Na⁺] by 13 mEq/L as follows:

$$40 / 5 \times 1.6 = 13$$

If hyponatremia is entirely due to dilution, her serum [Na⁺] should have been 126 mEq/L. Instead, her [Na⁺] was 120 mEq/L. This difference of 6 mEq/L may have accounted for translocation of water from ICF to ECF compartment.

Five hours later, she woke up but remained drowsy and confused. No seizure activity was noticed. Repeat serum chemistry: Na⁺ 130 mEq/L, K⁺ 4.0 mEq/L, BUN 18 mg/dL, and glucose 100 mg/dL. Serum osmolality was 276 mOsm/kg H_2O.

Question 3 What caused her altered mental status?

Answer Glycine enters the cell after 2 h, where it is metabolized to water, glucose, CO_2, urea, and most importantly NH_3. It has been shown that neurologic changes associated with glycine infusion are related to NH_3. Thus, her drowsiness and confusion may be attributed to NH_3 production.

The osmolal gap is normal, which is common after few hours of glycine infusion. Hyponatremia (130 mEq/L) is entirely due to dilutional rather than translocational because of water generation from glycine metabolism.

Case 10 A 32-year-old woman with AIDS was referred to the renal clinic for evaluation of persistent hyponatremia. There was no history of recent infections, but admits to daily intake of beer and at times depression. The patient is thin but not cachectic. BP is 120/80 mmHg with a pulse rate of 78 beats/min. There are no orthostatic changes. Lung and heart examination are normal. No peripheral edema is appreciated. Serum and urine chemistries:

Serum	Urine
Na^+ = 126 mEq/L	Osmolality = 578 mOsm/kg H_2O
K^+ = 4.2 mEq/L	Na^+ = 80 mEq/L
Cl^- = 94 mEq/L	K^+ = 40 mEq/L
HCO_3^- = 23 mEq/L	
BUN = 12 mg/dL	
Creatinine = 0.5 mg/dL	
Glucose = 104 mg/dL	
Albumin = 3.4 g/dL	
Normal liver function tests and cortisol	
Osmolality = 264 mOsm/kg H_2O	

Question 1 Which one of the following treatments is INAPPROPRIATE in this patient?

(A) Water restriction
(B) Lithium
(C) Demeclocycline
(D) Selective serotonin reuptake inhibitor (SSRI)
(E) Dilantin

The answer is D Except for SSRI, other treatment modalities have been tried to improve chronic asymptomatic hyponatremia in patients with ectopic production or stimulation of ADH. SSRIs such as sertraline, paroxetine, and duloxetine inhibit the reuptake of serotonin, thus causing hyponatremia. SSRIs induce SIDAH by several mechanisms that include (1) stimulation of ADH secretion, (2) augmentation of ADH action in the renal medulla, (3) resetting the osmostat that lowers the threshold for ADH secretion, and (4) interaction of SSRIs with other medications via p450 enzymes, resulting in enhanced action of ADH. Dilantin inhibits ADH secretion, so that it will improve hyponatremia.

Case 11 A 65-year-old man with small cell cancer of the left lung is found to have hyponatremia due to SIADH. He is seen by a nephrologist, who started him on a fluid restriction of 1 L/day. Patient refused to take demeclocycline because of his alcohol use and urea for gastrointestinal upset. For a while, his serum [Na^+] was maintained between 130 and 135 mEq/L. The patient was given a follow-up visit in 3 months, at which time he presented with weakness, fatigue, and inability to concentrate during conversation. He also complained that he had a sense of falling. He checked his BP which was 140/78 mmHg. He admitted to drinking >1 L of fluids/day because of increased thirst. His serum [Na$^+$] is 124 mEq/L and euvolemic. Other laboratories are consistent with SIADH.

Question 1 What is the appropriate step in the management of his hyponatremia?

Answer The patient is symptomatic from his chronic hyponatremia. Impairment in cognitive function and falls with fractures are not uncommon in patients with chronic hyponatremia. The patient should be admitted to the hospital for two reasons: (1) to improve symptoms with an increase in serum [Na$^+$] to 128–130 mEq/L in a 24-h period and (2) consideration for an oral vaptan, as the patient is noncompliant to fluid restriction. Tolvaptan is the oral form that is available as 15, 30, and 60 mg tablets.

Question 2 How is tolvaptan started?

Answer Tolvaptan should be started in a hospital setting for monitoring of serum [Na$^+$] during the dosage-titration phase. The drug is started at 15 mg once daily and titrated up to 60 mg daily without fluid restriction. Once this patient's symptoms improve, he can be discharged in 2–3 days on a fixed dose of tolvaptan.

Tolvaptan is indicated in patients with euvolemic and hypervolemic hyponatremic patients. It should not be used in patients with hypovolemic hyponatremia.

Question 3 Are there clinical studies that support the use of tolvaptan chronically?

Answer Yes. The SALT trials, which included patients with SIADH, CHF, and cirrhosis, showed that tolvaptan increased serum [Na$^+$] by 4.5 mEq/L on day 4 and 7.4 mEq/L over a 30-day period compared with fluid restriction alone. The patients were also followed up for a mean of 701 days. Mean serum [Na$^+$] increased from 131 to >135 mEq/L.

Question 4 Discuss the properties of the available vaptans.

Answer To date, five vaptans are available; however, only conivaptan (IV form) and tolvaptan (oral form) are available in the USA. As shown in Table 12.8, conivaptan is a combined V1$_a$/V$_2$ receptor antagonist. V1$_a$ receptors are present in hepatocytes and splanchnic circulation. The use of conivaptan in cirrhotic patient is expected to cause splanchnic vasodilation and cause an increase in portal pressure. Also, vaptans are contraindicated in patients with cirrhosis. As evident from Table 12.8, all vaptans can be taken orally other than conivaptan.

Table 12.8 Properties of vaptans

Drug	Receptor antagonism	Daily dose (mg)	Route of administration	Urine volume	Urine osmolality	Urine Na$^+$ excretion/day
Conivaptan	V1$_a$/V$_2$	20–40	IV	↑	↓	No change
Tolvaptan	V$_2$	15–60	Oral	↑	↓	No change
Lixivaptan	V$_2$	100–200	Oral	↑	↓	No change with low dose, but ↑ at high dose
Satavaptan	V$_2$	12.5–50	Oral	↑	↓	No change
Mozavaptan	V$_2$	60–120	Oral	↑	↓	No change

IV intravenous

Case 12 A 52-year-old woman was admitted with weakness and confusion for 2 days. She admits to drinking alcohol for the last 6 days. She has the history of central diabetes insipidus and on desmopressin. One week prior to admission, she was euvolemic and her serum chemistry was normal. She weighs 70 kg. Admitting labs:

Serum	Urine
Na$^+$ = 114 mEq/L	Na$^+$ = <20 mEq/L
K$^+$ = 2.2 mEq/L	K$^+$ = 30 mEq/L
Cl$^-$ = 92 mEq/L	Osmolality = 100 mOsm/kg H$_2$O
HCO$_3^-$ = 22 mEq/L	Ethanol = 0 mg/dL
Creatinine = 0.5 mg/dL	
BUN = 6 mg/dL	
Glucose = 90 mg/dL	
Osmolality = 238 mOsm/kg H$_2$O	

Question 1 Which one of the following is an APPROPRIATE initial fluid management in this patient?

(A) D5W
(B) Normal saline
(C) 3% saline
(D) KCl
(E) KCl and D5W

The answer is D This patient has profound hypokalemia. D5W and normal saline would lower K$^+$ even further; therefore, these are not appropriate fluids for this patient. Three percent saline increases serum [Na$^+$] but does not improve serum [K$^+$]. Therefore, 3% saline is not an appropriate choice of fluid. KCl and D5W is not an appropriate fluid for this patient, as this fluid may not normalize serum [K$^+$]. The appropriate fluid is administration of KCl, which improves both K$^+$ and Na$^+$ levels. Thus, D is correct.

Question 2 The patient received a total of 250 mEq of KCl (both IV and oral) in a 24-h period. What are the expected increases in serum osmolality and Na$^+$ level?

Answer It should be noted that K$^+$ is as osmotically active as Na$^+$. Therefore, infusion of KCl should raise both osmolality and Na$^+$. The expected increases are calculated as follows:

$$\text{Calculate total body water} \left(\text{TBW}\right): \text{Wt} \times 0.5 \text{ or } 70 \times 0.5 = 35 \text{ L}$$

$$\text{Calculate total osmoles in 250 mEq of KCl} = 500 \left(250 \text{ from K}^+ \text{and 250 from Cl}^-\right)$$

$$\text{Contribution of KCl to osmolality} = \text{Total osmoles} / \text{TBW or } 500 / 35 = 14 \text{ mOsm}$$

$$\text{Raise in serum Na}^+ \text{ level} = \text{Total K}^+ / \text{TBW or } 250 / 35 = 7 \text{ mEq} / 24 \text{ h}$$

Thus, KCl alone can increase serum Na$^+$ level without infusion of saline. Serum [K$^+$] was 4.1 mEq/L. Diet and normal saline improved Na$^+$ level by 5 mEq/L during the next 24 h period to serum [Na$^+$] of 126 mEq/L in 48 h (see case 5) .

Case 13 A 32-year-old man was referred to the renal clinic for evaluation of persistent hyponatremia (130 mEq/L) despite fluid restriction. The patient has been paraplegic for 4 years following a gunshot wound. He is alert, oriented, and not in any distress. He is on regular diet with 1.5 L fluid restriction. He is on 10 mg of oxycodone, as needed. His only complaint is occasional weakness, which he attributes to immobility. His labs: Na$^+$ 130 mEq/L, K$^+$ 4.5 mEq/L, Cl$^-$ 96 mEq/L, HCO$_3^-$23 mEq/L, BUN 14 mg/dL, creatinine 0.8 mg/dL, and glucose 90 mg/dL. Total protein and lipids are normal. Liver, thyroid, and adrenal function tests are normal. Urine osmolality is 580 mOsm/kg H$_2$O, and Na$^+$ is 80 mEq/L. Following 1 L of normal saline, his serum Na$^+$ remains at 129 mEq/L. In order to understand the etiology of his hyponatremia, a water loading test is performed by giving 1 L of water orally. The results of the test are shown in the following table.

Time (min)	Serum Na$^+$ (mEq/L)	Urine Na$^+$ (mEq/L)	Urine osmolality (mOsm/kg H$_2$O)	Urine volume (mL)
0	130	80	580	0
30	129	58	480	100
90	130	30	240	350
120	129	20	90	450

Based on the above data, which one of the following is the **MOST** likely diagnosis in this patient?

(A) Pseudohyponatremia
(B) Poor oral intake
(C) Syndrome of inappropriate antidiuretic hormone secretion (SIADH)
(D) Nephrogenic syndrome of inappropriate antidiuresis (NSIAD)
(E) Reset osmostat

The answer is E Pseudohyponatremia is unlikely, because glucose, total protein, and lipids are normal. Thus, answer A is incorrect. Patients with poor oral intake are unable to concentrate their urine to 580 mOsm/kg H_2O, although they can dilute to 100 mOsm/kg H_2O. Also, high urine Na excretion rules out poor solute intake. Patients with SIADH and NSIAD are unable to dilute their urine osmolality to <100 mOsm/kg H_2O. Also, these patients cannot excrete the water load in a short period of time because of ADH activity. Thus, answers B–D are incorrect. This patient has the diagnosis of reset osmostat, as he can concentrate or dilute his urine appropriately. Because of this ability, patients with reset osmostat can excrete most of the water load in <4 h and maintain their serum [Na^+] at their preset level despite changes in water intake. Thus, answer E is correct.

Case 14 A 65-year-old man with long history of smoking was admitted initially for treatment of non-small cell lung cancer and chemotherapy. His chemotherapy regimen includes cisplatin, gemcitabin, paclitaxel, and bevacizumab. He started having polyuria and weakness with orthostatic BP and pulse changes. His labs:

Serum	Urine
Na^+ = 124 mEq/L	Na^+ = 90 mEq/L
K^+ = 2.8 mEq/L	K^+ = 60 mEq/L
Cl^- = 112 mEq/L	Osmolality = 500 mOsm/kg H_2O
HCO_3^- = 22 mEq/L	
Creatinine = 1.5 mg/dL	
BUN = 36 mg/dL	
Glucose = 90 mg/dL	

Which one of the following is the *MOST* likely cause of his hyponatremia?

(A) Syndrome of inappropriate antidiuretic hormone secretion (SIADH)
(B) Nephrogenic syndrome of inappropriate antidiuresis (NSIAD)
(C) Reset osmostat
(D) Cisplatin-induced hyponatremia
(E) Cerebral salt wasting (CSW)

The answer is D This patient developed cisplatin-induced nephrotoxicity. Polyuria develops 24–48 h after cisplatin dose, which is related to defective concentrating ability of the kidneys. Cisplatin also induces proximal tubular injury and Fanconi syndrome. As a result, Na^+ is lost in the urine with other ions, and the patient develops volume depletion and hyponatremia. Thus, answer D is correct. Increase in creatinine is related to both volume depletion and cisplatin-induced proximal tubular injury. SIADH, NSIAD, and reset osmostat can be excluded based on orthostatic changes, as these conditions are associated with euvolemia. Thus, answers A–C are incorrect. CSW causes volume depletion, orthostatic changes, hyponatremia, elevation in creatinine, and urinary Na^+ loss, but not hypokalemia and kaliuresis. Thus, answer E is incorrect.

Suggested Reading

1. Adroguè HJ, Madias NE. Hyponatremia. N Engl J Med. 2000;342:1581–9.
2. Adroguè HJ, Madias NE. The challenge of hyponatremia. J Am Soc Nephrol. 2012;23:1140–8.
3. Berl T. Impact of solute intake on urine flow and water excretion. J Am Soc Nephrol. 2008;19:1076–8.

4. Buckley MS, Patel SA, Hattrup AE, et al. Conivaptan for treatment of hyponatremia in neurological and neurosurgical adults. Ann Pharmacother. 2013;47:1194–200.
5. Fenske WK, Christ-Crain M, Hörning A, et al. A copeptin-based classification of the osmoregulatory defects in the syndrome of inappropriate antidiuresis. J Am Soc Nephrol. 2014;25:2376–83.
6. Furst H, Hallows KR, Post J, et al. The urine/plasma electrolyte ratio: a predictive guide to water restriction. Am J Med Sci. 2000;319:240–4.
7. Garimella S, Bowden SA. Cerebral salt-wasting syndrome workup. 2016; emedicine. Medscape article 919609.
8. Liamis G, Milionis H, Elisaf M. A review of drug-induced hyponatremia. Am J Kidney Dis. 2008;52:144–53.
9. Lien Y-HH, Shapiro JI. Hyponatremia: clinical diagnosis and management. Am J Med. 2007;120:653–8.
10. Maesaka JK, Imbriano LJ, Ali NM, et al. Is it cerebral or renal salt wasting. Kidney Int. 2009;76:934–8.
11. Robertson GL. Regulation of arginine vasopressin in the syndrome of inappropriate antidiuresis. Am J Med. 2006;119:S36–42.
12. Sterns RH, Hix JK, Silver S. Treating profound hyponatremia: a strategy for controlled correction. Am J Kidney Dis. 2010;56:774–9.
13. Sterns RH. Disorders of plasma sodium-causes, consequences, and correction. N Engl J Med. 2015;372:55–65.
14. Sterns RH, Silver SM. Complications and management of hyponatremia. Curr Opin Nephrol Hypertens. 2016;25:114–9.
15. Thurman JM, Berl T. Disorders of water metabolism. In: Mount DB, Sayegh MH, Singh AJ, editors. Core concepts in the disorders of fluid, electrolytes and acid-base balance. New York: Springer; 2013. p. 29–48.

Disorders of Water Balance: Hypernatremia

13

Hypernatremia is defined as serum or plasma [Na⁺] >145 mEq/L and hyperosmolality (serum osmolality >295 mOsm/kg H₂O).

As discussed in the previous chapter, serum [Na⁺] is determined by total body Na⁺, K⁺, and water content:

$$\text{Serum}\left[\,Na^{+}\,\right] = Na^{+} + K^{+} / TBW$$

where Na⁺ and K⁺ are total quantities of these cations, and TBW is total body water. Therefore, hypernatremia can develop by a deficit in total body water and/or a gain of Na⁺ or a combination of both.

Mechanisms of Hypernatremia

In a healthy individual, two mechanisms defend against hypernatremia: (1) thirst, and (2) excretion of a concentrated urine. An increase in serum [Na⁺] and associated hyperosmolality create thirst, and water intake lowers serum [Na⁺] to a normal level (Chap. 11). By excreting a concentrated urine, the kidneys try to conserve water. Thus, hypernatremia and hyperosmolality are prevented. Hypernatremia develops when patients:

1. Cannot experience or respond to thirst
2. Have no access to water
3. Have salt loading
4. Excretion of dilute urine with no or resistance to ADH

Patients at Risk for Hypernatremia

1. Elderly
2. Children

© Springer Science+Business Media LLC 2018
A.S. Reddi, *Fluid, Electrolyte and Acid-Base Disorders*,
DOI 10.1007/978-3-319-60167-0_13

3. Diabetics with uncontrolled glucose
4. Patients with polyuria
5. Hospitalized patients

Lack of adequate free water intake or administration
Impaired water conservation due to concentrating inability
Lactulose administration
Osmotic diuretics (mannitol)
Normal or hypertonic saline administration
Tube feedings or hyperalimentation
Mechanical ventilation

Approach to the Patient with Hypernatremia

Step 1: Estimate Volume Status

Based on volume status, classify hypernatremia into (Fig. 13.1):

1. Hypovolemic hypernatremia (relatively more water than Na^+ loss)
2. Hypervolemic hypernatremia (relatively more Na^+ than water gain)
3. Normovolemic (euvolemic) hypernatremia (water loss with normal Na^+)

Step 2: History and Physical Examination

History
- Assess water intake and urine volume. Identify the cause of water loss. Is polyuria present? Polyuria is generally defined as urine volume >3 L/day.

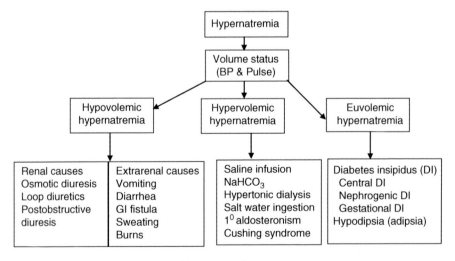

Fig. 13.1 Classification and causes of hypernatremia

Table 13.1 Diagnostic characteristics of hypernatremia

Volume status	Orthostatic changes	U_{Na} (mEq/L)	Urine osmolality (mOsm/kg H_2O)	Edema
Hypovolemic	Yes (renal)	>20 (renal)	>100 (both renal and extrarenal)	No
	Yes (extrarenal)	<20 (extrarenal)		
Hypervolemic	No	>20	>100	Yes
Euvolemic	No	>20	<100 (central DI)	No
			>100 (nephrogenic DI)	

- Look for infusions of hypertonic saline, hyperalimentation, or mannitol, including hyperglycemia for osmotic diuresis.
- Obtain history of diabetes, excessive sweating, or diarrhea that gives an idea of volume depletion.
- Take dietary history of high protein and electrolyte intake.
- Look for medications such as lactulose, loop diuretics, lithium, demeclocycline, and analgesics causing tubulointerstitial nephritis.

Physical Examination
- Vital signs and orthostatic changes (very important and mandatory). Record body weight.
- Examination of the neck, lungs, and heart for fluid overload and lower extremities for edema.
- Evaluation of mental status is extremely important.
- Diagnostic characteristics of various hypernatremic conditions are shown in Table 13.1.

Step 3: Diagnosis of Hypernatremia (See Table 13.1)

The most important tests besides urine volume are:

1. Plasma and urine osmolalities.
2. Urine Na^+ and K^+.
3. Other laboratory tests such as serum K^+, creatinine, BUN, and Ca^{2+} are also helpful.
4. Brain imaging studies, as indicated.

Electrolyte-free water clearance is useful during treatment of hypernatremia.

Brain Adaptation to Hypernatremia

- When serum $[Na^+]$ increases, the brain volume decreases due to exit of water and electrolytes, resulting in a decrease in intracranial pressure.
- However, within few hours, adaptive changes occur by moving water, electrolytes, and organic osmolytes (see Chap. 12) into the brain, thereby returning brain volume to normal (Fig. 13.2).

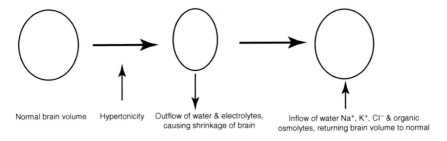

Fig. 13.2   Adaptation of brain volume to hypernatremia

Signs and Symptoms of Hypernatremia

- Mostly neurologic due to brain shrinkage and tearing of cerebral vessels.
- Acute hypernatremia: nausea, vomiting, lethargy, irritability, and weakness. These signs and symptoms may progress to seizures and coma.
- Chronic hypernatremia (present for >1–2 days): less neurologic signs and symptoms because of brain adaptation; however, weakness, nystagmus, and depressed sensorium may be seen.

Specific Causes of Hypernatremia

Polyuria

Polyuric syndromes constitute the most important causes of hypernatremia. These syndromes cause both water and solute (osmotic) diuresis. These patients usually have a urinary concentrating defect. Central DI, nephrogenic DI, and gestational DI cause water diuresis, whereas hyperalimentation and infusions of hypertonic saline, glucose, and mannitol cause solute diuresis. Solute diuresis also occurs in patients with high BUN or during post-obstructive period. In these patients, polyuria causes polydipsia. Psychogenic polydipsia is considered under polyuric syndromes; however, it causes hyponatremia. In these patients, polydipsia causes polyuria. Figure 13.3 provides a simple approach to a patient with polyuria.

Central DI
- Central DI is due to failure to synthesize or release ADH from hypothalamus.
- Two types of central DI: complete and partial.
- Thirst mechanism is intact in most except in patients with craniopharyngiomas (postoperative).
- Urine osmolality is usually ≤100 mOsm/kg H_2O in complete form.
- Distal nephron responds to ADH action.
- Patients usually prefer ice or ice water, and nocturia is common.
- Causes are both congenital and acquired.
- Post-traumatic, postsurgical, metastatic tumors, granulomas, and CNS infections are the most common causes of acquired central DI.
- Treatment (see later text).

Fig. 13.3 Diagnostic approach to the patient with polyuria

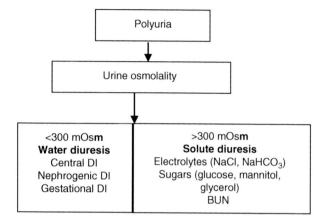

Nephrogenic DI
- Nephrogenic DI is defined as tubular resistance to ADH action despite adequate circulating levels of ADH.
- Thirst mechanism is intact.
- Urine osmolality is <300 mOsm/kg H_2O.
- Causes are both congenital and acquired.
- Two forms of congenital nephrogenic DI have been described:
  - X-linked form (90% of cases) due to loss-of-function mutation in vasopressin 2 receptor. Males with this mutation are characterized by dehydration, hypernatremia, and hyperthermia as early as the first week of life. Mental and physical retardation and renal failure are the consequences of late diagnosis.
  - The second form has either autosomal dominant or recessive inheritance (10% of cases). It is caused by loss-of-function mutation of AQP gene. Polyuria, dehydration, and hypernatremia are common. Carriers of AQP gene mutation are at risk for thromboembolism because of increased secretion of von Willebrand factor, the carrier protein for factor VIII.
- Treatment of both conditions includes hypotonic fluids to prevent dehydration. Hydrochlorothiazide alone or in combination with amiloride or indomethacin may be helpful in reducing urine output. Phosphodiesterase inhibitors, which prevent degradation of cAMP and cGMP, have been tried with variable success.
- Acquired nephrogenic DI: Important causes include CKD, hypokalemia, hypercalcemia, protein malnutrition, sickle cell disease, and lithium, or demeclocycline treatment. Table 13.2 describes the causes and mechanisms of acquired nephrogenic DI.

Gestational DI
- Occurs during late pregnancy and resolves after delivery.
- Caused by degradation of vasopressin (ADH) by the enzyme vasopressinase, and this enzyme is produced by the placenta.
- Treatment is desmopressin (DDAVP), which is not degraded by vasopressinase.

Table 13.2 Some causes and mechanisms of acquired nephrogenic DI

Cause	Urine concentrating ability	cAMP generation	AQP2 expression	Management
CKD	Decreased	Decreased	Decreased	Match daily intake and output
Hypercalcemia	Decreased	Decreased	Decreased	Correct hypercalcemia
Hypokalemia	Decreased	Decreased	Decreased	Correct hypokalemia
Lithium	Decreased	Decreased	Decreased	Amiloride[a]
Demeclocycline	Decreased	Decreased	Unknown	Discontinue the drug

[a]Inhibits lithium uptake by ENaC

Diagnosis of Polyuria

- The recommended test is water deprivation or dehydration test.
- Restrict fluid intake until urine osmolality reaches a plateau or until the patient loses 3–5% of body weight. Avoid excess weight loss.
- Measure the highest serum and urine osmolalities.
- Administer 5 units of aqueous vasopressin subcutaneously.
- Measure urine osmolalities 30 and 60 min later.
- Compare the last urine osmolality before vasopressin and the highest urine osmolality after vasopressin, and note the difference between the two values.

Table 13.3 provides the urine osmolality values after dehydration and following vasopressin in various polyuric conditions.

- Other test that is going to be useful in the differential diagnosis of polyuria is measurement of copeptin levels before water deprivation. The baseline levels were <2.6 pmol/L in central DI and ≥21.4 pmol/L in nephrogenic DI. However, baseline copeptin levels could not differentiate partial central DI from primary polydipsia. Insulin-stimulated copeptin test is required to differentiate between these two conditions when serum Na^+ level fails to differentiate them. Stimulated copeptin levels will be <4.9 pmol/L in partial central DI compared to ≥4.9 pmol/L in primary polydipsia.

Solute Diuresis

- Occurs mostly in hospitalized patients except in those with uncontrolled hyperglycemia.
- Hospitalized patients develop solute diuresis because of infusion of normal or hypertonic saline, glucose, mannitol, or hyperalimentation.
- Note that glucose and mannitol initially cause hyponatremia; however, continued osmotic diuresis results in water deficit and hypernatremia.
- Starvation ketosis, which is rather common in hospitalized patients, also causes osmotic natriuresis.

Table 13.3 Urine osmolalities (mmol/kg) in subjects with polyuric conditions in relation to normal subjects

Subjects	Urine osmolality after dehydration	Urine osmolality increase after vasopressin (%)	Comment
Normal	1,000–1,137	0 to −9	Normal subjects do not respond to exogenous vasopressin, as these subjects have maximal release of vasopressin following dehydration
Complete central DI	155–181	50–500	These patients respond adequately to vasopressin, as they lack vasopressin
Partial central DI	404–472	15–50	These patients respond partially, as they have some circulating vasopressin
Nephrogenic DI	124	0–42	These patients respond partially, as they have high levels of circulating vasopressin
Psychogenic polydipsia[a] (compulsive water drinkers)	685–791	0–6	These subjects washed out their medullary hypertonicity due to polydipsia. As a result, they do not respond to vasopressin

Data adapted from Miller et al. [1]
[a]Causes hyponatremia, and its inclusion completes polyuric conditions

- Urine osmolality is greater than plasma osmolality (>300 mOsm/kg H_2O), and urine osmoles (urine osmolality×urine volume) are >900 mosmol/day.
- High BUN due to high protein intake can also cause solute diuresis and water deficit.
- Post-obstructive diuresis can also cause hypernatremia with sufficient water loss.
- Measurement of solute is the only way to recognize the cause of solute diuresis.

Hypernatremia in the Elderly

- Chronic hypotonic hypernatremia is rather common in long-term care facility residents.
- Four factors account for hypernatremia in the elderly: (1) decreased water intake due to inaccessibility to water, (2) lack of thirst or relative hypodipsia, (3) use of loop diuretics, and (4) supplemental protein intake and urea-induced water loss.
- Hypertonic hypernatremia is rather uncommon, unless the patient has prolonged saline or $NaHCO_3$ infusion.
- Euvolemic hypernatremia is also common because of medications, such as lithium. Also, elderly subjects have decreased urine concentrating ability compared to young individuals.
- Altered mental status (lethargy, confusion) is common with mild hypernatremia, and seizures and coma can occur with severe hypernatremia.
- Treatment is prevention in hospitalized patients.

Hypodipsic (Adipsic) Hypernatremia

Hypodipsic conditions are characterized by absent or inadequate sensation of thirst with decreased water intake despite water availability. It arises as a result of complete or partial destruction of osmoreceptors for thirst. ADH release to osmotic stimuli may be normal or blunted, but response to nonosmotic stimuli (hypotension, nausea) is preserved. Previously, patients with hypodipsia or adipsia were described under the names of essential hypernatremia and primary hypodipsia. Because these patients are characterized by defective thirst, they are grouped under hypodipsic or adipsic hypernatremia or under osmoreceptor dysfunction. These hypodipsic patients develop not only hypernatremia but also hyperosmolality, a decrease in blood volume, and elevated blood urea nitrogen. Patients with mild hypernatremia can present with confusion and drowsiness, whereas those with severe hypernatremia can develop seizures, rhabdomyolysis, and coma. Hypodipsic patients have been shown to have pathologic lesions in the brain such as neoplastic, nonneoplastic, granulomatous, vascular, and other lesions. Based on hypertonic saline infusion, four types of osmoreceptor dysfunction (thirst and ADH release) have been described in hypodipsic patients: (1) reset osmostat, (2) decreased osmoreceptor function, (3) complete thirst osmoreceptor dysfunction, and (4) absence of thirst with intact ADH release. Among these four types, only types A and C are common, and these are described below.

- Type A hypodipsic patients (previously named essential hypernatremia) have an upward resetting threshold for thirst and ADH release. In other words, these patients do not have either thirst or ADH release until their plasma osmolality is >300 mOsm/kg H_2O (normal osmotic threshold is 284 mOsm/kg H_2O). Once they reach their higher set point, they can concentrate their urine. When water-loaded, they can suppress their thirst and ADH and can dilute their urine. Therefore, they do not develop hyponatremia but maintain mild chronic hypernatremia. Treatment is daily water intake of 2–3 L. Interestingly, some patients may not have any hypothalamic-pituitary lesion on CT scan or MRI.
- Type C patients have complete destruction of their osmoreceptors for thirst. Thirst is totally absent even at very high plasma osmolality, and these patients have no motivation to drink spontaneously. ADH secretion is low without any response to hypertonic saline. However, ADH response is seen in response to nonosmotic stimuli such as hypotension. Surgery to ruptured aneurysm of the anterior communicating artery of the circle of Willis seems to produce type C hypodipsia. These patients can develop severe hypernatremia easily unless they are forced to drink water. Since type C patients have low rate of ADH release, intake of large quantities of water for prolonged period may cause severe hyponatremia. Because these patients are prone to develop either hyper- or hyponatremia, frequent measurement of serum Na^+ is needed.

Treatment of Hypernatremia

Treatment of hypernatremia depends on six factors:

1. Correction of the underlying cause
2. Calculation of water deficit
3. Selection and route of fluid administration
4. Volume status
5. Onset of hypernatremia (acute or chronic)
6. Rate of correction

Correction of the Underlying Cause

Causes of hypernatremia, such as diarrhea, hyperglycemia, diuretic use, hypokalemia, hypercalcemia, and saline or mannitol infusion, should be addressed and treated, if possible.

Calculation of Water Deficit

Several formulas can be used.

Formula 1

$$\text{Water deficit} = \text{Previous total body water}\,(\text{TBW}) \times \text{Actual}\left[\text{Na}^+\right]$$

$$= \text{Desired}\left[\text{Na}^+\right] \times \text{New TBW}$$

$$\text{New TBW} = \frac{\text{Previous TBW} \times \text{Actual}\left[\text{Na}^+\right]}{\text{Desired}\left[\text{Na}^+\right]}$$

Example :

Weight $= 70\,\text{kg}$

Previous TBW $= 70 \times 0.6 = 42\,\text{L}$

Actual$\left[\text{Na}^+\right] = 160\,\text{mEq/L}$

Desired$\left[\text{Na}^+\right] = 140\,\text{mEq/L}$

New TBW $= 42 \times 160/140 = 48\,\text{L}$

Water deficit $=$ New TBW $-$ Previous TBW

Water deficit $= 48 - 42 = 6\,\text{L}$

Formula 2

$$\text{Water deficit} = \text{Previous TBW} \times \left(\frac{\text{Actual}\left[\text{Na}^+\right]}{\text{Desired}\left[\text{Na}^+\right]} - 1\right)$$

By using the above example, we obtain:

$$42 \times \left(\frac{160}{140} - 1 \right) = 6\,L$$

Formula 3 (a rough estimate)

- An editorial by Sterns and Silver [2] suggests that administration of 3–4 mL/kg of electrolyte-free water can lower serum $[Na^+]$ by 1 mEq/L in a lean individual. Total water deficit can be calculated as weight in kilogram × milliliters to be administered (3 or 4 mL) × the difference between the actual and desired $[Na^+]$.
- If we apply 4 mL/kg to a 70 kg individual to reduce serum $[Na^+]$ from 160 to 140 mEq/L, the water deficit would be $70 \times 4 \times 20$ or $280 \times 20 = 5.6$ L.

Selection and Route of Fluid Administration

- Selection of fluid is based on the blood pressure. If the patient is hypotensive, normal saline is the fluid of choice despite hypernatremia. Note that normal saline is relatively hypotonic in a patient with severe hypernatremia.
- If possible, oral intake of water is preferred to correct hypernatremia; however, most of the patients require IV administration.
- Fluids that are commonly used are D5W, 0.45%, or 0.225% saline.
- Infrequently, hemodialysis is used in patients with salt loading.

Volume Status

As mentioned previously, estimation of volume status is extremely important to select the appropriate fluid.

Treatment of Acute Hypernatremia

- Prevention of hypernatremia in hospitalized patients is important, as its development is mostly iatrogenic, resulting from inadequate and inappropriate prescription of fluids to patients whose water deficits are large and their thirst mechanism is impaired.
- Hypernatremia developed over a period of hours due to salt overload or following hypothalamic-pituitary surgery can be fully corrected with appropriate fluid (oral fluids or IV D5W or 0.225% saline) to the baseline value without causing cerebral edema, because accumulated electrolytes (Na^+, K^+, and Cl^-) are extruded from brain cells.
- The consequences of acute hypernatremia are shrinkage of brain cells and intracranial hemorrhage.

- The rate of correction is 1 mEq/h.
- Administration of volume includes the amount of water deficit and ongoing fluid losses (insensible loss and loss from other sources).

Treatment of Chronic Hypernatremia

- Hypernatremia developed 24–48 h later is considered chronic, and brain adaptation is complete by that time. Therefore, slow correction is warranted.
- The rate of correction is 6–8 mEq/L in a 24-h period with full correction in 2–3 days.
- Studies in children showed that outcomes were better when the rate of correction was ≤ 0.5 mEq/h.
- Electrolyte-free water clearance, urine volume (V) $\left(1 - \dfrac{U_{Na} + U_K}{P_{Na}}\right)$, is useful during correction of hypernatremia.

Treatment of Specific Causes

Hypovolemic Hypernatremia

- Administer normal saline until hemodynamic stability is established.
- Once the patient is euvolemic, give D5W or 0.45% saline to correct the water deficit and ongoing water losses.

Hypervolemic Hypernatremia

- Not uncommon in intensive care units because of saline or mannitol infusion.
- Administer loop rather than thiazide diuretics.
- Use of loop diuretics may increase water deficit; therefore, the need for free water is increased.
- In some situations, consider hemodialysis.

Normovolemic (Euvolemic) Hypernatremia

Central DI
- DDAVP is the drug of choice for central DI.
- Available as nasal spray or oral form.
- Use the lowest dose 5–10 µg nasally or 0.1 or 0.2 mg orally at bedtime to avoid nocturia and hyponatremia.
- Duration of therapy depends on the cause of central DI. Idiopathic disease requires permanent use, and acquired form may require transiently.

- Other drugs such as chlorpropamide, carbamazepine, or clofibrate can be used in patients with partial central DI, as they can stimulate release of ADH.
- Induction of mild volume depletion with salt restriction and thiazide use (25 mg daily) can be effective in some patients with central DI, but more effective in nephrogenic DI.

Nephrogenic DI

- Congenital DI patients should receive enough water to prevent dehydration.
- Thiazide diuretics may be helpful.
- Removal of the cause, water intake, thiazide, and amiloride are the mainstay of therapy in acquired nephrogenic DI (Table 13.2).

Study Questions

Case 1 A 74-year-old man is admitted from the nursing home for lethargy, disorientation, and confusion. The nursing record shows that the patient had cerebrovascular accident 5 years ago. The patient did not have any fever, diarrhea, or fluid loss. Urine output is recorded as 700 mL/day.

On admission, the blood pressure is 100/70 mmHg with a pulse rate of 100 (supine) and 80/60 mmHg with a pulse rate of 110 (sitting). Physical examination is normal except for dry mucous membranes. He weighs 70 kg. Laboratory results are as follows:

Serum	Urine
Na^+ = 168 mEq/L	Na^+ = 12 mEq/L
K^+ = 4.6 mEq/L	Osmolality = 600 mOsm/kg H_2O
Cl^- = 114 mEq/L	
HCO_3^- = 26 mEq/L	
Creatinine = 1.9 mg/dL	
BUN = 64 mg/dL	
Glucose = 110 mg/dL	

Question 1 Is the patient's hypernatremia related to water deficit or gain of Na^+?

Answer The patient's hypernatremia is due to water deficit rather than Na^+ gain, as the patient has orthostatic changes. Hypernatremia due to Na gain presents with high blood pressure.

Question 2 Calculate his water deficit for serum [Na^+] of 140 mEq/L?

Answer Any one of the three formulas given previously can be used to calculate water deficit. One such formula is:

$$\text{Water deficit} = \text{Previous TBW} \times \left(\frac{\text{Actual}\left[Na^+ \right]}{\text{Desired}\left[Na^+ \right]} - 1 \right).$$

By using the above example, we obtain:

$$42 \times \left(\frac{168}{140} - 1 \right) = 8.4\,L.$$

Question 3 Assuming the patient had no oral intake and daily urine output of 700 mL, how many days it would have taken to develop serum [Na⁺] of 168 mEq/L?

Answer To answer this question, one needs to calculate the total daily fluid loss. This can be calculated from daily urine output and insensible loss (approximately 500 mL/day). Thus, the patient's daily fluid loss is 700 mL+500 mL=1200 mL (1.2 L).

The patient's total water deficit is 8.4 L; dividing 8.4 by 1.2 gives 7. Thus, it would have taken approximately 7 days for this patient to increase serum [Na⁺] from 140 mEq/L to 168 mEq/L.

Question 4 What is your initial choice of fluid administration?

Answer Normal saline because of volume depletion. Note that normal saline is hypotonic to patient's serum osmolality.

Question 5 Estimate the reduction in serum [Na⁺], if 1 L of normal saline is infused in 1 h?

Answer Change in serum [Na⁺] can be estimated by the following formula:

$$\text{Change in serum}\ \left[Na^+ \right] = \frac{\text{Infusate}\ \left[Na^+ \right] - \text{Serum}\ \left[Na^+ \right]}{\text{Total body water} + \text{Volume of infusate}}$$

$$= \frac{154 - 168}{42 + 1} = -0.33$$

Thus, serum [Na⁺] decreases only by 0.33 mEq/L.

Question 6 What is your further management of this patient?

Answer The patient requires free water repletion. In a mentally alert patient, oral ingestion of water is strongly advised. In other patients, IV administration of D5W is preferred. In a diabetic patient, 0.45 % (half-normal saline) is preferable. The rate of correction should not exceed 6–8 mEq/24 h. This patient has chronic hypernatremia. Therefore, serum [Na⁺] should be lowered from 168 to 160 mEq/L in a 24-h period. Full correction requires 2–3 days.

If the serum [Na⁺] does not improve with replacement of calculated water deficit, you have not adequately assessed the total water deficit.

Case 2 A 50-year-old man with history of hypertension, type 2 diabetes, chronic kidney disease stage 3, and coronary artery disease underwent surgery for abdominal aortic aneurysm. He received normal saline to maintain blood pressure and urine output. Normal saline was continued until the patient developed hypertension (156/90 mmHg) and peripheral edema. The patient is alert and oriented. Renal consult was requested for evaluation of hypernatremia (developed over a period of 4 days).The patient weighs 74 kg. Chest X-ray showed mild vascular congestion. Laboratory results are as follows:

Serum	Urine
Na^+ = 154 mEq/L	Na^+ = 90 mEq/L
K^+ = 4.1 mEq/L	K^+ = 48 mEq/L
Cl^- = 124 mEq/L	Osmolality = 560 mOsm/kg H_2O
HCO_3^- = 19 mEq/L	
Creatinine = 2.0 mg/dL	
BUN = 52 mg/dL	
Glucose = 110 mg/dL	

Question 1 Is his hypernatremia related to water deficit, Na gain, or both?

Answer In this patient, hypernatremia is due to both Na gain and water deficit.

Question 2 Calculate his water deficit.

Answer He weighs 74 kg; therefore, his total body water is 44.4 $L(74 \times 0.6 = 44.4\,L)$. The total body water deficit is 4.4 L (see the question 2 in case 1).

Question 3 How would you manage his hypernatremia?

Answer Since hypernatremia is due to Na^+ gain, promotion of urinary excretion of Na^+ with furosemide should be started. This would also improve pulmonary congestion. However, furosemide promotes both Na^+ and free water (hypotonic fluid), resulting in worsening of hypernatremia. Therefore, both furosemide and free water (either oral or IV) should be started concurrently. Since this patient is alert and oriented and able to drink water, oral fluid intake is the preferred route of administration.

Question 4 Estimate the reduction in serum [Na^+], if 1 L of D5W is infused in 4 h?

Answer The reduction in serum [Na^+] is 3.4 mEq/L (see question 5 in case 1).

Case 3 A 55-year-old obese woman is admitted for frequent urination, thirst, and poor appetite for 2-week duration. She has no previous history of diabetes or hypertension. She complains of blurred vision for 1 week. She is not on any medications. Her blood pressure is 110/70 mmHg with a pulse rate of 102 beats/min. Orthostatic changes were noted. She weighs 100 kg. Initial laboratory results are as follows:

Serum	Urine
Na^+ = 140 mEq/L	Na^+ = 50 mEq/L
K^+ = 5.2 mEq/L	K^+ = 36 mEq/L
Cl^- = 98 mEq/L	Glucose 4+
HCO_3^- = 27 mEq/L	Ketone = negative
Creatinine = 1.8 mg/dL	
BUN = 60 mg/dL	
Glucose = 1,100 mg/dL	

Question 1 Does this patient have hypernatremia?

Answer Yes. Hyperglycemia causes hyponatremia by translocation of water from intracellular to extracellular compartment. As discussed in the previous chapter, serum [Na^+] decreases by 1.6 mEq/L for each 100 mg/dL glucose above normal glucose level (i.e., 100 mg/dL). Therefore, the actual serum [Na^+] in this patient is 156 mEq/L ($10 \times 1.6 = 16$ mEq/L).

Question 2 Calculate her water deficit.

Answer Based on total body water of 50 L ($100 \times 0.5 = 50$ L; obese individuals have 50% rather than 60% of water), the water deficit is 5.71 L (see case 1).

Question 3 What is the nature of urine composition in this patient?

Answer The patient has hyperglycemic hyperosmolar syndrome. This causes osmotic diuresis (glucosuria). Each liter of urine contains 1 L of water and 150 mOsm of non-reabsorbed solute (glucose) as well as 150 mOsm of Na^+, K^+, and their anions (Cl^-, HCO_3^-, and phosphate). Since urine contains 150 mEq/L of Na^+ and its anions, it is hypotonic to serum; therefore, the fluid loss is considered hypotonic.

Question 4 How are her extracellular fluid (ECF) and intracellular fluid (ICF) compartments compared to those in a normal subject?

Answer Initially, water moves from ICF to ECF compartment due to hyperglycemia and hyperosmolality. As a result, the ECF compartment expands and ICF compartment contracts. This results in hyponatremia. As glucose levels increase, osmotic diuresis continues to increase, and both water and electrolytes are lost from the ECF compartment. This results in the return of ECF compartment to normal. With osmotic diuresis, water loss occurs from both the ICF (two-third loss) and ECF (one-third loss) compartments. This results in further contraction of the ICF.

Question 5 What happens to the fluid compartments when insulin is administered without adequate fluid repletion?

Answer Insulin administration promotes glucose transport from ECF to ICF. Since ICF glucose is high, its osmolality is also high. This causes water movement from ECF to ICF compartment. As a result, the ECF compartment contracts, while the ICF compartment returns to normal as glucose is metabolized to CO_2 and water. Because of contracted ECF, serum [Na^+] increases. Thus, adequate intravascular volume should be maintained with Na^+-containing fluids prior to administration of insulin.

Question 6 How would you manage her fluid and electrolyte balance?

Answer Correction of water deficit is the immediate step in the management of this patient. Since the patient is volume depleted, the fluid of choice is normal saline. Infusing 1–2 L of normal saline in 1–2 h raises blood pressure and urination. Then half-normal saline should be started. As a result of hydration, blood glucose levels fall substantially. The patient should then receive insulin. Once serum glucose levels reach approximately 250 mg/dL, the fluid should be changed to D5W. With fluid and glucose improvement, serum [Na^+] returns toward normal.

Case 4 A 50-year-old hypertensive man is admitted for headache and altered mental status. A CT scan of the head shows subarachnoid hemorrhage. He is receiving hyperalimentation, and his urine output is 4 L/day. Also, the nurse notices diarrhea of 1-day duration. His serum [Na^+] is 149 mEq/L, K^+ 3.3 mEq/L, HCO_3^- 26 mEq/L, BUN 44 mg/dL, creatinine 1.6 mg/dL, and glucose 200 mg/dL. His urine Na^+ is 70 mEq/L, and urine osmolality 380 mOsm/kg H_2O. His volume status is adequate.

Question Which one of the following is the MOST likely cause of his hypernatremia?

(A) Nephrogenic diabetes insipidus (NDI)
(B) Partial central diabetes insipidus
(C) Osmotic diarrhea
(D) Osmotic diuresis
(E) 7.5% NaCl administration to improve brain edema

The answer is D Patients with either NDI or partial central diabetes insipidus have mostly water diuresis rather than high solute diuresis. The osmolal excretion is normal in diabetes insipidus. Patients with diabetes insipidus have low urine osmolality despite a high serum osmolality or hypernatremia. The patient is excreting a total of 1,520 mOsm/day (380×4 L=1,520). Therefore, the patient has solute diuresis. Thus, options A and B are unlikely in this patient. Option C is also unlikely because the urinary [Na^+] is 70 mEq/L, which is high in conditions such as diarrhea. In a patient with diarrhea, the kidneys conserve rather than excrete Na^+. Option E is also unlikely because the patient does not have any volume expansion due to hypertonic saline infusion, and the patient should have Na^+ diuresis. The patient has osmotic diuresis because of hyperalimentation, which is the cause of his hypernatremia. In general, the urine osmolality in osmotic diuresis is relatively higher than serum osmolality.

Case 5 A 1-week-old boy was brought to the emergency department for irritability, polyuria, vomiting milk soon after ingestion, dehydration, hypernatremia, and hyperthermia. The patient responds adequately to volume replacement.

Question Which of the following statements regarding this infant is FALSE?

(A) The clinical presentation is consistent with the diagnosis of X-linked nephrogenic diabetes insipidus (NDI).
(B) X-linked NDI is due to loss-of-function mutation in vasopressin V2 receptor (AVPR2).
(C) Dehydration in infants with X-linked NDI can be so severe that can lead to low BP and impairment in oxygenation to the kidneys, brain, and other organs.
(D) The clinical presentation is consistent with NDI due to mutations in the aquaporin 2 (AQP2) gene.
(E) Combination of a thiazide diuretic and indomethacin is the most effective therapy to improve polyuria.

The answer is D All options other than D are consistent with the diagnosis of X-linked NDI. The other form of congenital NDI has either autosomal dominant or recessive inheritance (10% of cases). It is caused by loss-of-function mutation of AQP gene. Polyuria, dehydration, and hypernatremia are also common in this form of congenital DI.

Case 6 A 46-year-old woman is admitted for polyuria, polydipsia, and nocturia. She fulfills her thirst mostly with ice water. Her serum $[Na^+]$ is 158 mEq/L with urine osmolality of 98 mOsm/kg H_2O.

Question Which one of the urine osmolalities (mOsm/kg H_2O) is consistent with her diagnosis?

	Osmolality (mOsm) before dehydration	Osmolality (mOsm) after 12 h dehydration	Osmolality (mOsm) after vasopressin
A	600	1,100	1,080
B	100	120	360
C	180	350	500
D	300	310	314
E	120	500	520

The answer is B Based on the history and urine osmolality, the patient has central diabetes insipidus (CDI). Option B is consistent with CDI. Options A, C, D, and E are consistent with normal subject, partial CDI, nephrogenic DI, and psychogenic polydipsia, respectively.

References

1. Miller M, et al. Recognition of partial defects in antidiuretic hormone secretion. Ann Intern Med. 1970;73:721–9.
2. Sterns RH, Silver SM. Salt and water: read the package insert. QJM. 2003;96:549–52.

Suggested Reading

3. Adroguè HJ, Madias NE. Hypernatremia. N Engl J Med. 2000;342:1493–9.
4. Arieff AI, Ayus CJ. Strategies for diagnosing and managing hypernatremic encephalopathy. When to suspect and how to correct fluid deficits safely. J Crit Care. 1996;11:720–7.
5. Baylis PH, Thompson CJ. Osmoregulation of vasopressin secretion and thirst in health and disease. Clin Endocrinol. 1988;29:349–76.
6. Christ-Crain M, Morgenthaler NG, Fenske W. Copeptin as a biomarker and a diagnostic tool in the evaluation of patients with polyuria-polydipsia and hyponatremia. Best Pract Res Clin Endocrinol Metab. 2016;30:235–47.
7. Feig PU, McCurdy DK. The hypertonic state. N Engl J Med. 1977;297:1444–54.
8. Oster JR, Singer I, Thatte L, et al. The polyuria of solute diuresis. Arch Intern Med. 1997;157:721–9.
9. Sands JM, Bichet DG. Nephrogenic diabetes insipidus. Ann Intern Med. 2006;144:186–94.
10. Sterns RH. Disorders of plasma sodium-causes, consequences, and correction. N Engl J Med. 2015;372:55–65.
11. Thurman JM, Berl T. Disorders of water metabolism. In: Mount DB, Sayegh MH, Singh AJ, editors. Core concepts in the disorders of fluid, electrolytes and acid-base balance. New York: Springer; 2013. p. 29–48.
12. Verbalis JG. Disorders of water balance. In: Skorecki K, et al., editors. Brenner & Rector's the kidney. 10th ed. Philadelphia: Elsevier; 2016. p. 460–510.

Disorders of Potassium: Physiology

14

General Features

Potassium (K^+) is the predominant intracellular cation in the body. The intracellular [K^+] is 140–150 mEq/L; in blood it is 3.5–5 mEq/L. Serum contains a slightly higher concentration of K^+ than plasma because K^+ is released from red blood cells during clot formation. Maintenance of a high cellular concentration of K^+ is necessary for several cellular functions, including growth, nucleic acid and protein synthesis, and regulation of cell volume, as well as pH and enzyme activation. In addition, a high intracellular concentration of K^+ is essential to the maintenance of the resting membrane potential for cellular excitability and contraction. The high intracellular K^+ concentration is maintained by the Na/K-ATPase located in the cell membranes of all animal cells. The activity of this enzyme is influenced by a variety of hormones.

The kidney is the primary route for K^+ excretion. In general, K^+ excretion in the urine, called *kaliuresis*, parallels dietary intake. The other route for K^+ excretion is the colon. Under conditions of decreased renal function, K^+ excretion by the colon is enhanced.

Renal Handling of K⁺ Transport

Renal handling of K^+ involves filtration, reabsorption, and secretion. Most of the filtered K^+ is reabsorbed in segments of the proximal nephron, and the K^+ that is found in the urine is secreted by the distal segments of the nephron (Fig. 14.1).

© Springer Science+Business Media LLC 2018
A.S. Reddi, *Fluid, Electrolyte and Acid-Base Disorders*,
DOI 10.1007/978-3-319-60167-0_14

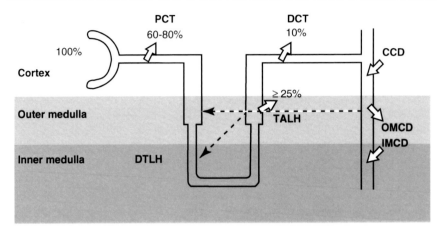

Fig. 14.1 Handling of K$^+$ by various segments of the nephron; 60–80% of K$^+$ is reabsorbed by the proximal convoluted tubule (PCT) and about 25% by the medullary thick ascending limb of Henle's loop (TALH). Only 10% of filtered K$^+$ is delivered to the distal convoluted tubule (*DCT*). CCD, OMCD, and IMCD refer to cortical collecting, outer medullary collecting, and inner medullary collecting ducts, respectively. *Broken arrows* denote K$^+$ secretion into the late segment of the proximal tubule and descending thin limb of Henle's loop (*DTHL*)

Proximal Tubule

K$^+$ is freely filtered at the glomerulus. About 60–80% of this filtered K$^+$ is reabsorbed by the proximal tubule. Reabsorption of K$^+$ is mostly passive and occurs via a K$^+$ transporter. Also, passive reabsorption of K$^+$ occurs through the paracellular pathway. This passive transport of K$^+$ is coupled with Na$^+$ and water transport. Volume expansion and osmotic diuretics (e.g., mannitol) inhibit this passive diffusion of Na$^+$-coupled K$^+$ transport.

Loop of Henle

In this segment of the nephron, both secretion and reabsorption of K$^+$ occur. K$^+$ enters the late segment of the proximal tubule and the descending thin limb of the Henle's loop. This observation is based on evidence that the [K$^+$] is higher in the lumen of the hairpin turn of the Henle's loop than the plasma [K$^+$], suggesting that K$^+$ enters passively from the medullary interstitium.

The thick ascending limb of Henle's loop actively reabsorbs K$^+$. This segment also reabsorbs Na$^+$ and Cl$^-$. K$^+$ reabsorption occurs mostly in the medullary thick ascending limb and could account for as much as 25% of the filtered K$^+$. The K$^+$ transport in this segment of the nephron occurs by secondary active transport, as well as by passive diffusion through the paracellular pathway. The secondary active transport mechanism involves the cotransport of 1 Na$^+$, 1 K$^+$, and 2 Cl$^-$ ions (Fig. 14.2). The driving force for this cotransport is provided by the Na/K-ATPase

Fig. 14.2 Cellular model for transepithelial K⁺ transport in the thick ascending limb of Henle's loop. *Thick broken arrows* indicate diffusion of K⁺ via renal outer medullary K (ROMK) channels, and Cl⁻ channel

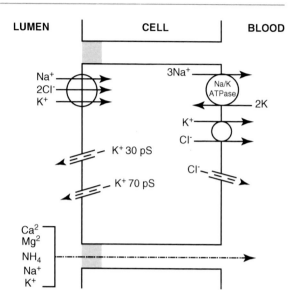

located in the basolateral membrane. This enzyme decreases the intracellular concentration of Na^+, thereby creating a steep Na^+ gradient across the apical membrane. In order to stimulate Na^+ entry, K^+ must leak back into the lumen. Indeed, K^+ diffuses back into the lumen through K^+ conductance channels, called renal outer medullary K (ROMK) channels, to provide a continuous supply of K^+ ions for cotransport with Na^+ and Cl^-. Without this back-leak of K^+, the low luminal K^+ concentration would limit the reabsorption of Na^+ and Cl^-. This cotransport system is inhibited by the loop diuretics (furosemide, bumetanide, etc.).

Three types of K^+ channels have been identified: a low or small-conductance (SK) 30 pS channel, an intermediate 70 pS (picosiemens) channel, and a high conductance calcium-activated maxi-K^+ or BK (150 pS) channel. Only 30 pS and 70 pS channels make up the ROMK and account for most of the K^+ that diffuses into the lumen in the thick ascending Henle's loop. The BK channel pumps out K^+ in A (α) intercalated cells.

Distal Nephron

Distal Tubule

About 10% of the filtered K^+ reaches the distal tubule. The K^+ secretion occurs in this segment because of low luminal Cl^- and high luminal Na^+ concentration. In this segment, a luminal K/Cl cotransporter is responsible for K^+ secretion (Fig. 14.3). This cotransporter operates in cooperation with a luminal Na/Cl cotransporter. It has been shown that delivery of Na^+ to the distal tubule promotes secretion of K^+ via the K/Cl cotransporter. Also, K^+ secretion occurs via the ROMK channel. Thiazide diuretics (hydrochlorothiazide) inhibit Na/Cl cotransporter.

Fig. 14.3 Cellular model for transepithelial K⁺ transport in the distal tubule. ROMK channel is not shown in the figure. *Broken arrow* indicates diffusion of K through conductance channel

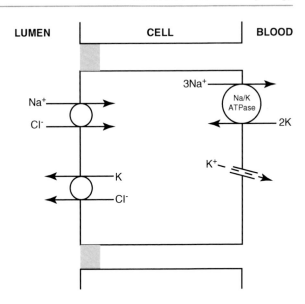

Connecting Tubule

The apical membrane of the connecting tubule cells contains Na⁺ (ENaC) and K⁺ (ROMK) conductance channels. The entry of Na⁺ via the ENaC creates a lumen-negative potential difference, which promotes K⁺ secretion via ROMK. The connecting tubule cells secrete K⁺ at a higher rate than the rate at which it is excreted in the urine. K⁺ secretion is sensitive to aldosterone.

Cortical Collecting Duct

The collecting duct is considered the major site for K⁺ secretion, although the early distal tubule and connecting tubule cells play an important role in K⁺ secretion. Two types of cells are found in this segment: principal cells and intercalated cells. Principal cells are the primary cells for K⁺ secretion. K⁺ enters the cell via Na/K--ATPase. The principal cell possesses two secretory pathways for K⁺ in the apical membrane (Fig. 14.4a). One pathway is the ROMK channel and the other is the K/Cl cotransporter. As stated above, K⁺ secretion into the lumen occurs in association with a Na/K-ATPase located in the basolateral membrane, which pumps 2 K⁺ into and 3 Na⁺ ions out of the cell. This cellular K⁺ is secreted into the lumen when Na⁺ is reabsorbed via the Na⁺ channel (ENaC). Blockage of Na⁺ uptake by amiloride inhibits K⁺ secretion. Similarly, K⁺ secretion is inhibited by decreased delivery of Na⁺ to the cortical collecting duct due to dehydration or low salt diet. Thus, K⁺ secretion is dependent on Na⁺ uptake from the lumen. The A-type intercalated cell is involved in K⁺ reabsorption. This cell reabsorbs K⁺ in exchange for H⁺ secretion via an H/K-ATPase (Fig. 14.4b). For each H⁺ secreted, one HCO₃⁻ is generated. Thus, the H/K-ATPase may participate in acid-base balance.

Fig. 14.4 Cellular model for transepithelial K⁺ transport in the cortical collecting duct. (**a**) Principal cell; (**b**) intercalated cell. *Broken arrows* indicate diffusion of respective ions through specific conductance channels. *ENaC* epithelial Na⁺ channel, *ROMK* renal outer medullary K⁺ channel, *Maxi-K* calcium-activated BK channel

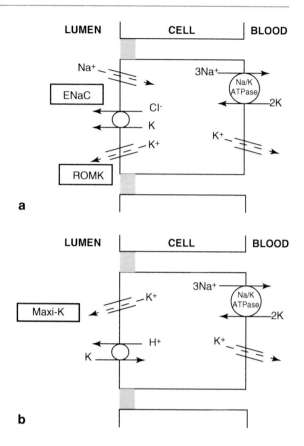

Outer Medullary Collecting Duct

The lumen of this segment contains a high concentration of K⁺ because of K⁺ secretion in the cortical collecting duct. The lumen, therefore, becomes electro-positive. The combination of a high concentration of K⁺ in the lumen and its electropositivity creates a driving force for passive reabsorption of K⁺.

Inner Medullary Collecting Duct

Under normal conditions, this segment plays only a minor role in K⁺ secretion. However, in K⁺-loaded animals, the inner medullary collecting duct secretes significant amounts of K⁺. Aldosterone potentiates the secretion of K⁺ in this segment.

In summary, K⁺ secretion in the nephron is mediated by the following mechanisms:

1. Ion transporters
2. ROMK channels
3. Active reabsorption of Na via ENaC
4. Paracellular pathways

Table 14.1 Factors that influence K$^+$ excretion	Dietary K$^+$ intake and plasma [K$^+$]
	Urine flow rate and Na$^+$ delivery
	Hormones
	Acid-base balance
	Anions
	Diuretics

Factors Affecting K$^+$ Excretion

As stated earlier, K$^+$ secretion occurs in the cortical collecting ducts which accounts for the K$^+$ excreted in the urine. A number of factors (Table 14.1) influence K$^+$ excretion.

Dietary Intake and Plasma [K$^+$]

An increase in K$^+$ intake has been shown to raise plasma as well as intracellular [K$^+$]. This increase in plasma [K$^+$] stimulates aldosterone synthesis and secretion, which enhances K$^+$ secretion and excretion. Increased K$^+$ excretion by the kidney is due to decreased reabsorption by Henle's loop and enhanced secretion by the cortical and inner medullary collecting ducts. A decrease in K$^+$ intake for 2–3 days lowers urinary K$^+$ excretion to 10–15 mEq/day without lowering its plasma concentration. Reduced K$^+$ excretion is due to increased activity of H/K-ATPase in A-type intercalated cells and decreased expression of ROMK channels in principal cells. Thus, severe hypokalemia does not occur, if dietary intake of K$^+$ is reduced for few days.

The above description suggests that K$^+$ excretion in response to dietary K$^+$ intake is dependent on aldosterone levels. This type of mechanism is called feedback control. A different mechanism called feedforward control suggests that high K$^+$ diet promotes its renal excretion independent of plasma K$^+$ levels. This acute response appears to be independent of aldosterone. After a K$^+$ diet, a gut factor is induced which promotes renal and extrarenal excretion of K$^+$. This excretion occurs without any changes in plasma [K$^+$]. Thus, this new kind of K$^+$ homeostasis is under feedforward control. The gut factor, a component of the feedforward mechanism, seems to be protective against acute changes in plasma [K$^+$].

Urine Flow Rate and Na$^+$ Delivery

K$^+$ secretion depends on the urine flow rate to the distal nephron. In d little is delivered to the distal nephron. Delivery of Na$^+$ therefore decreases, and thus exchange of Na$^+$ for K$^+$ also decreases. As a result, K$^+$ is retained.

Increase in Na$^+$ intake or intravenous infusion of saline tends to expand the extracellular fluid volume. Both GFR and Na$^+$ delivery to the distal nephron are increased, which stimulate K^+ excretion. This kaliuresis is independent of aldosterone effect or increase in plasma $[K^+]$ but can be attributed to increased Na^+ delivery to the distal nephron. In this situation, Na^+ excretion is also increased.

Hormones

Four important hormones are involved in K^+ secretion and excretion: (1) aldosterone, (2) antidiuretic hormone (ADH), (3) angiotensin II (AII), and (4) tissue kallikrein.

Aldosterone

Hyperkalemia and hypovolemia stimulate aldosterone secretion, which, in turn, stimulates ENaC and Na/K-ATPase. The net effect of aldosterone is an increase in K^+ entry from the basolateral membrane and its secretion into the lumen due to lumen-negative potential difference. Enhanced ENaC occurs via aldosterone-induced serum-glucocorticoid-induced kinase-1 (SGK-1). Also, aldosterone potentiates ROMK with an interaction between SGK-1 and WNK, a family of serine-threonine protein kinases.

Antidiuretic Hormone

This hormone has been shown to promote K^+ secretion despite a reduction in urine flow rate. ADH stimulates AQP 2 receptors, which, in turn, activate ENaC in principal cells, causing K^+ secretion. Also, ADH activates ROMK channels in these principal cells. This is particularly important in volume-depletion states to prevent severe hyperkalemia.

Angiotensin II

Under hypovolemic conditions. AII has been shown to inhibit apical ROMK channels in principal cells of connecting tubule and collecting duct, causing decreased secretion of K^+ and hyperkalemia.

Tissue Kallikrein

TK is a serine protease that is involved in the generation of kinins (bradykinin). It is secreted by connecting tubule cells by oral KCl loading. TK enhances ENaC, which causes K^+ secretion.

Other hormones have also been shown to influence K^+ secretion. Epinephrine decreases and norepinephrine increases K^+ secretion in the cortical collecting duct.

Acid-Base Balance

A number of studies have shown that changes in systemic pH alter K^+ excretion. Infusion of NH_4Cl causes metabolic acidosis (pH<7.20) acutely, which reduces K^+ excretion. This reduction may be related to inhibition of K^+ secretion by the cortical collecting duct, possibly by closing pH-sensitive K^+ channels in the luminal membrane. In contrast, chronic acidosis promotes K^+ secretion due to increased fluid delivery to the cortical collecting duct.

Induction of metabolic alkalosis (pH>7.50) acutely by infusion of $NaHCO_3$ increases K^+ excretion. Chronic alkalosis also augments K^+ excretion. This augmented excretion is presumably due to enhanced K^+ entry into the principal cell across the basolateral membrane and by accelerated exit across the apical membrane through K^+ channels into the lumen.

Acute respiratory acidosis decreases and respiratory alkalosis increases K^+ excretion. However, chronic acidosis may increase K^+ excretion. In chronic respiratory acidosis, the plasma $[HCO_3^-]$ is elevated, which increases the distal delivery of $NaHCO_3$, and thus promotes K^+ excretion.

Anions

When Na^+ with nonchloride anions such as sulfate or bicarbonate is infused into the body, K^+ excretion by the cortical collecting duct can be markedly augmented. Delivery of impermeant anions (sulfate, some penicillins) to the distal nephron creates a lumen-negative voltage gradient favoring K^+ secretion. K^+ secretion can also be augmented when the luminal $[Cl^-]$ is decreased independently of the transepithelial potential difference. This effect suggests the presence of a K/Cl cotransporter that is stimulated by the increased cellular luminal gradient.

Diuretics

In general, diuretics promote K^+ excretion by increasing distal delivery of fluid and Na^+. Osmotic diuretics, such as mannitol, inhibit Na^+ and water reabsorption by the proximal tubule and increase distal rates of flow. Acetazolamide, a carbonic anhydrase inhibitor, reduces $NaHCO_3$ reabsorption by the proximal tubule and thus creates a lumen-negative potential difference in the distal nephron that promotes K^+ secretion. Loop diuretics, such as furosemide or bumetanide, inhibit the Na/K/2Cl cotransporter in the thick ascending limb of Henle's loop and thus promote kaliuresis. Thiazide diuretics act on the distal tubule and inhibit NaCl reabsorption. Kaliuresis occurs due to increased fluid delivery to the cortical collecting duct.

Spironolactone, triamterene, and amiloride inhibit secretion and thus inhibit urinary loss of K^+. Spironolactone antagonizes the effects of aldosterone, whereas triamterene and amiloride inhibit Na^+ conductance channels (ENaC) and impede the entry of Na^+. Because Na^+ entry is blocked, the luminal membrane of the principal cells becomes hyperpolarized, resulting in decreased K^+ secretion.

Suggested Reading

1. Giebisch G, Krapf R, Wagner C. Renal and extrarenal regulation of potassium. Kidney Int. 2007;72:397–410.
2. Mount DB. Transport of sodium, chloride, and potassium. In: Skorecki K, et al., editors. Brenner & Rector's the kidney. 10th ed. Philadelphia: Elsevier; 2016. p. 144–84.
3. Malnic M, Giebisch G, Muto S. et al. In: Alpern RJ, Moe OW, Caplan M, editors. Seldin and Giebisch's the kidney. Physiology and pathophysiology. 5th ed. San Diego: Academic Press (Elsevier); 2013. p. 1659–715.
4. Segal A. Potassium and the dyskalemias. In: Mount DB, Sayegh MH, Singh AJ, editors. Core concepts in the disorders of fluid, electrolytes and acid-base balance. New York: Springer; 2013. p. 49–102.

Disorders of Potassium: Hypokalemia

15

Hypokalemia is defined as a serum $[K^+] <3.5$ mEq/L. The important causes of hypokalemia can be divided into five major categories: (1) dietary, (2) K^+ uptake by cells (transcellular), (3) renal loss, (4) gastrointestinal loss, and (5) skin loss (Table 15.1).

Table 15.1 Causes of hypokalemia

Cause	Mechanism
1. Dietary	
Low-K^+ diet	Combination of low dietary K^+ and its obligatory loss in urine
Eating disorders	Low oral intake and total body K^+ depletion
High-carbohydrate intake with alcohol	Low K^+ intake and shift into cells
2. Transcellular distribution	
Insulin	Shift of K^+ into cells
β_2-Agonists (albuterol, clenbuterol)	Same as above
Alkalosis	Same as above
Theophylline, caffeine	
B_{12} injections	Consumption of K^+ in protein synthesis
Familial hypokalemic periodic paralysis	Mutation in the gene encoding the α_1-subunit of skeletal muscle L-type Ca^{2+} channel (60–70% of cases) or mutation in the gene encoding skeletal muscle Na^+ channel
Thyrotoxic hypokalemic periodic paralysis	Hyperthyroidism
3. Renal loss	
Drugs (diuretics other than K^+-sparing diuretics, penicillins, amphotericin B, lithium, cisplatin, licorice, gentamicin, amikacin, tobramycin, mineralocorticoids, cetuximab)	Renal K^+ wasting

(continued)

© Springer Science+Business Media LLC 2018
A.S. Reddi, *Fluid, Electrolyte and Acid-Base Disorders*,
DOI 10.1007/978-3-319-60167-0_15

Table 15.1 (continued)

Cause	Mechanism
Hypokalemic-hypertensive disorders	Activation of renin–AII–aldosterone
Malignant hypertension	Same as above
Renovascular hypertension	Same as above
Renin-secreting tumors	Excess aldosterone production by adrenals
Primary aldosteronism	Mutation in ENaC
Liddle syndrome	Excess aldosterone production
Glucocorticoid-remediable aldosteronism	Deficiency of 11β-hydroxysteroid dehydrogenase enzyme
Apparent mineralocorticoid excess syndrome	Mutation in mineralocorticoid receptor
Activating mutations of the mineralocorticoid receptor	Deficiency of 11β- and 17α-hydroxylase enzymes
Congenital adrenal hyperplasia	Renal K^+ wasting
Hypokalemic-normotensive disorders	
Renal tubular acidosis (types 1 and 2)	Renal K^+ wasting
Bartter syndrome	Mutations in Na/K/2Cl cotransporter and ROMK channel
Gitelman syndrome	Mutation in distal tubule Na/Cl cotransporter
Hypomagnesemia	Renal K^+ wasting
Cushing's syndrome	Same as above
4. Gastrointestinal loss	
Diarrhea	K^+ loss in stools
Vomiting	Renal K^+ wasting
5. Skin loss	
Excessive heat	Skin loss
Strenuous exercise	Renal loss

ENaC epithelial sodium channel, *ROMK* renal outer medullary potassium channel

Some Specific Causes of Hypokalemia

Hypokalemic Periodic Paralysis (HypoPP)

There are two major types of hypokalemic periodic paralysis: familial and thyrotoxic.

Familial
Familial HypoPP is an autosomal dominant form. A genetic test in the context of symptoms is the gold standard for diagnosis.

- The most familial form of HypoPP results in 60–70% of cases from mutation in the gene encoding the α_1-subunit of skeletal muscle L-type Ca^{2+} channel. In the remaining 10–20% of cases, the mutation occurs in the gene that codes for muscle Na^+ channel.
- Hypokalemia is entirely due to movement of K^+ from extracellular fluid (ECF) to intracellular fluid (ICF) compartment.
- Onset is usually before 20 years of age, and the prevalence is 1 per 100,000 people.

- Symptoms include severe muscle weakness, progressing at times to flaccid paralysis. A discrete attack may last hours to days.
- Triggers or stimuli of attacks are high-carbohydrate meal (insulin release), cold exposure during rest period following strenuous exercise (β_2-adrenergic surge), and administration of glucocorticoids.
- Treatment:
  - In acute attacks, patients are treated with either oral or IV KCl. The rate of administration should not exceed 10 mEq/h, as there is a risk for rebound hyperkalemia.
  - Acetazolamide (250–750 mg/day) to prevent the frequency of attacks. The mechanism is unrelated to inhibition of carbonic anhydrase.
  - Diet that is high in K^+ and low in Na^+ and carbohydrate may reduce the frequency and severity of attacks.

Thyrotoxic
- Thyrotoxic HypoPP is the acquired form that is precipitated by subclinical or clinical hyperthyroidism.
- Excess stimulation of Na/K-ATPase activity by thyroid hormones and reduced K^+ efflux from the skeletal muscle seem to be responsible for acute attacks of HypoPP.
- Asian and Hispanic males (20–50 years of age) are at increased risk for this disorder.
- Symptoms and triggers are similar to the familial type.
- Treatment includes KCl (oral or IV, as indicated) and propranolol. Antithyroid medications are part of long-term management in these patients.

Hypokalemic-Hypertensive Disorders

Malignant Hypertension
- A disorder of high renin–AII–aldosterone levels.
- Characterized by hypertension (HTN), hypokalemia, and metabolic alkalosis.
- Hyponatremia due to pressure natriuresis is occasionally seen.

Renal Artery Stenosis
It is similar to malignant HTN with high renin–AII–aldosterone levels.

- Patients present with severe hypokalemia, HTN, and metabolic alkalosis.
- Stenosis is caused by fibromuscular dysplasia in the young and atherosclerosis in the elderly.
- Removal of stenosis by stents or surgery improves hypokalemia and HTN.
- Hyponatremia due to pressure natriuresis is occasionally seen.

Primary Aldosteronism
- Caused by autonomous secretion of aldosterone by adrenal adenoma or hyperplasia of the adrenal gland.
- Characterized by hypokalemia, HTN, and metabolic alkalosis.

- Plasma renin levels are low because of aldosterone-induced Na^+ reabsorption and volume expansion. Despite volume expansion, aldosterone levels are high.
- Removal of adenoma or treatment with K^+-sparing diuretics (spironolactone) corrects metabolic abnormalities and HTN.

Liddle Syndrome
- An autosomal dominant disorder, caused by mutations in the ENaC.
- Characterized by Na^+ reabsorption, hypokalemia, and HTN with low renin–aldosterone levels.
- Amiloride is the drug of choice (see questions in case 3 for more details).

Glucocorticoid-Remediable Hyperaldosteronism (GRH)
- Also called familial hyperaldosteronism type 1.
- Caused by fusion of two enzymes: aldosterone synthase and 11β-hydroxylase.
- Patients with GRA may have hypokalemia, HTN, and metabolic alkalosis.
- Plasma renin is suppressed, but aldosterone levels are increased.
- Aldosterone secretion is stimulated by adrenocorticotropic hormone (ACTH) and not by angiotensin II. Therefore, administration of glucocorticoid suppresses excessive aldosterone secretion and improves hypokalemia and HTN (see questions in case 3 for more details).

Apparent Mineralocorticoid Excess (AME) Syndrome
- Cortisol, in addition to aldosterone, binds to mineralocorticoid receptor (MR) and promotes Na^+ reabsorption. Therefore, endogenous cortisol is converted into inactive cortisone by the enzyme 11β-hydroxysteroid dehydrogenase type 2.
- Mutations in 11β-hydroxysteroid dehydrogenase type 2 reduce its activity and prevent the conversion from cortisol to cortisone. As a result, cortisol exerts mineralocorticoid actions.
- Patients with AME present with hypokalemia, metabolic alkalosis, HTN, and low plasma renin–aldosterone levels.
- Treatment with spironolactone or amiloride improves hypokalemia and HTN (see questions in case 3 for more details).
- AME can also be acquired. Ingestion of licorice, chewing tobacco, bioflavonoids, or carbenoxolone can cause AME. These agents contain glycyrrhetinic acid, which is a competitive inhibitor of 11β-hydroxysteroid dehydrogenase type 2.
- Clinical manifestations are similar to the genetic type of AME.
- Glycyrrhetinic acid has been suggested as a potential therapy for hyperkalemia in dialysis patients.

Activating Mutations of the Mineralocorticoid Receptor

- A mutation in an MR gene causes conformational change that allows nonmineralocorticoids such as progesterone or spironolactone to act as potent agonists.
- Subjects with this mutation develop HTN before the age of 20 with hypokalemia and low renin–aldosterone levels.

Table 15.2 Plasma renin and aldosterone levels in hypokalemic-hypertensive states

Disorder	Renin	Aldosterone
Malignant hypertension	↑	↑
Renovascular hypertension	↑	↑
Renin-secreting tumor	↑	↑
Primary aldosteronism	↓	↑
Liddle syndrome	↓	↓
GRA	↓	↑
AME	↓	↓
Licorice ingestion	↓	↓
Activating mutations of MR receptor	↓	↓

GRA glucocorticoid-remediable hyperaldosteronism, *AME* apparent mineralocorticoid excess syndrome, ↑ increase, ↓ decrease

- Pregnancy exacerbates HTN without proteinuria, edema, or neurologic changes because of high progesterone levels.
- Spironolactone is contraindicated for hypertensive management in nonpregnant subjects (see questions in case 3 for more details).

Table 15.2 summarizes plasma renin and aldosterone levels in hypokalemic conditions associated with HTN.

Hypokalemic-Normotensive Disorders

Renal Tubular Acidosis (RTA)
Both type 1 (distal) and type 2 (proximal) RTAs cause hypokalemia because of K^+ wasting in the urine due to high aldosterone levels.

Bartter Syndrome
- As shown in Table 3.1, there are five types of Bartter syndrome, which are caused by genetic defects in the apical or basolateral membrane transport systems of the thick ascending limb of Henle's loop.
- Bartter syndrome behaves similar to a patient on loop diuretics.
- All of them are characterized by hypokalemia, metabolic alkalosis, and normal blood pressure (BP) or at times hypotension.
- Bartter syndromes occur in perinatal period or early in life.
- Treatment includes supplementation of K^+. Spironolactone, amiloride, ACE inhibitors, and nonsteroidal anti-inflammatory drugs have been tried with variable results.

Gitelman Syndrome

- As shown in Tables 3.1 and 15.1, Gitelman syndrome is caused by mutations in distal tubule Na/Cl cotransporter.
- Gitelman syndrome behaves similar to a patient on thiazide diuretic.

- Characterized by hypokalemia, hypomagnesemia, metabolic alkalosis, and normal BP. Although these manifestations are similar to Bartter syndrome, Gitelman syndrome occurs at any age (1–70 years) but is diagnosed in young adults.
- The only way one can distinguish Gitelman syndrome from Bartter syndrome is urinary Ca^{2+} excretion. In Gitelman syndrome, urinary excretion of Ca^{2+} is *low* (hypocalciuria), whereas in Bartter syndrome it is *normal* or *high* (hypercalciuria).
- Hypocalciuria is due to proximal tubule reabsorption of Ca^{2+}, and hypomagnesemia is probably related to downregulation of Mg^{2+} channel in the distal collecting tubule.
- Treatment includes lifelong liberal salt intake, K^+ and Mg^{2+} supplementation (KCl, $MgCl_2$), as well as K^+-sparing diuretics (spironolactone, amiloride, spironolactone-receptor blocker).

Hypokalemia Due to Aminoglycosides

- Gentamicin, amikacin, and tobramycin are cationic drugs that bind to the Ca^{2+}-sensing receptor on the basolateral membrane of the thick ascending limb of Henle's loop and inhibit Na/K/2Cl cotransporter with resultant inhibition of ROMK channel. As a result, K^+ secretion into the lumen is inhibited, causing renal salt, K^+, Ca^{2+}, and Mg^{2+} wasting. Other cationic drugs, such as cisplatin, can act in a similar fashion.
- Discontinuation of these drugs improves the electrolyte abnormalities.

Diagnosis

Step 1

History and physical examination is essential. BP is extremely important, as high or low BP gives clues to the etiology of hypokalemia (Fig. 15.1).

Step 2

Rule out pseudohypokalemia. Patients with leukemia and leukocyte count > 100,000/μl can present with hypokalemia because of K^+ uptake by these leukocytes.

Step 3

Exclude poor oral intake and transcellular distribution of K^+ (Table 15.1). Note that the total body K^+ is normal in conditions of transcellular distribution.

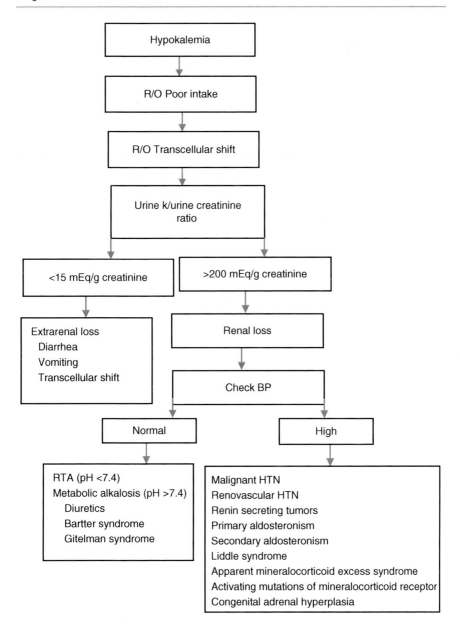

Fig. 15.1 Approach to the patient with hypokalemia

Step 4

In true hypokalemia, total body K^+ is depleted.

Determination of 24 h urine Na^+ and K^+ concentration is important.

Spot urine K^+ determination is not useful, as K^+ excretion is variable in the day.

If 24 h urine collection is not feasible, urine K^+/creatinine ratio in a spot urine can be performed. A urine ratio <15 mEq/g creatinine is suggestive of extrarenal loss, whereas a ratio >200 mEq/g creatinine suggests renal loss.

Normal urine K^+ in HypoPP and others that cause transcellular distribution.

If urinary Na^+ is <100 mEq/day and urinary K^+ <20 mEq/day (i.e., 24 h urine), suspect extrarenal losses from either the gastrointestinal tract or the skin.

Note that K^+ loss from diarrhea, malabsorption, or fistulas causes normal anion gap metabolic acidosis as opposed to hypokalemic metabolic alkalosis due to vomiting.

Step 5

If urinary Na^+ is >100 mEq/day and urinary K^+ >20 mEq/day (i.e., 24 h urine), suspect renal loss.

At this time, determination of BP most likely establishes the diagnosis of hypokalemia.

High BP and high plasma renin and aldosterone levels suggest malignant HTN, renovascular HTN, or renin-secreting tumor.

High plasma aldosterone and low renin levels are characteristic of primary aldosteronism.

Determine serum HCO_3^- in patients with hypokalemia and normal BP.

Low serum HCO_3^- suggests renal tubular acidosis.

High serum HCO_3^- suggests metabolic alkalosis.

In patients with metabolic alkalosis, determination of urinary Cl^- distinguishes renal from extrarenal causes of hypokalemia. Urine Cl^- <10 mEq/L is suggestive of extrarenal loss, whereas >10 mEq/L indicates renal loss.

Clinical Manifestations

The clinical manifestations of hypokalemia are mostly neuromuscular and cardiac that warrant immediate attention. In addition, hypokalemia causes several metabolic and renal effects (Table 15.3).

Treatment

Treatment of hypokalemia depends on the following factors:

Table 15.3 Clinical and physiologic manifestations of hypokalemia

Neuromuscular
Skeletal muscle: weakness, tetany, cramps, paralysis (flaccid)
Smooth muscle: ileus, constipation, urinary retention
Cardiovascular
Abnormal EKG changes (U waves, prolonged Q-T interval, ST depression) and arrhythmias
Abnormal contractility
Potentiation of digitalis toxicity
Metabolic
Decreased insulin release
Abnormal tolerance to glucose causing diabetes
Impaired hepatic glycogen and protein synthesis
Decreased aldosterone and growth hormone secretion
Growth retardation
Maintenance of metabolic alkalosis
Renal
Decreased renal blood flow and glomerular filtration rate (GFR)
Impaired urine concentration (nephrogenic diabetes insipidus)
Increased renal ammonia genesis, precipitating encephalopathy
Increased renal HCO_3 reabsorption
Chronic tubulointerstitial disease
Cyst formation
Proximal tubular vacuolization
Rhabdomyolysis

Severity

Mild to moderate hypokalemia (3–3.5 mEq/L) can be treated with oral KCl (40–80 mEq/day). Oral route is the preferred way of administering KCl. Severe hypokalemia (<2.5 mEq/L) can be life-threatening in a patient with cardiac disease and thus warrants immediate treatment. Intravenous (IV) administration of KCl is preferred to oral administration. Generally, 10–20 mEq of KCl in 100 mL of normal or one-half normal saline given over an hour is considered safe via the peripheral vein. Higher concentrations of KCl may lead to hyperkalemia, pain, and sclerosis of peripheral veins. KCl should not be given with dextrose solution for initial therapy because of exacerbation of dextrose-induced hypokalemia through insulin release.

Underlying Cause

If hypokalemia is due to cellular shift, treating underlying causes is preferred. However, if severe weakness, paresis, or paralysis occurs, IV administration of KCl (10 mEq/h) should be given with EKG and plasma K^+ monitoring. If cellular shift is

Table 15.4 Monitoring of serum [K⁺]

Serum [K⁺] (mEq/L)	K⁺ deficit (mEq)/70 kg
3.5	125–250
3.0	150–400
2.5	300–600
2.0	500–750

Data from Sterns et al. [1]

caused by thyrotoxicosis or excessive β-adrenergics, a nonselective β-blocker, such as propranolol, should be given. Causes of diarrhea should be sought and treated appropriately. Long-term use of K⁺-sparing diuretics is recommended for certain diseases.

Degree of K⁺ Depletion

It is not easy to estimate total body K⁺ depletion, because it is largely stored in the muscle. As muscle mass decreases with age in both males and females, more in the former, and everybody does not have the same weight, estimation of total body K⁺ depletion should be individualized. However, Table 15.4 provides a rough estimate of total body K⁺ deficiency in relation to serum [K⁺]. Treatment includes oral KCl alone or combination of KCl and K⁺-sparing diuretics. Frequent monitoring of serum [K⁺] is indicated to avoid hyperkalemia.

Study Questions

Case 1 Hypokalemic periodic paralysis (HypoPP) may be familial or acquired. Which one of the following statements is FALSE for this disorder?

(A) The most common familial form (60–70%), an autosomal dominant disorder, is due to mutations in the muscle Ca²⁺ channel α1-subunit gene.
(B) A smaller number (10–20%) of the familial form of the disorder is due to mutations in the skeletal muscle Na⁺ channel.
(C) Carbonic anhydrase inhibitor frequently reduces the number of paralysis attacks in patients with familial HypoPP.
(D) Hyperthyroidism or high-carbohydrate intake precipitates paralytic attacks in many Asian populations.
(E) Paralytic attacks are best treated with IV infusion of KCl at the rate of 20 mEq/h.

The answer is E All of the above statements except for E are correct with HypoPP. It is prudent to infuse KCl at a rate of 10 mEq/h in order to avoid rebound hyperkalemia.

Case 2 An 18-year-old man comes to the emergency department with a complaint of severe muscle weakness and dizziness. His systolic BP is 94 mmHg with orthostatic change. He says that he craves for Chinese food with added salt. He is not on any medications, and he does not use any illicit drugs. He complains of arthritic-like knee pain. X-rays of the knees show Ca^{2+} deposition. Pertinent labs:

Serum	Urine (24 h)
Na^+ = 137 mEq/L	Na^+ = 120 mEq/L
K^+ = 2.9 mEq/L	K^+ = 80 mEq/L
Cl^- = 84 mEq/L	Ca^{2+} = 50 mg/dL
HCO_3^- = 30 mEq/L	pH = 6.2
Ca^{2+} = 8.5 mg/dL	Osmolality = 300 mOs/kg H_2O
Mg^{2+} = 0.8 mg/dL	Diuretic screening = negative
Blood pH = 7.48	

Question 1 Which one of the following disorders is the most likely diagnosis in this patient?

(A) Bartter syndrome with mutation in ROMK channel (type 2)
(B) Liddle syndrome
(C) Gitelman syndrome
(D) Hereditary mineralocorticoid excess syndrome
(E) Acquired mineralocorticoid excess syndrome

The answer is C Based on the BP, options B, D, and E can be excluded, as these disorders are characterized by HTN. Type 2 Bartter syndrome and Gitelman syndrome are characterized by hypokalemia, metabolic alkalosis, and hypo- or normal BP. Type 2 Bartter syndrome is usually present in neonates, whereas Gitelman syndrome occurs in adolescents. Thus, the patient described in this case has Gitelman syndrome, as his urine Ca^{2+} excretion is low. In Bartter syndrome, Ca^{2+} excretion is normal to high. Patients with Gitelman syndrome have hypomagnesemia due to increased loss of Mg^{2+} in the urine. The patient's dizziness is related to volume depletion caused by Na^+ diuresis.

Question 2 How would you manage this patient?

Answer This patient needs lifelong supplementation of high-salt intake, KCl, and $MgCl_2$ (magnesium sulfate or magnesium oxide, which causes more diarrhea than magnesium chloride). Eplerenone (spironolactone-receptor blocker) seems to be better than either spironolactone or amiloride to maintain serum $[K^+]$.

Question 3 Why did the patient have Ca^{2+} deposition in his knees?

Answer Patients with Gitelman syndrome occasionally present with arthropathy due to deposition of calcium pyrophosphate dihydrate (CPPD) crystals in knees and other joints. This condition is referred to as chondrocalcinosis, which is thought to be due to hypomagnesemia. Mg^{2+} is a cofactor for various pyrophosphatases, including alkaline phosphatase. Decreased alkaline phosphatase activity due to hypomagnesemia causes increased plasma levels of ionic inorganic pyrophosphate (PPi). PPi is generally hydrolyzed to inorganic phosphate by alkaline phosphatase and inorganic pyrophosphatase. In the presence of hypomagnesemia, chondrocytes synthesize increased levels of PPi, and this PPi combines with Ca^{2+} to form CPPD. Correction of hypomagnesemia prevents CPPD crystal deposition.

Case 3 Match the following clinical histories of patients with the molecular defects:

(A) An 18-year-old man with low renin–aldosterone levels, hypokalemia, and severe hypertension, who responds to amiloride but is unresponsive to spironolactone	1. Mutations in the cytoplasmic COOH-terminus of the β- and γ-subunits of the epithelial sodium channel (ENaC)
(B) A child with low renin–aldosterone levels, hypokalemia, severe hypertension, poor growth, short stature, and nephrocalcinosis	2. Loss-of-function mutations in 11β-hydroxysteroid dehydrogenase type 2 (11β-HSD2) enzyme
(C) A 16-year-old man with mild hypertension, mild hypokalemia (3.4 mEq/L), and HCO_3^- concentration of 29 mEq/L. His hypertension is unresponsive to angiotensin-converting enzyme inhibitors (ACE-Is) and β-blockers but responsive to glucocorticoids	3. A chimeric gene duplication from unequal crossover between 11β-hydroxylase and aldosterone synthase genes
(D) A 20-year-old pregnant woman develops severe hypertension without proteinuria during her third trimester. Her 17-year-old brother is also hypertensive whose blood pressure rises on spironolactone	4. A missense mutation in mineralocorticoid receptor

Answers A = 1, B = 2, C = 3, D = 4

The patient described in choice A has Liddle syndrome, which is an autosomal dominant disorder. It is caused by mutations in the cytoplasmic COOH-terminus of the β- and γ-subunits of the ENaC. Activation of this channel results in increased Na^+ reabsorption with blunted Na^+ excretion, hypokalemia, and HTN with low renin–aldosterone levels. HTN responds to triamterene or amiloride, but not to spironolactone. Affected patients are at increased risk for cerebrovascular and cardiovascular disease.

The child described in choice B carries the diagnosis of the syndrome of AME, which is a rare autosomal recessive disorder. It is due to a loss-of-function mutation in the gene encoding the enzyme 11β-hydroxysteroid dehydrogenase type 2 (11β-HSD2). This enzyme converts cortisol to the inactive cortisone. As a consequence of the mutation, the 11β-HSD2 enzyme activity is decreased with resultant accumulation of cortisol. Cortisol acts like a mineralocorticoid by occupying its receptor, causing Na^+ reabsorption, hypokalemic metabolic alkalosis, and HTN with low renin–aldosterone levels. Suppression of renin and aldosterone is due to volume excess caused by Na^+ and water retention. Children with AME demonstrate low birth weight and nephrocalcinosis; the latter is due to hypokalemic nephropathy. HTN responds to salt restriction, amiloride, or triamterene but not to regular doses of spironolactone. Licorice ingestion induces a similar syndrome. Complications include cardiac events, including stroke and renal failure.

The clinical history described in choice C is consistent with the diagnosis of GRA. This disorder, also called familial hyperaldosteronism type 1, is caused by a chimeric gene duplication from unequal crossover between aldosterone synthase and 11β-hydroxylase. Some patients with GRA may have severe HTN, hypokalemia, and metabolic alkalosis. Some other patients may have mild HTN, normal to low serum K^+, and mild increase in serum HCO_3 concentrations. Plasma renin is suppressed, but aldosterone levels are increased. Aldosterone secretion is stimulated by ACTH and not by angiotensin II. Therefore, administration of glucocorticoid suppresses excessive aldosterone secretion and improves HTN.

The possible diagnosis of the patient presented in choice D is a case of early-onset HTN with severe exacerbation during pregnancy. This disorder is caused by an activating heterozygous missense mutation in the MR gene called S810 L mutation. Clinically the patient presents with HTN before age 20 years with low plasma K^+, renin, and aldosterone levels. Pregnancy exacerbates HTN without proteinuria, edema, or neurologic changes. Aldosterone levels, which are elevated during pregnancy, are extremely low in MR gene mutation. MR antagonists, such as spironolactone, become agonists and increase BP in patients with mutation in MR gene. Therefore, spironolactone is contraindicated in these patients. Progesterone also increases BP in patients with MR gene mutation, since this hormone level is extremely high in these patients. It should be remembered that heterozygous loss-of-function mutations in the MR gene (locus symbol NR3C2) result in pseudohypoaldosteronism type I (PHA I), an autosomal disorder that causes salt wasting and hypotension. This disease remits with age.

Case 4 A 30-year-old man visits the emergency department with acute exacerbation of asthma.

Which one of the following drugs does NOT cause hypokalemia?

(A) Insulin
(B) β₂-Agonists
(C) Clenbuterol
(D) Propranolol
(E) Gentamicin

The answer is D Insulin, β₂-agonists, and clenbuterol promote K^+ from extracellular to intracellular compartment, whereas gentamicin binds to Ca^{2+}-sensing receptor located at the basolateral membrane of the thick ascending limb of Henle's loop, causing inhibition of ROMK channel. This results in urinary K^+ loss and hypokalemia. Propranolol is a nonspecific β-adrenergic antagonist, causing elevation in serum $[K^+]$. Thus, choice D is correct.

Case 5 A 26-year-old man is seen in the emergency department for anxiety, palpitations, and tachypnea following heroin intake with his friends. He is alert, oriented, and afebrile without any respiratory distress. His pupils are normal. BP and pulse rate are 110/70 mmHg and 114 beats per minute, respectively. Labs: Na^+ 140 mEq/L, K^+ 2.6 mEq/L, Cl – 106 mEq/L, HCO_3–24 mEq/L, creatinine 0.9 mg/dL, BUN 16 mg/dL, and glucose 164 mg/dL. EKG shows prolonged QT interval and Q waves without ST segment changes. Troponin levels are normal. Urine drug screen is positive only for opiates. He refuses naloxone, as he says that his symptoms are not related to heroin alone.

   Which one the following is the MOST likely cause of his hypokalemia?

(A) Caffeine
(B) Theophylline
(C) Clenbuterol-tainted heroin
(D) Cocaine and heroin
(E) None of the above

The answer is C The patient does not demonstrate classic symptoms of heroin abuse, such as CNS and respiratory depression, miosis, or bradycardia. Although caffeine and theophylline can cause hypokalemia by cellular shift, urine toxicology was negative for these substances. Clenbuterol is a β_2-agonist that is approved to treat bronchospasm in the horse. In addition, clenbuterol has been shown to increase muscle mass while simultaneously decreasing fat mass in lambs, horses, broiler chickens, and steers. Clenbuterol is similar to salbutamol, and it has been used as a bronchodilator in humans in Europe. Because of its anabolic and lipolytic effects, clenbuterol has been used by body builders illicitly to gain muscle mass. In the USA, foods containing clenbuterol have been banned.

   In 2005, the CDC reported 26 suspected or confirmed cases of clenbuterol-tainted heroin in New Jersey, New York, Connecticut, and North and South Carolina. Because of its β_2-adrenergic effects, clenbuterol causes profound hypokalemia by shifting K^+ into the cell. It is not known whether heroin is sold in the street as heroin tainted with clenbuterol or clenbuterol sold as heroin. Thus, choice C is correct.

   The combination of cocaine and heroin rarely causes hypokalemia unless a β_2-adrenergic drug is contaminated. Thus, answers D and E are incorrect.

Case 6 Match the following serum values of patients with the clinical diagnoses:

Case	Na^+	K^+	HCO_3^-	Renin	Aldosterone
A	↑	↓	↑	↓	↑
B	N/↑	↓	↑	↓	↑
C	↓	↓	↑	↑	↑
D	N/↑	↓	↑	↓	↓

↑ increase, ↓ decrease, *N* normal

1. Primary aldosteronism
2. Glucocorticoid-remediable aldosteronism (GRA)
3. Renal artery stenosis
4. Liddle syndrome

Answers A = 1, B = 2, C = 3, D = 4
   Primary aldosteronism is the most common hypertensive disorder that is associated with low renin and high aldosterone levels. High levels of aldosterone are due

to increased secretion of this hormone by either adrenal cortical adenoma or bilateral hyperplasia of the gland. Aldosterone promotes Na^+ reabsorption and K^+ secretion in the distal nephron. As a result, plasma volume is increased with an increase in serum Na concentration and volume-dependent HTN. Hypernatremia may also be caused by relative suppression of ADH due to volume expansion. Plasma renin level is low because of volume expansion; however, aldosterone levels are high due to autonomous secretion of this hormone by the adenoma or bilateral hyperplasia of the adrenal gland. Primary aldosteronism is commonly seen in young patients with refractory HTN, hypokalemia, hypernatremia, and saline-resistant metabolic alkalosis. Spironolactone or amiloride is the drug of choice for HTN management. Labs shown in A are consistent with primary aldosteronism. Labs shown in B are consistent with GRA (see case 3).

Patients with renal artery stenosis present with severe HTN, hyponatremia, hypokalemia, and saline-resistant metabolic alkalosis. Hyponatremic hypertensive syndrome is characteristic of unilateral renal artery stenosis, but this syndrome has also been described in patients with bilateral renal artery stenosis. The pathophysiology involves that renal ischemia causes an increase in renin–AII–aldosterone levels, which in turn raises BP. This increase in BP causes pressure natriuresis through the nonstenosed kidney, resulting in volume depletion and orthostatic hypotension. High levels of AII stimulate thirst and water consumption, finally leading to hyponatremia. Hyponatremic hypertension can also be seen in patients with malignant hypertension and renin-secreting tumors, by the same mechanism. In young patients, renal artery stenosis is predominantly due to fibromuscular dysplasia, and, in subjects aged >50 years, it is the atherosclerosis of the renal artery that causes HTN. Labs shown in C are consistent with renal artery stenosis. Labs shown in D are consistent with Liddle syndrome (see case 3).

Case 7 A 45-year-old man visits his family primary care physician for headache and weakness for 10 days. He thought that both symptoms are related to his work as a construction worker. He has been healthy all his life and denies taking any medications or illicit drugs. Both his parents are hypertensive. Physical examination reveals a well-built man with a BP of 194/98 mmHg with a pulse rate of 64 beats per minute. Except for trace edema, the physical examination is otherwise normal. Serum chemistry is normal except for low K^+ (1.8 mEq/L) and high HCO_3^- (30 mEq/L).

Question 1 What is the differential diagnosis of his hypokalemic hypertension?

Answer There are at least nine clinical conditions that are associated with hypokalemia, elevated HCO_3^-, and HTN (Table 15.1).

Question 2 What laboratory tests are useful in the evaluation of his condition?

Answer Determination of plasma renin and aldosterone levels is the most useful test to make the diagnosis.

Plasma levels of renin and aldosterone were ordered and both were low (less than reference range).

Question 3 What are the conditions that would give low renin and aldosterone levels in this patient?

Answer From Table 15.2, it is evident that Liddle syndrome, AME, licorice ingestion, and activating mutations of MR receptor are the conditions that are characterized by hypokalemia, metabolic alkalosis, HTN, and low renin and aldosterone levels.

The patient was started on KCl supplements with spironolactone and was asked to come to the office in 7 days for follow-up. Repeat labs showed K^+ 3.6 mEq/L and HCO_3^- 25 mEq/L. BP was 144/78 mmHg with a pulse rate of 74 beats per minute.

Question 4 Based on the above BP and electrolyte response, what disease conditions can be excluded?

Answer Liddle syndrome and activating mutations of MR receptor can be excluded because patients with Liddle syndrome do not respond to spironolactone, and, in patients with activating mutations of MR receptor, it aggravates BP.

Question 5 What is the diagnosis in this patient?

Answer The other conditions that are associated with low renin and aldosterone levels are hereditary AME and licorice ingestion. Generally, hereditary AME is present during childhood. However, this condition has been reported in a 23-year-old subject. Upon further history taking, the patient admits to chewing tobacco, which contains glycyrrhetinic acid. Millions of individuals chew tobacco, and several cases with paralysis have been reported. The diagnosis of licorice ingestion was made and stopping chewing tobacco improves BP.

Case 8 A 70-year-old woman with chronic kidney disease (CKD) stage 4 fell and sustained hip fracture. Following hip surgery, she developed watery diarrhea, which did not respond to fasting for 24 h. She complained of abdominal pain. An abdominal X-ray shows dilatation of the colon, and acute pseudo-obstruction (Ogilvie syndrome) was diagnosed. Her stool volume was 876 mL/day. Over a period of 4 days, her serum $[K^+]$ fell from 4.2 to 2.2 mEq/L.

Question 1 Which one of the following is MOST likely overexpressed in the colon?

(A) Na/K/2Cl cotransporter
(B) Na/Cl cotransporter
(C) Big K (BK) channel
(D) Epithelial Na channel (ENaC)
(E) None of the above

The answer is C The patient has secretory diarrhea, as it did not respond to fasting (osmotic diarrhea responds to fasting). Several case reports suggest that secretory diarrhea develops following the development of pseudo-obstruction and loss of K^+ in the stool in the order of 130–170 mEq/L. This extensive loss of K^+ is attributed to overexpression of BK channels in the colon. Thus, option C is correct.

References

1. Sterns RH, Cox M, Feig PU, et al. Internal potassium balance and the control of the plasma potassium concentration. Medicine. 1981;60:339–54.

Suggested Reading

2. Asmar A, Mohanda R, Wingo CS. A physiologic-based approach to the treatment of a patient with hypokalemia. Am J Kidney Dis. 2012;60:492–7.
3. Gennari FJ. Hypokalemia. N Engl J Med. 1998;339:451–8.
4. Lin S-H, Huang C-L. Mechanism of thyrotoxic periodic paralysis. J Am Soc Nephrol. 2012;23:985–8.
5. Mount DB. Disorders of potassium balance. In: Skorecki K, et al., editors. Brenner & rector's the kidney. 10th ed. Philadelphia: Elsevier; 2016. p. 559–600.
6. Segal A. Potassium and dyskalemias. In: Mount DB, Sayegh MH, Singh AJ, editors. Core concepts in the disorders of fluid, electrolytes and acid-base balance. New York: Springer; 2013. p. 49–102.
7. Trepiccione F, Zacchia M, Capasso G. Physiopathology of potassium deficiency. In: Alpern RJ, Moe OW, Caplan M, editors. Seldin and Giebisch's the kidney. Physiology and pathophysiology. 5th ed. San Diego: Academic Press (Elsevier); 2013. p. 1717–39.
8. Unwin RJ, Luft FC, Shirley DG. Pathophysiology and management of hypokalemia: a clinical perspective. Nat Rev Nephrol. 2011;7:75–84.

Disorders of Potassium: Hyperkalemia

16

Hyperkalemia is defined as a serum [K$^+$] >5.5 mEq/L. It is common in both outside and in-hospital patients. Hyperkalemia can be fatal if not recognized and treated. Proper treatment of hyperkalemia depends on the underlying cause. True hyperkalemia is caused by an excessive exogenous load of K$^+$; it can also result from a decrease in cellular uptake, a massive release following cell lysis, or a decrease in renal excretion. A number of drugs also cause hyperkalemia (Table 16.1). *Pseudohyperkalemia* refers to a condition in which K$^+$ is released from cells during venipuncture following prolonged application of a tourniquet in the arm. Hemolysis of red blood cells and an increased number of white blood cells (>100,000 cells) and platelets (>1,000,000 platelets) also release K$^+$ and cause pseudohyperkalemia. A benign form of familial pseudohyperkalemia due to leakage of K$^+$ from blood cells has been described in some families.

Table 16.1 Causes of hyperkalemia

Cause	Mechanism
1. *Exogenous intake*	
Oral	Excess oral intake
High K$^+$—containing foods (fruits, salt substitutes, KCl supplements, riverbed clay, burnt match heads, raw coconut juice)	
Herbal medications (horsetail, noni juice, dandelion, alfalfa)	
Endogenous	K$^+$ release from cell lysis
Gastrointestinal bleeding	
Hemolysis	
Exercise	
Catabolic states	
Red cell transfusion	
Rhabdomyolysis	
Tumor lysis syndrome	
Thalidomide	

(continued)

© Springer Science+Business Media LLC 2018
A.S. Reddi, *Fluid, Electrolyte and Acid-Base Disorders*,
DOI 10.1007/978-3-319-60167-0_16

Table 16.1 (continued)

Cause	Mechanism
2. Transcellular shift (transfer of K⁺ from ICF to ECF)	
Insulin deficiency	Decreased cell uptake
Hyperglycemia and hyperosmolality	Movement of K^+ from ICF to ECF compartment by solvent drag
β-Adrenergic blockers (propranolol, labetalol, carvedilol)	Inhibit cellular K^+ uptake and also inhibition of renin–AII–aldosterone axis
Digoxin	Inhibition of Na/K-ATPase
Chinese medicines (Dan Shen, Asian ginseng, Chan Su, Lu-Shen-Wan)	Inhibition of Na/K-ATPase
Herbal remedies prepared from foxglove, lily of the valley, yewberry, oleander, red squill, dogbane, toad skin	Inhibition of Na/K-ATPase
Succinylcholine	K^+ efflux from skeletal muscle via K^+ channels
Arginine, lysine, ε-aminocaproic acid	K^+ efflux from ICF to ECF
Acute metabolic mineral acidosis (HCl or citric acid)	K^+ efflux from ICF to ECF
Hyperkalemic periodic paralysis	Mutations in skeletal muscle Na^+-channel
3. Decreased renal excretion	
Advanced renal failure (CKD 5) and decreased delivery of filtrate to distal tubule	Diminished ability to secrete K^+
Hypoaldosteronism	
Addison disease	Lack of glucocorticoid production
Congenital adrenal hyperplasia	21α-hydroxylase deficiency
Pseudohypoaldosteronism type I (PHA I)	Autosomal dominant form: mutations in mineralocorticoid receptor Autosomal recessive form: mutations in all subunits of ENaC
Pseudohypoaldosteronism type II (PHA II)	Mutations in "with no lysine" (WNK) 1 and 4 kinases
Syndrome of hyporeninemic hypoaldosteronism	Many diseases (diabetes, lupus, multiple myeloma, tubulointerstitial disease, AIDS) and drugs (see below) are associated with hyporeninemic hypoaldosteronism
4. Drugs	
ACE inhibitors, ARBs, renin inhibitors, NSAIDs, COX-2 inhibitors, heparin, ketoconazole	↓ aldosterone synthesis
Amiloride, triamterene, trimethoprim, pentamidine	Block ENaC
Spironolactone, eplerenone	Block aldosterone receptors
Drospirenone	A progestin derived from spironolactone (used as a combined oral contraceptive)
Cyclosporine, tacrolimus	(1) Hyporeninemic hypoaldosteronism, (2) blocks K^+ channels in distal nephron, (3) inhibits Na/K-ATPase, (4) inhibits ROMK channel, (5) increases Cl^- shunt in DCT
Cocaine, statins	Indirect effect by causing rhabdomyolysis

ICF intracellular fluid, *ECF* extracellular fluid, *CKD 5* chronic kidney disease stage 5, *ENaC* epithelial sodium channel, *NSAIDs* nonsteroidal anti-inflammatory drugs, *AII* angiotensin II, *COX-2* cyclooxygenase-2, *ARB* angiotensin II receptor blocker, *ACE* angiotensin-converting enzyme, DCT distal convoluted tubule

Some Specific Causes of Hyperkalemia

Hyperkalemic Periodic Paralysis (HyperPP)

- HyperPP is an autosomal dominant disorder, characterized by episodic muscle weakness.
- It is caused by mutations in the skeletal muscle Na^+ channel (α-subunit).
- It is generally precipitated by exposure to cold, rest following exercise, high-K^+ intake, or glucocorticoids.
- Treatment includes β_2-agonists (salbutamol) and acetazolamide (250–750 mg/day).

Chronic Kidney Disease Stage 5 (CKD5)

- CKD patients are able to maintain serum $[K^+]$ near normal until glomerular filtration rate (GFR) is <20 mL/min. Under certain conditions such as metabolic acidosis or severe tubulointerstitial disease, hyperkalemia develops even under moderate decrease in GFR (>30 mL/min).
- Some of the causes of hyperkalemia in patients with GFR <20 mL/min include decreased nephron mass, low lumen-negative voltage in the distal tubule because of low Na^+ reabsorption via the epithelial sodium channel (ENaC), metabolic acidosis, defective renin–aldosterone axis, and concomitant intake of medications that interfere with K^+ secretion.
- Treatment includes diuretics, correction of acidosis, and underlying cause of CKD.
- Acute kidney injury with severe decrease in GFR may also cause hyperkalemia.

Decreased Effective Arterial Blood Volume

- Occasionally mild hyperkalemia is seen in patients with congestive heart failure, cirrhosis, and nephrotic syndrome who have decreased effective blood volume. This hyperkalemia is due to the decreased delivery of filtrate to the distal tubule. Judicious use of ACE-Is, ARBs, or aldosterone antagonists is warranted in these patients.
- Also, patients with severe volume depletion related to lack of water intake, particularly the elderly, may have hyperkalemia with decreased GFR. Correction of volume deficit in these patients improves both GFR and hyperkalemia.

Addison Disease

- Autoimmune adrenalitis is the most common cause of Addison disease.
- Lack of aldosterone is the primary cause of hyperkalemia due to low ENaC activity and lack of lumen-negative voltage.
- Electrolyte abnormalities besides hyperkalemia include hyponatremia, hyperchloremia, hypobicarbonatemia, and at times hypercalcemia.

- Patients are hypovolemic because of Na^+ loss in urine.
- Plasma renin is high. Aldosterone and cortisol levels are high.
- Adrenal crisis is a medical emergency.
- Normal saline and hydrocortisone restore volume and other electrolytes toward normal.

Adrenal Hyperplasia

- Rare disorders of aldosterone deficiency. Glucocorticoid deficiency also occurs.
- One of the most common disorders of adrenal hyperplasia is caused by the deficiency of 21α-hydroxylase. This enzyme converts progesterone to 11-deoxycorticosterone in the biosynthetic pathway of aldosterone.
- Affected patients present with salt wasting, hyponatremia, hyperkalemia, volume depletion, and high renin levels.
- Treatment in children includes supplementation of fludrocortisones and a glucocorticoid.

Syndrome of Hyporeninemic Hypoaldosteronism (SHH)

- SHH is a common disorder, which is associated with many disease conditions (Table 16.1).
- It is characterized by low renin and aldosterone levels, adequate GFR (CKD stages 2–3), hyperchloremic metabolic acidosis, and hyperkalemia.
- Volume expansion and associated increase in atrial natriuretic peptide seem to be responsible for low renin and aldosterone levels.
- Fludrocortisone therapy and discontinuation of the causative agent normalize plasma $[K^+]$.

Pseudohypoaldosteronism Type I (PHA I)

- PHA I occurs during infancy. It is characterized by salt wasting, hypovolemia, hyponatremia, hyperkalemia, metabolic acidosis, and normal blood pressure (BP).
- Plasma renin and aldosterone levels are elevated.
- PHA I is inherited as autosomal dominant or autosomal recessive forms.
- *Autosomal dominant form*: caused by mutations in the mineralocorticoid receptor. The disease is limited to the kidney. Salt supplementation for 1–3 years and carbenoxolone are recommended to improve electrolyte abnormalities.
- *Autosomal recessive form*: caused by mutations in α-, β-, or γ-subunit of ENaC.

- PHA I affects multiorgans, including the skin.
- Treatment includes lifelong salt supplementation and K^+-restricted diet. Carbenoxolone is not helpful.

Pseudohypoaldosteronism Type II (PHA II)

- It is an autosomal dominant disease, usually called familial hyperkalemic hypertension or Gordon syndrome.
- It is considered a "mirror image" of Gitelman syndrome.
- It is caused by mutations in the genes that encode WNK family of serine–threonine kinases, WNK1, and WNK4. Both kinases are expressed in the distal nephron.
- WNK4 downregulates the expression of Na/Cl cotransporter as well as renal outer medullary potassium (ROMK) channel.
- WNK1 inhibits WNK4 as well as ROMK.
- When mutations occur in WNK4 or its activity is suppressed by WNK1, NaCl reabsorption is increased in the distal tubule, leading to fluid overload and hypertension. WNK4 mutations further inhibit ROMK channel, causing hyperkalemia.
- Plasma renin and aldosterone levels are reduced to a variable degree.
- Thiazide diuretic is the treatment of choice.

Posttransplant Hyperkalemia

- Hyperkalemia develops in 44–73% of transplant recipients who are treated with cyclosporine or tacrolimus. Several mechanisms have been implicated, including (1) type 4 RTA due to hyporeninemic hypoaldosteronism, (2) activation of NaCl cotransporter in the distal tubule so that NaCl delivery to ENaC is decreased with resultant decreased secretion of K^+, (3) inhibition of ROMK channel, and (4) inhibition of basolateral Na/K-ATPase in the collecting duct so that K^+ does not enter the cell for secretion into the renal tubular lumen.
- Aldosterone agonists improve hyperkalemia.
- Chronic use of ACE-Is and ARBs worsens hyperkalemia.

Diagnosis

Step 1

- Check electrocardiogram (EKG), as hyperkalemia is an emergency (see Figs. 16.1 and 16.2). If there are no EKG abnormalities, proceed to step 2.

Fig. 16.1 EKG changes in hyperkalemia. A normal EKG is also shown for comparison. The earliest change in hyperkalemia is the peaked (tented) T wave. With an increase in plasma [K⁺], the QRS complex widens, the P wave disappears, and finally a sine wave pattern appears, leading to asystole.

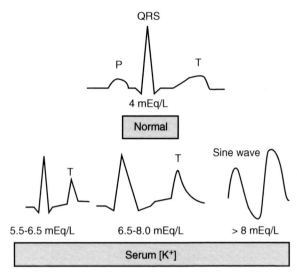

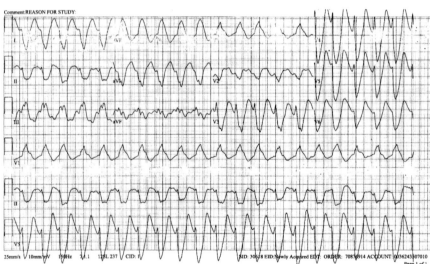

Fig. 16.2 EKG changes in a dialysis patient with serum [K⁺] of 8.5 mEq/L

Step 2

History
- Inquire about diet and dietary supplements.
- Check medications that cause hyperkalemia.
- Review risk factors and disease conditions that predispose to hyperkalemia (Table 16.2).

Table 16.2 Factors and conditions that predispose to hyperkalemia	CKD 4–5
	AKI
	Congestive heart failure and other conditions with decreased effective arterial blood volume
	Diabetes
	Volume depletion
	Elderly subjects
	White race
	Metabolic acidosis
	Dietary intake of foods and medications that contain K^+ (see Table 16.1)
	Concomitant use of ACE-Is, ARBs, or renin inhibitors with the following drugs:
	K^+-sparing drugs
	NSAIDs
	β-Adrenergic blockers
	Cyclosporine or tacrolimus
	Heparin
	Ketoconazole
	Trimethoprim
	Amiloride
	Pentamidine

Physical Examination

- Check blood pressure, pulse rate, and orthostatics, if indicated.
- Evaluate respiratory status for any weakness.
- Evaluate volume status.
- Evaluate muscle tenderness (rhabdomyolysis) and muscle weakness.

Step 3

- Obtain serum chemistry, complete blood count, and ABG (if needed).
- Measure $U_K/U_{Creatinine}$ ratio. The expected ratio in a patient with hyperkalemia and normal renal function is >200 mEq/g or >20 mmol/mmol. This ratio will be low in patients with decreased K^+ excretion (CKD, volume depleted, or hyporeninemic hypoaldosteronism patients). A 24-h urine collection for K^+ excretion is needed for such patients.
- Establish true hyperkalemia after excluding pseudohyperkalemia and transcellular shift of K^+. A $U_K/U_{Creatinine}$ ratio far less than 200 mEq/g is suggestive of transcellular distribution.
- Obtain estimated GFR. Based on the estimated GFR, rule out defective K^+ excretion.
- Obtain plasma aldosterone and renin levels. Obtain plasma cortisol levels as indicated.
- Follow Fig. 16.3 to delineate the cause of hyperkalemia.

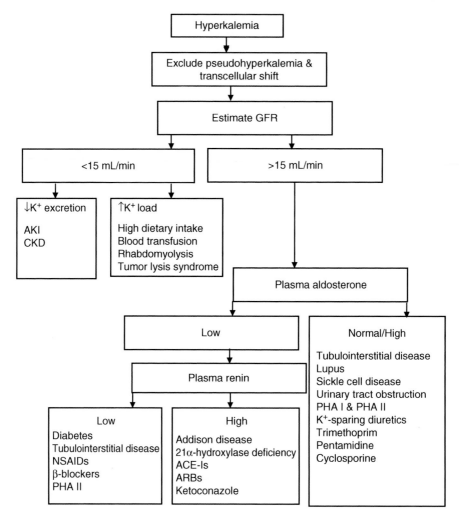

Fig. 16.3 A simplified approach to hyperkalemia. *PHA* pseudohypoaldosteronism, *ARB* angiotensin II receptor blocker, *ACE-Is* angiotensin-converting enzyme inhibitors, *NSAIDs* nonsteroidal anti-inflammatory drugs

Clinical Manifestations

Like hypokalemia, hyperkalemia also causes neuromuscular, cardiac, and metabolic effects. Table 16.3 summarizes these manifestations, and Fig. 16.1 shows some EKG changes in hyperkalemia.

Table 16.3 Clinical manifestations of hyperkalemia

Effects	Mechanism
Neuromuscular	
Muscle weakness	Reduced membrane potential caused by reduction in the ratio of intracellular to extracellular $[K^+]$
Paralysis (ascending)	Reduction in membrane potential from -90 mV to threshold potential, causing generation of an action potential
Cardiac (EKG changes related to serum $[K^+]$)[a]	
5.5–6.5 mEq/L	
Peaked T waves with narrow base	
6.5–8.0 mEq/L	
Peaked T waves, prolonged PR interval, widening of QRS complex	
> 8.0 mEq/L	
Absence of P waves, further widening of QRS complex, bundle branch blocks, sine wave, ventricular fibrillation, asystole	
Metabolic	
Hyperchloremic (nonanion gap) metabolic acidosis with hyperkalemia (hyperkalemic distal renal tubular acidosis)	Urinary tract obstruction is the major cause. Decreased H^+ secretion due to decreased cortical and medullary collecting duct H-ATPase activity. Urine pH is alkaline. However, combined hyperkalemic distal renal tubular acidosis with low aldosterone has been reported
Type 4 renal tubular acidosis (RTA)	Occurs in diseases and conditions with hyporeninism and hypoaldosteronism. Urine pH is usually acidic. The major defect is suppression of NH_4^+ synthesis by hyperkalemia. Drugs that cause aldosterone resistance also induce type 4 RTA

[a]Not every patient demonstrates these EKG changes. A large interpatient variability occurs in EKG changes. Patients on hemodialysis may not have any EKG changes at serum $[K^+]$ >6–6.5 mEq/L.

Treatment

Acute Treatment

Hyperkalemia is an acute emergency. Its management depends on serum $[K^+]$ and EKG changes. In many cases, hyperkalemia without EKG changes warrants treatment. The goals of acute therapy are threefold: (1) counteracting the membrane effects of hyperkalemia, (2) promoting cellular uptake of K^+, and (3) removing K^+ from the body slowly by cation exchange resin (sodium polystyrene sulfonate, Kayexalate) or a new approved nonreabsorbable polymer (patiromer) or rapidly by hemodialysis using either 1 or 2 mEq/L K^+ dialysate bath (Table 16.4). Kayexalate should be used cautiously, as it may alone or in sorbitol can cause bowel necrosis. It should not be used in patients with GI problems such as constipation, ischemic colitis, intestinal vascular atherosclerosis, and inflammatory bowel disease. Recently, two new oral K^+-binding drugs have been introduced: patiromer (Veltassa, Relypsa) and sodium zirconium cyclosilicate (ZS-9). Patiromer is a nonreabsorbable polymer that binds K^+ in exchange for Ca^{2+}. It binds K^+ throughout the GI tract but preferentially in the distal colon. Patiromer reduces serum K^+ level in patients with CKD, cardiovascular disease, and diabetes who are on ACE-Is or ARBs and is well tolerated. GI-related adverse effects are most common with patiromer. ZS-9 is under FDA review process and is effective in lowering serum K^+ level. It binds to K^+ in exchange for Na^+ and H ion. It is 125 more selective for K^+ than kayexalate.

Table 16.4 Acute treatment of hyperkalemia

Treatment	Dose	Onset	Duration of effect	Mechanism
Antagonism of membrane effects				
Calcium gluconate (10%)	10–20 mL	1–3 min	30–60 min	Counteract the membrane effects of K^+
Hypertonic (3%) saline	50 mL	Immediate	Unknown	Membrane antagonism
Promote cellular uptake				
Insulin and glucose	20–50 g of glucose +10–20 U of rapid-acting insulin	<30 min	4–6 h	K^+ uptake by cells
$NaHCO_3$ (only when significant acidosis is present)	44–88 mEq	5–10 min	1–6 h	K^+ uptake by cells
Albuterol	10–20 mg by nebulizer	15–20 min	2–3 h	K^+ uptake by cells
Salbutamol	10 mg by nebulizer	15–20 min	2 h	K^+ uptake by cells
Removal of K^+ from body				
Kayexalate (sodium polystyrene sulfonate) in 30% sorbitol (cation exchange resin)[a]	Oral (30–45 g) or enema (50–100 g)	≥ 2 h	2–6 h	Exchange of Na^+ for K^+
Patiromer[b]	Oral (8.4 g in water) once or twice	>4 h	24 h	Exchange of Ca^{2+} for K^+
Hemodialysis	–	Immediate	2–8 h	Immediate removal of K^+ from ECF

[a]Avoid in patients at risk for bowel necrosis, ileus, and volume depletion and in the first postoperative week. Oral treatment is preferable than enema (see FDA safety information).
[b]Dose may be increased to 16.8 g.

Chronic Treatment

- Patients with diabetes, tubulointerstitial disease, heart failure, and CKD 4–5 are at risk for hyperkalemia.
- Estimate GFR and inquire about diet and dietary supplements.
- Review all the medications, including over-the-counter medications.
- Patients with chronic hyperkalemia have a defect (low lumen-negative voltage in the distal nephron) in eliminating their daily intake of K^+ until they develop a new steady state.
- After a steady state, they excrete their intake of K^+ very slowly at the expense of higher plasma $[K^+]$.
- Use a loop diuretic (furosemide) or a thiazide diuretic, depending on GFR, to increase the delivery of Na^+ to the distal nephron to increase the excretion of K^+.
- Use kayexalate judiciously, if necessary.
- Alternatively, patiromer 8.4 g mixed in water can be taken once daily with food and 3 h before or 3 h after ingestion of all other medications.
- Use loop diuretics and/or fludrocortisone (0.05–0.1 mg orally) for patients with hyporeninemic hypoaldosteronism. Taper fludrocortisones as needed.
- Use $NaHCO_3$ tablets to correct acidosis.
- In a patient with heart failure, use low doses of an ACE-I or ARB (do not use both). Follow serum creatinine and $[K^+]$ in 3–5 days. If creatinine increases by >30% and K^+ is 6.0 mEq/L, hold ACE-I or ARB. If both measurements remain stable, repeat them in 7–14 days. If spironolactone is required, start with 12.5 mg, and go up to 25 mg/day. Some authors prefer to go up to 100 mg/day.

Study Questions

Case 1 A 32-year-old man is referred to you for evaluation of persistent hyperkalemia (5.9 mEq/L) and hypertension. Two members in his family have similar clinical presentation. Other laboratory results are as follows: Na^+ 140 mEq/L, Cl^- 114 mEq/L, HCO_3^- 16 mEq/L, creatinine 0.8 mg/dL, and glucose 90 mg/dL. Minor workup reveals low renin and aldosterone levels. Urinary Na^+ levels were 30 mEq/L. Arterial blood gas shows hyperchloremic metabolic acidosis. He is not on any medications.

Which one of the following therapeutic regimens is APPROPRIATE for this patient?

(A) Furosemide (Lasix)
(B) Hydrochlorothiazide (HCTZ)
(C) Spironolactone
(D) Acetazolamide (Diamox)
(E) Salt substitute

The answer is B In any young male, the presence of hyperkalemia, hypertension, hyperchloremic metabolic acidosis, low renin with low or normal aldosterone levels, and normal renal function should suggest pseudohypoaldosteronism type II (PHA II) (Gordon syndrome) as the most likely diagnosis. PHA II is considered a "mirror image" of Gitelman syndrome. Overexpression and activity of NaCl cotransporter in the distal tubule results in PHA II, which is an autosomal dominant disease. It is caused by mutations in genes that encode WNK kinases. Only mutations in WNK1 and WNK4 cause PHA II.

Under normal conditions, WNK4 inhibits the activities of NaCl cotransporter and ROMK, but enhances the paracellular Cl transport. The activity of WNK4 is suppressed by WNK1. When mutations occur in WNK1, there is an abundance of WNK1, which then removes the inhibitory effect of WNK4 on NaCl cotransporter activity. This results in excessive reabsorption of NaCl and thus volume-dependent hypertension. Mutations in WNK4 also result in similar enhancement of NaCl reabsorption.

As mentioned earlier, WNK4 inhibits ROMK by endocytosis of the channel. Mutations in WNK4 enhance the inhibitory effect of ROMK and thus hyperkalemia. Also, long WNK1 (L-WNK1) suppresses ROMK, thus contributing to hyperkalemia. Therefore, hyperkalemia is related to the combined effect of both WNK4 and WNK1.

WNK4 has also been shown to phosphorylate claudins, which are tight junction proteins involved in paracellular Cl^- transport. Thus, mutations in WNK4 cause enhanced transcellular NaCl and paracellular Cl^- transport with inhibition of K^+ secretion, resulting in volume expansion, hyperkalemia, and hypertension as seen in PHA II. Volume expansion leads to suppression of renin and at times aldosterone levels. Urine Na^+ concentration decreases because of its enhanced reabsorption in the distal tubule.

PHA II responds to thiazide diuretics such as HCTZ, as overactivity of NaCl cotransporter is suppressed. Therefore, option B is correct. Furosemide is a loop diuretic, and it does not act on NaCl cotransporter that is localized in the distal tubule. Spironolactone is a K^+-sparing diuretic, which increases serum K^+ levels even further. Diamox is a carbonic anhydrase inhibitor, which inhibits HCO_3^- regeneration in the proximal tubule. Hyperchloremic metabolic acidosis is further exacerbated by Diamox. Generally, salt substitutes contain K^+ and is not indicated in this subject. Therefore, options A, C, D, and E are incorrect.

Case 2 A 55-year-old man with multiple myeloma is admitted for paraparesis. A magnetic resonance imaging (MRI) of the spinal cord is normal. Neurologic examination shows muscle weakness of the lower limbs with tendinous areflexia and absence of pyramidal symptoms. His medications at the time of admission include dexamethasone 4 mg q6 h and thalidomide 200 mg/day. Blood pressure and pulse rate are normal. Except for serum K^+ of 8.4 mEq/L, other laboratory results are normal.

What is the MOST likely cause of his hyperkalemia and sudden paraparesis?

(A) Hyperkalemia due to steroid use
(B) Hyperkalemia due to remission of multiple myeloma
(C) Hyperkalemia due to thalidomide
(D) Hyperkalemia due to volume depletion
(E) Pseudohyperkalemia

The answer is C Thalidomide is being used by some investigators as the first-line treatment of multiple myeloma. In both dialysis and CKD patients, thalidomide has been shown to cause severe hyperkalemia, which may be related to either cell lysis or cellular shift. Thus, option C is correct. Both steroid use and remission of multiple myeloma are unlikely causes of hyperkalemia. Also, pseudohyperkalemia has not been reported with thalidomide. Severe volume depletion may cause hyperkalemia by limiting delivery of glomerular filtrate to the distal nephron, but this patient does not have either renal insufficiency or volume depletion.

Case 3 Which one of the following is NOT associated with hyperkalemic periodic paralysis (HyperPP) compared with hypokalemic periodic paralysis (HypoPP)?

(A) The familial form of HyperPP is due to the mutations in skeletal muscle Na^+ channel.
(B) The secondary form of HyperPP can mimic Guillain–Barré syndrome with respiratory failure and diaphragmatic paralysis.
(C) The familial form of HyperPP predominantly presents with myopathic weakness during high-K^+ intake or rest after exercise compared with the secondary form of HyperPP.
(D) Younger age (<10 year or infancy to childhood) of onset, greater frequency of attacks with faster recovery, and frequent attacks during fasting distinguish the familial form of HyperPP from that of HypoPP.
(E) High-carbohydrate intake, insulin stimulation, and epinephrine release are the frequent causes of attacks in HyperPP.

The answer is E Except for option E, all the other options characterize HyperPP, which is precipitated by exposure to cold, rest after exercise, and high-K^+ diet.

Case 4 A 32-year-old woman with tubulointerstitial disease has serum [K^+] of 5.1 mEq/L without any EKG changes.
Which one of the following is NOT associated with the exacerbation of her serum [K^+]?

(A) Trimethoprim
(B) Amiloride
(C) Pentamidine
(D) Nafamostat (a serine protease inhibitor)
(E) Licorice

The answer is E Except for licorice (causes hypokalemia), all other medications inhibit ENaC and cause hyperkalemia. Nafamostat is a serine protease inhibitor that is used in acute pancreatitis and disseminated intravascular coagulation.

Case 5 A 50-year-old man is brought to the emergency department by the family for weakness and fatigue. He missed two hemodialysis treatments. His serum [K$^+$] is 7.6 mEq/L. EKG shows widened peaked T waves.

Which one of the following is NOT indicated in the management of his hyperkalemia with EKG changes?

(A) Calcium gluconate
(B) Hypertonic (3%) saline
(C) Albuterol
(D) Hemodialysis
(E) Peritoneal dialysis

The answer is E Calcium antagonizes the membrane effects of hyperkalemia without lowering serum [K$^+$] by reducing the threshold potential of cardiac myocytes. Calcium gluconate (10%) is preferred than calcium chloride because the latter causes necrosis if it extravasates into the tissue. Calcium salts can be given over a 10–15-min period in an individual not on digitalis. However, in a patient on digitalis and hyperkalemic EKG changes, calcium can be given slowly over a period of 30 min. It is of interest to note that a patient with unrecognized digitalis toxicity and hyperkalemia was successfully treated with calcium chloride.

Hypertonic (3%) saline has been shown to reverse the EKG changes due to hyperkalemia in a patient with hyponatremia. It is given as a bolus of 50 mL. Whether this treatment is effective in normonatremic individuals is unknown. The effect is due to changes in the electrical properties of cardiac myocytes rather than a change in serum [K$^+$].

Albuterol (10 mg) by nebulization has been shown to lower plasma [K$^+$] by 0.6 mEq/L in patients with normal or decreased renal function. An additive effect of insulin/glucose has been reported with albuterol. Plasma K$^+$-lowering effect of albuterol is due to its transport into the cell.

Hemodialysis is the most effective way of removing K$^+$ from the body. Rapid removal of K$^+$ may precipitate ventricular arrhythmias in some patients; therefore, continuous EKG monitoring is recommended.

Peritoneal dialysis (PD) also removes K$^+$ in maintenance PD patients with modest hyperkalemia; however, it is not the choice of treatment for severe hyperkalemia with EKG changes. It should be noted that glucose in the peritoneal fluid can transport K$^+$ into the cell without affecting total body K$^+$ stores. Thus, option E is correct.

Case 6 A 46-year-old Indian woman with type 2 diabetes for 12 years is found to have a serum [K$^+$] of 5.8 mEq/L, HCO$_3^-$ 24 mEq/L, and glucose 100 mg/dL on a follow-up visit. One month ago, her serum [K$^+$] was 4.2 mEq/L. Her eGFR is 48 mL/min, which is stable for the last 1 year. She is on glipizide (5 mg/day) and sitagliptin (50 mg/day). She denies taking any dietary supplements or NSAIDs. The only complaint is fatigue.

Question 1 Which one of the following is an UNLIKELY cause of her hyperkalemia?

(A) Noni juice
(B) Raw coconut juice
(C) COX-2 inhibitors
(D) Oral hypoglycemic agents
(E) Alfalfa

The answer is D Except for oral hypoglycemic agents, all other food supplements cause hyperkalemia. Noni juice contains 56 mEq/L, and raw coconut juice contains 44.3 mEq/L of K^+. COX-2 inhibitors cause hypoaldosteronism, whereas alfalfa is rich in K^+. Thus, option D is correct.

Question 2 Is low GFR responsible for her new-onset hyperkalemia?

The answer is no Hyperkalemia occurs with GFR <20 mL/min. However, type 4 RTA in a diabetic patient is a possibility due to hypoaldosteronism, but her serum [HCO_3^-] of 24 mEq/L rules out this possibility.

Question 3 How can we explain her hyperkalemia?

Answer Upon further questioning, she admits to drinking fresh coconut juice (12 oz) everyday for the last 3 weeks. Thus, exogenous intake of K^+ is responsible for hyperkalemia in this patient who has compromised GFR.

Case 7 A 22-year-old female student presents to her student health clinic for fatigue and weakness of her lower extremities following her routine jogging. Her complaints started 6 weeks ago when her physician started a new oral contraceptive (OC). She has no significant medical history and is not on any medication other than OC. Serum chemistry other than K^+ (5.9 mEq/L) is normal.

  Which one of the following oral contraceptives predisposes to hyperkalemia?

(A) Ethinyl estradiol and norethindrone
(B) Ethinyl estradiol and norgestrel
(C) Ethinyl estradiol and desogestrel
(D) Ethinyl estradiol and drospirenone
(E) None of the above

The answer is D Millions of women worldwide use combined OCs (COCs). COCs contain both estrogen and progestin. Ethinyl estradiol is the estrogen component of the COCs; however, the progestin component varies and may include a first-generation progestin (option A), a second-generation progestin (option B), a third-generation progestin (option C), or a newly added progestin (option D), which is a spironolactone derivative. Review of her COC confirmed drospirenone, which was discontinued with return of her serum [K^+] to normal.

Case 8 A 22-year-old type 1 diabetic man is admitted for diabetic ketoacidosis with pH of 7.1. Clinically, he is volume depleted with a blood pressure of 100/72 mmHg, a pulse rate of 100 beats/min, and orthostatic changes. Laboratory results: Na^+ 132 mEq/L, K^+ 6.2 mEq/L, Cl^- 92 mEq/L, HCO_3^- 12 mEq/L, creatinine 1.6 mg/dL, blood urea nitrogen (BUN) 82 mg/dL, and glucose 440 mg/dL. In the emergency department, he was started on normal saline and rapid-acting insulin. After 6 h, his serum $[K^+]$ dropped to 3.4 mEq/L.

Question 1 What are the causes of hyperkalemia in this patient?

Answer Lack of insulin and hyperglycemia are the potential causes of hyperkalemia in this diabetic patient.

Question 2 Does his metabolic acidosis contribute to his hyperkalemia?

The answer is no Diabetic ketoacidosis is due to the accumulation of acetoacetate and β-hydroxybutyrate, which are organic acids. Lactic acid is also an organic acid. Infusion of these acids does not cause transcellular shift (from intracellular fluid (ICF) to extracellular fluid (ECF)) of K^+, whereas that of inorganic acids (NH_4Cl or HCl) causes transcellular shift and hyperkalemia. This difference between inorganic and organic acidoses is related to the cell permeability of their anions.

In metabolic acidosis, H^+ moves into the cell to raise ECF pH. Along with H^+, the corresponding anions also permeate. For example, the anion of HCl is Cl^-, which is relatively impermeable. Consequently, for each H^+ that enters the cell, one K^+ ion leaves the cell in order to maintain electroneutrality. This causes hyperkalemia. On the other hand, organic anions such as β-hydroxybutyrate or lactate move readily with H^+, so that electroneutrality is maintained and K^+ does not exit. Therefore, hyperkalemia does not usually occur with organic acidoses.

Question 3 What would be the total body K^+ in this patient?

The answer is low Osmotic diuresis due to hyperglycemia causes large urinary losses of Na^+, K^+, and water. Generally, the reabsorption of these electrolytes and water in the proximal tubule is decreased. As a result, more filtrate is delivered to the distal nephron, and K^+ secretion is enhanced. Secondary hyperaldosteronism due to volume loss and delivery of nonreabsorbable ketoanions further augment K^+ excretion. Thus, a large K^+ deficit occurs in diabetic subjects. Hypokalemia occurred in this patient because of insulin and volume administration.

Since phosphate is also lost in the urine and transcellularly exported following insulin, K-phosphate is usually administered during the treatment of diabetic ketoacidosis.

Question Match the following drugs that cause hyperkalemia and their mechanism of action (use all applicable answers).

Drug	Mechanism of action
1. Digitalis intoxication	(A) Transports K$^+$ out of cells
2. Arginine	(B) Inhibits Na/K-ATPase activity
3. Amiloride, trimethoprim, pentamidine	(C) Decrease aldosterone synthesis
4. ACE-Is	(D) Decrease renin/aldosterone
5. Nonsteroidal anti-inflammatory drugs	(E) Inhibits Na$^+$ channel in principal cells
6. Salt substitutes	(F) Increase K$^+$ intake
7. Heparin	(G) Decrease K$^+$ channel activity
8. Cyclosporine and tacrolimus	
9. Chan Su, toad skin, oleander	

ACE-Is angiotensin-converting enzyme inhibitors

Answers $1 = B, 2 = A, 3 = E, 4 = C, 5 = D, 6 = F, 7 = C, 8 = B, C$, and G, and $9 = B$. A large number of drugs have been shown to cause hyperkalemia by a variety of mechanisms. Na/K-ATPase transports three Na$^+$ ions out and two K$^+$ ions into the cell. Inhibition of this transport mechanism causes mild hyperkalemia in a euvolemic subject. Infusion of arginine causes shift of K$^+$ out of cells. Amiloride, trimethoprim, and pentamidine block Na$^+$ uptake by Na$^+$ channel (ENaC) in principal cells of the cortical collecting duct with resultant decrease in K$^+$ secretion by K$^+$ channel (ROMK). ACE-Is and heparin cause hypoaldosteronism and hyperkalemia. Nonsteroidal anti-inflammatory drugs inhibit renin production, resulting in decreased aldosterone synthesis and hyperkalemia. Hypertensive individuals who take salt substitutes develop hyperkalemia because of K$^+$ overload. Cyclosporine and tacrolimus commonly cause hyperkalemia by a variety of mechanisms, including a decrease in Na/K-ATPase activity and aldosterone synthesis as well as inhibition of K$_{ATP}$ channel activity by cyclosporine. Herbal medications such as Chan Su, toad skin, and oleander inhibit Na/K-ATPase activity and increase serum [K$^+$], particularly in CKD patients.

Suggested Reading

1. Evans KJ, Greenberg A. Hyperkalemia: a review. J Intens Care Med. 2005;20:272–90.
2. Mount DB. Disorders of potassium balance. In: Skorecki K, et al., editors. Brenner & Rector's the kidney. 10th ed. Philadelphia: Elsevier; 2016. p. 559–600.
3. Lehnhardt A, Kemper MJ. Pathogenesis, diagnosis and management of hyperkalemia. Pediatr Nephrol. 2011;26:377–84.
4. Nyirenda M, Tang JI, Padfield PL, et al. Hyperkalemia. BMJ. 2009;339:1019–24.
5. Palmer BF. A physiologic-based approach to the evaluation of a patient with hyperkalemia. Am J Kidney Dis. 2010;56:387–93.
6. Segal A. Potassium and dyskalemias. In: Mount DB, Sayegh MH, Singh AJ, editors. Core concepts in the disorders of fluid, electrolytes and acid-base balance. New York: Springer; 2013. p. 49–102.

7. Shingarev R, Allon M. A physiologic-based approach to the treatment of acute hyperkalemia. Am J Kidney Dis. 2010;56:578–84.
8. Weir MR. Current and future treatment options for managing hyperkalemia. Kidney Int Suppl. 2016;6:29–34.
9. Weisberg LS. Management of severe hyperkalemia. Crit Care Med. 2008;36:3246–51.

Disorders of Calcium: Physiology

17

General Features

Calcium (Ca^{2+}) is the most abundant divalent ion in the body. Approximately 1.2–1.3 kg of Ca^{2+} is present in a 70 kg individual. Of this amount, 99% is present in the bone in the form of hydroxyapatite ($Ca_{10}(PO_4)_6 (OH)_2$), and the remaining 1% is found in the teeth, soft tissues, plasma, and cells. The plasma (serum) Ca^{2+} concentration (abbreviated as [Ca^{2+}]) is 10 mg/dL (range 8.5–10.2 mg/dL) and circulates in three forms. About 50% of Ca^{2+} exists as free or ionized form. Approximately 40% of Ca^{2+} is bound to proteins, mostly to albumin and to some extent globulins. The remaining 10% is complexed with anions such as phosphate, bicarbonate, and citrate (Table 17.1). Only the ionized and anion-complexed Ca^{2+} is filtered at the glomerulus. Protein-bound Ca^{2+} is not filtered. Only the ionized (free) Ca^{2+} is physiologically active. The free intracellular [Ca^{2+}] is about 10,000-fold lower than the extracellular free [Ca^{2+}]; this concentration gradient is maintained by Ca^{2+}-specific channels, Ca-ATPase, and a Na/Ca exchanger.

Ca^{2+} plays a significant role in cellular metabolic functions, such as muscle and nerve contraction, activation of enzyme, blood coagulation, and cell growth. Consequently, low plasma [Ca^{2+}] (hypocalcemia) or high plasma [Ca^{2+}] (hypercalcemia) may lead to severe cellular dysfunction.

Table 17.1 Circulating form of Ca^{2+} in the body

Form	mg/dL	Percentage of total
Total	10	100
Ionized	5	50
Protein-bound	4	40
Complexed	1	10

© Springer Science+Business Media LLC 2018
A.S. Reddi, *Fluid, Electrolyte and Acid-Base Disorders*,
DOI 10.1007/978-3-319-60167-0_17

Ca²⁺ Homeostasis

The plasma [Ca²⁺] is maintained within narrow limits by the interplay between resorption and formation of Ca²⁺ by the intestine, bone, and kidney (Fig. 17.1). The daily intake of Ca²⁺ is approximately 1,000 mg. Of this amount, about 400 mg are absorbed by the intestine, and 200 mg are secreted into the intestine from the extracellular Ca²⁺ pool. This 200 mg of secreted Ca²⁺ plus the nonreabsorbed Ca²⁺ from the diet (600 mg) to a total of 800 mg are eliminated in the feces. Formation (deposition) and resorption (mobilization) of 500 mg also occur in the bone. Therefore, the bone does not lose Ca²⁺ in a normal state. In the kidney, the filtered Ca²⁺ amounts to 60% of the total Ca²⁺. If the GFR is 180 L per day and filterable Ca²⁺ is 60% (6 mg/dL or 60 mg/L), the filtered load of Ca²⁺ is 10,800 mg (60 mg/L × 180 L = 10,800 mg). In order to maintain Ca²⁺ balance, 98% of the filtered Ca²⁺ must be reabsorbed by the kidney, and only 200 mg are excreted in the urine. Thus, the interplay among the three organs maintains plasma Ca²⁺ level within a narrow range.

Three hormones and a Ca²⁺-sensing receptor system maintain Ca²⁺ homeostasis:

1. Ca²⁺-sensing receptor
2. Parathyroid hormone (PTH)
3. Active vitamin D_3 (1,25-dihydroxycholecalciferol, or calcitriol or $1,25(OH)_2D_3$)
4. Calcitonin

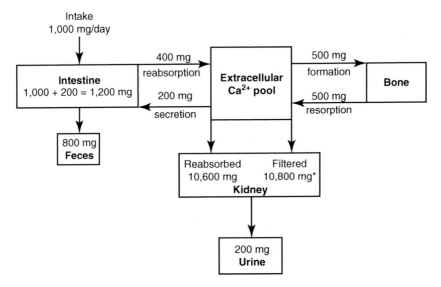

Fig. 17.1 Processes involved in Ca²⁺ homeostasis in an adult subject. (*Of 10 mg/dL plasma Ca²⁺, only 6 mg/dL are filtered which amount to the filtered load of 10,800 mg/day (60 mg/L × 180 L = 10,800 mg) (Modified with permission from Nordin [8])

Ca²⁺-Sensing Receptor (CaSR)

Ca^{2+}-sensing receptor (CaSR) is expressed in the plasma membranes of cells that are involved in Ca^{2+} homeostasis. Its expression is highest in parathyroid glands and kidneys. The presence of CaSR has also been demonstrated in the bone cells, thyroid, brain, gut, and other organs.

The CaSR exerts three important functions on parathyroid glands: (1) PTH synthesis, (2) PTH secretion, and (3) parathyroid cellular proliferation. In humans, the CaSR senses the circulating levels of Ca^{2+} and translates this information via a complex of signaling pathways either to inhibit or stimulate secretion of PTH by chief cells of the parathyroid gland. Low serum Ca^{2+} levels inhibit the CaSR so that PTH is secreted, whereas high levels of Ca^{2+} activate the CaSR and inhibit PTH secretion.

In the kidney, activation of CaSR in the thick ascending limb of Henle's loop inhibits paracellular transport of Ca^{2+}, resulting in hypercalciuria. In the inner medullary collecting duct, CaSR is localized in the endosomes that contain vasopressin-regulated water channel, aquaporin 2. Activation of CaSR causes a reduction in vasopressin-stimulated water absorption, resulting in defective urinary concentration. This results in polyuria, particularly in conditions of hypercalcemia due to which the development of nephrocalcinosis and nephrolithiasis is prevented.

In the bone, CaSR inhibits the formation and activity of osteoclasts and stimulates the osteoblasts. In thyroid C cells, activation of CaSR by high serum Ca^{2+} stimulates the secretion of calcitonin, which promotes bone formation by taking up Ca^{2+}. Thus, CaSR plays an important role in Ca^{2+} homeostasis.

PTH

Active PTH is a large polypeptide containing 84 amino acids. PTH is secreted by the parathyroid gland. The secretion of PTH is primarily regulated by extracellular ionized Ca^{2+}. As little as a 10% increase or a decrease in plasma $[Ca^{2+}]$ either inhibits or stimulates PTH secretion. This response of PTH to changes in Ca^{2+} is mediated, as stated earlier, by CaSR. Other modulators of PTH secretion are calcitriol and Mg^{2+}. Calcitriol and hypomagnesemia inhibit both the secretion and synthesis of PTH. PTH regulates plasma $[Ca^{2+}]$ by three mechanisms: (1) it stimulates bone resorption (demineralization) by activating osteoclasts (cells that break down bone mineral); (2) it increases the synthesis of calcitriol by enhancing the activity of 25-hydroxycholecalciferol-1α–hydroxylase (1,α-hydroxylase); and (3) it increases Ca^{2+} reabsorption in the distal convoluted tubule. Calcitriol increases bone resorption in concert with PTH and also promotes Ca^{2+} absorption from the intestine.

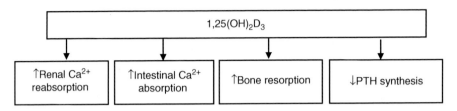

Fig. 17.2 Effects of 1,25(OH)$_2$D$_3$ on Ca^{2+} homeostasis

Active Vitamin D$_3$ (1,25-Dihydroxycholecalciferol or 1,25(OH)$_2$D$_3$ or Calcitriol)

As stated earlier, calcitriol is an active form of vitamin D$_3$. It is formed from 25-dihydroxyvitamin D (25(OH)D$_3$) by the enzyme 1,α-hydroxylase in the proximal tubule cells. PTH stimulates the activity of 1,α-hydroxylase, whereas hypercalcemia and hyperphosphatemia inhibit this enzyme. In the intestine, calcitriol promotes Ca^{2+} absorption.

Active vitamin D$_3$ regulates Ca^{2+} metabolism by four mechanisms: (1) it stimulates renal Ca^{2+} reabsorption in distal convoluted tubule (see below); (2) it increases intestinal absorption of Ca^{2+}; (3) it increases the release of Ca^{2+} from bone (resorption); and (4) it inhibits PTH synthesis independent of serum [Ca^{2+}]. Figure 17.2 shows these effects of active vitamin D$_3$ on Ca^{2+} homeostasis.

Intestinal absorption of Ca^{2+} is influenced by certain physiologic conditions. Normal pregnancy and growth are associated with increased absorption, whereas aging causes decreased absorption. Foods containing oxalates and phytates also decrease intestinal absorption of Ca^{2+}.

Calcitonin

Calcitonin is a 32-amino acid peptide synthesized by the parafollicular or C cells of the thyroid gland. It is released in response to elevated plasma [Ca^{2+}]. Calcitonin inhibits bone resorption directly by inhibiting the activity of osteoclasts.

Thus, it is the coordinated interactions between hormones, CaSR and the intestinal absorption, bone turnover, and renal reabsorption that maintain the plasma [Ca^{2+}] within narrow limits.

Defense Against Low and High Plasma [Ca^{2+}]

Several physiologic adaptations occur during low or high plasma [Ca^{2+}] to maintain normocalcemia. When plasma [Ca^{2+}] is low, CaSR on the parathyroid glands senses hypocalcemia and stimulates PTH synthesis and secretion. In turn, PTH acts on the bone, kidney, and intestine to increase plasma [Ca^{2+}] to normal. The opposite sequence of events occurs when plasma [Ca^{2+}] is increased. CaSR plays a significant role in hypercalcemia, as its stimulation by hypercalcemia enhances hypercalciuria by the kidney.

Renal Handling of Ca^{2+}

As stated earlier, only ionized and anion-complexed Ca^{2+} is filtered. Approximately 65% of the filtered Ca^{2+} is reabsorbed by the proximal tubule, 25% by the thick ascending limb of Henle's loop, 5–10% by the distal convoluted tubule, and 5% by the collecting duct. Less than 2% of Ca^{2+} is excreted in the urine. The thin descending and ascending limbs of Henle's loop do not participate in Ca^{2+} transport.

Proximal Tubule

In the proximal tubule, Ca^{2+} reabsorption is mostly passive in conjunction with Na$^+$ and water reabsorption. Na$^+$ and water reabsorption creates a modest concentration gradient and lumen-positive potential difference that drive Ca^{2+} via the paracellular pathway.

Thick Ascending Limb

In the thick ascending limb of Henle's loop, the lumen is electropositive due to Na/K/2Cl cotransporter activity and backleak of K$^+$ via ROMK. This causes Ca^{2+} to diffuse passively via the paracellular pathway into the blood.

Distal and Connecting Tubule

In the distal convoluted and connecting tubules, Ca^{2+} transport is an active process and therefore occurs against an electrochemical gradient. These segments are the major regulatory sites for Ca^{2+} excretion in the urine. The mechanism of Ca^{2+} transport in these segments has recently been demonstrated. Ca^{2+} enters the cell through the apical transient receptor potential vanilloid 5 (TRPV5) Ca^{2+} channel. Inside the cell, calbindin-D$_{28K}$ binds Ca^{2+} and transports it to the basolateral membrane (Fig. 17.3). Another calbindin-D$_{9K}$ also participates in this transport. Both calbindins are dependent on vitamin D.

Fig. 17.3 Possible cellular
mechanisms for Ca²⁺ entry
into the cell via TRPV5
channel in the distal
convoluted and connecting
tubule. The transcellular
exit of Ca²⁺ seems to occur
via Ca-ATPase (*1*) and Na/
Ca exchanger (*2*). *Thick
broken arrow* indicates
Ca²⁺ entry via TRPV5

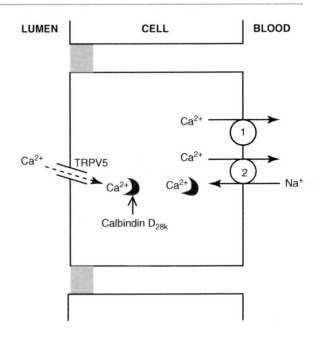

Ca²⁺ exit across the basolateral membrane is mediated by two transport systems:
Ca-ATPase and Na/Ca exchanger. Calbindin-D_{9K} stimulates Ca-ATPase.

Collecting Duct

Ca²⁺ transport in the collecting duct is minor compared to the other segments of the
nephron. The transport may be active in the cortical collecting duct and passive in
the medullary segment.

Factors Influencing Ca²⁺ Transport

A number of factors, as listed in Table 17.2, either decrease or increase Ca²⁺
reabsorption in various segments of the nephron. As a result, the urinary excretion of Ca²⁺ varies. Among the hormones, PTH is an important regulator. It promotes Ca²⁺ reabsorption by the thick ascending limb of Henle's loop and the
distal convoluted tubule. The effects of PTH on the proximal tubule are variable
(increase, decrease, or no effect). Calcitonin also has variable effects. Vitamin D

Table 17.2 Effect of various factors on Ca^{2+} reabsorption in the nephron

Factor	PCT	TALH	DCT	Urinary excretion
PTH	Variable	↑	↑	↓
Vitamin D	?	No effect	↑	↓
Hypercalcemia	↓	↓	↓	↑
Volume expansion	↓	?	↓	↑
Volume contraction	↑	?	?	↓
Metabolic acidosis	↓	?	↓	↑
Metabolic alkalosis	↑	?	↑	↓
Loop diuretics	?	↓	No effect	↑
Thiazide diuretics (acute)	?	?	↑	↑
Thiazide diuretics (chronic)	↑	No effect	?	↓
Amiloride	No effect	No effect	↑	↓

PCT proximal convoluted tubule, *TALH* thick ascending limb of Henle's loop, *DCT* distal convoluted tubule, *PTH* parathyroid hormone, ↑ increase, ↓ decrease

may stimulate Ca^{2+} reabsorption in the distal convoluted tubule by stimulating the production of Ca^{2+}-binding proteins (calbindins). Hypercalcemia decreases Ca^{2+} reabsorption via a decrease in PTH secretion and enhances Ca^{2+} excretion. Volume expansion reduces Ca^{2+} reabsorption, whereas volume contraction promotes Ca^{2+} reabsorption.

Metabolic acidosis inhibits Ca^{2+} reabsorption in the proximal and distal convoluted tubule and promotes Ca^{2+} excretion. Metabolic alkalosis has an opposite effect. Diuretics influence Ca^{2+} reabsorption and its excretion. Most importantly, loop diuretics such as furosemide and bumetanide inhibit Ca^{2+} reabsorption in the thick ascending limb of Henle's loop thereby promoting Ca^{2+} excretion. Acute administration of thiazides promotes Ca^{2+} reabsorption in the distal convoluted tubule. The urinary excretion of Ca^{2+} may transiently increase due to marked natriuresis. Conversely, chronic administration of thiazides causes hypocalciuria due to enhanced Ca^{2+} reabsorption in the proximal tubule caused by volume contraction. Amiloride also promotes Ca^{2+} reabsorption in the distal convoluted tubule.

Factors Influencing Ca²⁺ Channel (TRPV5)

Studies have shown that a number of factors influence TRPV5, resulting in changes in Ca^{2+} reabsorption in the distal convoluted and connecting tubule (Table 17.3).

Table 17.3 Factors that increase and decrease TRPV5 activity

Increased TRPV5 activity	Decreased TRPV5 activity
PTH	Hypercalcemia
Active vitamin D$_3$	Metabolic acidosis
KLOTHO (antiaging hormone) Metabolic alkalosis	
Hypocalcemia	
WNK4	

Suggested Reading

1. Berndt TJ, Thompson JR, Kumar R. The regulation of calcium, magnesium, and phosphate excretion by the kidney. In: Skorecki K, et al., editors. Brenner & Rector's the kidney. 10th ed. Philadelphia: Elsevier; 2016. p. 185–203.
2. Bindels RJM, Hoenderop GJ, Biber J. Transport of calcium, magnesium, and phosphate. In: Taal MW, Chertow GM, Marsden PA, editors. Brenner & Rector's the kidney. 9th ed. Philadelphia: Saunders; 2012. p. 226–51.
3. Hoenderrop JG, Nilius B, Bindels RJM. Calcium absorption across epithelia. Phys Rev. 2005;85:373–422.
4. Mensenkamp AR, Hoenderop JGJ, Bindels RJM. Recent advances in renal tubular calcium absorption. Curr Opin Nephrol Hypertens. 2006;15:524–9.
5. Riccardi D, Brown EM. Physiology and pathophysiology of the calcium-sensing receptor in the kidney. Am J Physiol Renal Physiol. 2010;298:F485–F99.
6. Riccardi D, Kemp PJ. The calcium-sensing receptor beyond extracellular calcium homeostasis: conception, development, adult physiology, and disease. Ann Rev Physiol. 2012;74:271–97.
7. Trepiccione F. Capasso G. Calcium homeostasis. In: Turner N, et al., editors. Oxford textbook of clinical nephrology. 4th ed. Oxford: Oxford University Press; 2016. p. 231–42.
8. Nordin BEC, editor. Calcium, phosphate, and magnesium metabolism. Edinburgh: Churchill Livingstone; 1976.

Disorders of Calcium: Hypocalcemia

18

As stated in Chap. 17, Ca^{2+} homeostasis is maintained by the interrelationship among intestinal absorption, bone turnover, and renal excretion. Alterations in any one of these functions may lead to changes in the extracellular $[Ca^{2+}]$. A plasma $[Ca^{2+}]$ <8.5 mg/dL defines hypocalcemia.

Hypocalcemia is less common than hypercalcemia, and the causes are shown in Table 18.1. Since Ca^{2+} is bound to albumin, a decrease in plasma albumin concentration may cause hypocalcemia. For each gram decrease of albumin from normal (i.e., 4.0 g/dL), $[Ca^{2+}]$ decreases by 0.8 mg/dL.

Table 18.1 Causes of hypocalcemia

Cause	Mechanism
Pseudohypocalcemia	MRI with contrast agents (gadodiamide and gadoversetamide) interferes with colorimetric determination of Ca^{2+}
Low serum albumin levels (for each gram decrease in serum albumin from 4.0 g/dL, serum Ca^{2+} decreases by 0.8 mg/dL)	Decreased synthesis (poor intake, liver disease, infection, or inflammation)
	Nephrotic syndrome
	Protein-losing enteropathy
Low or absent parathyroid hormone (PTH) levels	
Hypoparathyroidism	
Genetic	
Parathyroid agenesis	Branchial dysembryogenesis (DiGeorge's syndrome)
Autoimmune	Polyglandular autoimmune disorder type 1
Activating mutations of CaSR	An autosomal dominant disorder characterized by hypocalcemia, low PTH levels, neonatal seizures, and carpopedal spasm
Acquired	
Parathyroid destruction	Parathyroid surgery, infiltrative diseases, irradiation

(continued)

© Springer Science+Business Media LLC 2018
A.S. Reddi, *Fluid, Electrolyte and Acid-Base Disorders*,
DOI 10.1007/978-3-319-60167-0_18

Table 18.1 (continued)

Cause	Mechanism
Hypomagnesemia	Inhibition of PTH secretion and/or PTH resistance to bone resorption
Neonatal hypocalcemia	Functional maternal hypoparathyroidism; maternal hypercalcemia with suppression of PTH levels
High PTH levels	
Pseudohypoparathyroidism	Resistance to PTH action
Disturbance in vitamin D metabolism	
Decreased oral intake	Malnutrition
Decreased intestinal absorption	Gastrectomy, intestinal bypass
Decreased production of $25(OH)D_3$	Liver disease
Decreased synthesis of $1,25(OH)_2D_3$	Renal failure, hyperphosphatemia (inhibits 1α-hydroxylase)
Increased urinary loss of $25(OH)D_3$	Nephrotic syndrome
Drugs	
Anticonvulsants	Increased metabolism of $25(OH)D_3$, decreased Ca^{2+} release from bone, decreased intestinal absorption of Ca^{2+}
Bisphosphonates	Inhibit bone resorption ($\downarrow$ osteoclast activity)
Denosumab	Inhibits bone resorption
Calcitonin	Inhibits bone resorption
Citrate	Chelates Ca^{2+}
Foscarnet, fluoride	Chelate Ca^{2+}
Antibiotics	Hypocalcemia (consequence of hypomagnesemia)
Cinacalcet	Inhibition of PTH secretion by activation of CaSR
Phosphate binders (calcium acetate)	Bind phosphate in gut and decrease Ca^{2+} absorption
Miscellaneous	
Pancreatitis	Ca^{2+} deposition at sites of fat necrosis as Ca^{2+} soaps, relative hypoparathyroidism, high glucagon levels, hypomagnesemia, and shift of Ca^{2+} from extracellular to intracellular compartment by catecholaminess
Sepsis and toxic shock syndrome	Exact mechanism unknown (TNF, IL-2 may mediate)
Hungry bone syndrome	Ca^{2+} uptake by bones following parathyroid surgery
Increased osteoblastic activity	Hypocalcemia seen in breast and prostate cancer is due to consumption for bone formation and due to increased metastatic osteoblast activity
Chronic respiratory alkalosis or metabolic alkalosis	Binding of Ca^{2+} to albumin, resulting in hypocalcemia
Rhabdomyolysis or tumor lysis syndrome	Hyperphosphatemia-induced hypocalcemia

MRI magnetic resonance imaging, *PTH* parathyroid hormone, *TNF* tumor necrosis factor, *IL* interleukin, *CaSR* Ca^{2+}-sensing receptor

Some Specific Causes of Hypocalcemia

Hypoparathyroidism

- Hypoparathyroidism can be either genetic or acquired. Genetic hypoparathyroidism includes developmental and autoimmune hypoparathyroidism and mutations in Ca^{2+}-sensing receptor.
- Developmental hypoparathyroidism occurs in the neonates because of branchial dysembryogenesis, resulting in absent parathyroid glands and thymus.
- A common example is DiGeorges's syndrome, which is characterized by hypocalcemia, cardiac abnormalities, and a defect in T-cell-mediated immunity.
- Autoimmune hypoparathyroidism, called polyglandular autoimmune syndrome type I, is due to mutations in the autoimmune regulatory gene (AIRE) on chromosome 21q22.3.
- Characterized by a triad of hypothyroidism, hypoadrenalism, and mucocutaneous candidiasis.
- Activating mutations of Ca^{2+}-sensing receptor (CaSR) is characterized by autoantibodies to CaSR, hypocalcemia, hypomagnesemia, hypercalciuria, and low to normal parathyroid hormone (PTH) level.
- Treatment of the above three conditions of genetic hypoparathyroidism includes calcium supplements and sufficient vitamin D to suppress symptoms. Thiazide diuretics and injectable PTH have been used with variable results.
- Acquired hypoparathyroidism can be either surgical or nonsurgical.
- Surgical resection of thyroid (cancer, Grave's disease, head and neck cancer) or parathyroid (adenoma or hyperplasia) glands is the most common cause of hypoparathyroidism in adults.
- Transient hypocalcemia is extremely common after surgery because of Ca^{2+} uptake by bones (hungry bone syndrome). This syndrome is seen in hyperparathyroid patients with severe hypercalcemia. Patients need IV calcium gluconate or chloride and active vitamin D_3 to improve symptomatic hypocalcemia.
- Nonsurgical causes include infiltrative diseases such as hemochromatosis, thalassemia major, Wilson's disease, infections, or metastatic cancers. Irradiation to the neck also presents with hypoparathyroidism.

Pseudohypoparathyroidism (PsHPT)

- PsHPT is a condition of PTH resistance. The first documented cases were described by Albright and colleagues in 1942. These patients were hypocalcemic and hyperphosphatemic and failed to respond to infusion of bovine PTH. These patients had several facial and skeletal abnormalities, including obesity, short stature, brachydactyly, and mental retardation. Subsequent studies have shown that these patients have elevated PTH levels. These features are now considered characteristics of the disorder called *Albright's hereditary osteodystrophy* (AHO).

- AHO results from loss-of-function mutation of the GNAS1 gene, which encodes the stimulatory G protein α-subunit.
- PsHPT is considered heterogeneous with different clinical and biochemical features and is classified into types Ia, Ib, II, and pseudo-PsHPT.
- Patients with type Ia PsHPT are similar to those of AHO.
- Type Ib PsHPT patients have normal appearance but have resistance to PTH action.
- Patients with type II PsHPT have normal developmental features but hypocalcemic. PTH infusion causes normal excretion of cAMP, but urinary excretion of phosphate is decreased.
- Pseudo-PsHPT patients have characteristics similar to those of type Ia PsHPT, but without PTH resistance, because urinary excretions of cAMP and phosphate are normal to PTH infusion.
- Urinary cAMP response to the infusion of synthetic PTH is used to establish the diagnosis of PTH resistance.

Vitamin D Deficiency

- Vitamin D deficiency may be due to an absolute deficiency of vitamin D or an abnormality in vitamin D metabolism.
- Absolute deficiency is generally related to inadequate oral intake, lack of sun exposure, use of sunscreens, or fat malabsorption as vitamin D absorption is dependent on fat intake. Elderly are at particular risk for vitamin D deficiency.
- Altered metabolism due to medications and disease conditions seems to be the common cause of vitamin D deficiency (Table 18.1).
- Vitamin D-dependent rickets in children or osteomalacia in adults is a rare inborn error of vitamin D metabolism, resembling vitamin D deficiency.

Two types of vitamin D-dependent rickets have been described:

- Type I disease is inherited as an autosomal recessive disorder, which is due to defective activity of 1α-hydroxylase, caused by mutations in the gene of this enzyme. Patients are hypocalcemic with low calcitriol $(1,25(OH)_2D_3)$ levels and respond to calcitriol.
- Type II disorder is characterized by increased calcitriol levels but fails to respond to pharmacologic doses of calcitriol. These patients, therefore, have hypocalcemia due to calcitriol resistance. This resistance is caused by mutations in the vitamin D receptor.

Diagnosis

Step 1

- Obtain surgical history and good history regarding nutrition, medications, and inherited and developmental anomalies.

- Physical examination should focus on blood pressure (usually hypotension), bradycardia, and neurologic and ocular (cataracts) changes.

Step 2

- Rule out pseudohypocalcemia following magnetic resonance imaging (MRI) with contrast agents.

Step 3

- Establish true hypocalcemia by determining serum ionized Ca^{2+}.

Step 4

- Determine serum albumin, and correct Ca^{2+} for normal albumin concentration.

Step 5

- Measure serum Mg^{2+} and phosphate. Correct hypomagnesemia and hyperphosphatemia.

Step 6

- Review medications that alter $25(OH)D_3$ (calcifediol) metabolism, and change or choose alternative medications.

Step 7

- Check liver and renal functions.

Step 8

- Determine serum PTH and vitamin D status. Start vitamin D preparations for vitamin D deficiency.

Step 9

- If PTH is elevated, evaluate parathyroid glands. If PTH resistance is suspected, measure urinary cAMP levels in response to PTH infusion. Figure 18.1 shows the suggested diagnostic workup of a patient with hypocalcemia.

Table 18.2 shows some biochemical abnormalities found in various conditions of hypocalcemia.

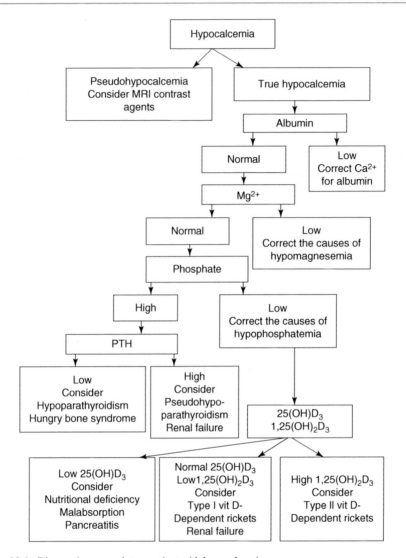

Fig. 18.1 Diagnostic approach to a patient with hypocalcemia

Table 18.2 Pertinent biochemical abnormalities in various hypocalcemic conditions

Disorder	Phosphate	PTH	25(OH)D₃	1,25(OH)₂D₃
Hypomagnesemia	$\uparrow$/N	$\downarrow$	N	$\downarrow$/N
Vitamin D deficiency	$\downarrow$	$\uparrow$	$\downarrow$	$\uparrow$/$\downarrow$/N
Hypoparathyroidism	$\uparrow$	$\downarrow$	N	$\downarrow$
Pseudohypoparathyroidism	$\uparrow$	$\uparrow$	N	$\downarrow$
Liver failure	$\downarrow$	$\uparrow$	$\downarrow$	$\downarrow$/N
Renal failure	$\uparrow$	$\uparrow$	N	$\downarrow$
Nephrotic syndrome	$\downarrow$	$\uparrow$	$\downarrow$	$\downarrow$/N
Vitamin D-dependent rickets I	$\downarrow$	$\uparrow$	$\uparrow$/N	$\downarrow$
Vitamin D-dependent rickets II	$\downarrow$	$\uparrow$	$\uparrow$/N	$\uparrow$/N

$\uparrow$ increased, $\downarrow$ decreased, *N* normal, *PTH* parathyroid hormone

Table 18.3 Clinical manifestations of hypocalcemia

Neuromuscular	Muscle weakness and fatigue
	Perioral, finger, and toe tingling
	Chvostek's sign (tapping over facial nerve next to ear elicits tetany or facial twitching)
	Trousseau's sign (carpopedal spasm: inflation of blood pressure cuff to 20 mm Hg above systolic pressure for 3 min elicits flexion of the wrist, thumb, and metacarpophalangeal joints with flexion of fingers)
Cardiovascular	Prolonged QT interval
	Arrhythmias
	Hypotension
	Cardiomyopathy with congestive heart failure
Central nervous system	Altered mental status
	Irritability
	Pseudotumor cerebri
	Tonic–clonic seizures
	Vascular calcification of basal ganglia

Clinical Manifestations

The clinical manifestations depend on the severity of hypocalcemia and the duration of its onset. Also, associated conditions such as alkaline pH, hypomagnesemia, and hypokalemia may precipitate the sudden onset of signs and symptoms of hypocalcemia. Usually, the symptoms are related to neuromuscular, cardiac, and central nervous systems. Table 18.3 summarizes the signs and symptoms of hypocalcemia.

Treatment

Acute Hypocalcemia

- Signs and symptoms of acute hypocalcemia usually occur in hospital settings: following thyroid, parathyroid, or neck surgery, during transfusion of citrated blood, and during plasma exchange.
- Intravenous *calcium gluconate* (1 g available as 10% in a 10 mL ampule) is the treatment of choice for symptomatic hypocalcemia.
- Each gram of calcium gluconate contains 93 mg of elemental Ca^{2+}.
- Initially, one to two ampules of calcium gluconate in 50 mL of 5% dextrose should be given over a period of 10–20 min, followed by 0.3–1 mg of elemental Ca^{2+}/kg/h, if necessary. Once symptoms improve, the patient can be started on oral Ca^{2+} tablets (Table 18.4).
- In order to increase total serum Ca^{2+} by 2–3 mg/dL, a 70 kg patient requires 1 g of elemental Ca^{2+} (approximately ten ampules of calcium gluconate).
- One gram of *calcium chloride* (10%) contains 273 mg of elemental Ca^{2+}; however, it is not always preferred because of its unbearable irritation to veins. However, it can be used to treat severe hypocalcemia in an extremely symptomatic patient.

Table 18.4 Oral calcium preparations

Compound	Tablet size (mg)	Elemental Ca²⁺ (mg)
Calcium gluconate	500	45
Calcium carbonate	1250	500
Calcium lactate	650	84
Calcium citrate	950	200
Calcium phosphate	1565	600
Calcium acetate	668	167
Calcium glubionate	5 mL	115 mg

Table 18.5 Oral vitamin D preparations

Name	Abbreviation	Trade name	Effective dose
Cholecalciferol	Vitamin D₃		400–1,000 U/day
Ergocalciferol	Vitamin D₂	Calciferol	Dietary deficiency: 400–1,000 U/day
			Vitamin D deficiency: 25,000–50,000 U 3×/week
Calcifediol	25(OH)D₃	Calderol	20–50 µg 3×/week or once a day
Dihydrotachysterol	DHT	Dihydrotachysterol	0.1–1 mg/day
Calcitriol	1,25(OH)₂D₃	Rocaltrol	0.25–2 µg/day
Paricalcitol	1-nor-1α-25(OH)₂D₃	Zemplar	1–2 µg/day
Doxercalciferol	1α-(OH)D₃	Hectorol	1–3.5 µg/day

- One gram of *calcium gluceptate* (22% solution in 5 mL ampule) contains 90 mg of elemental Ca^{2+}.
- If hypomagnesemia is the underlying cause for hypocalcemia, IV magnesium sulfate (8 mEq) should be given.
- Hyperphosphatemia-induced hypocalcemia responds to phosphate binders or hemodialysis.
- For patients immediately following parathyroid surgery owing to primary hyperparathyroidism or hyperparathyroidism with renal osteodystrophy in chronic kidney disease stage 5, either calcitriol (Rocaltrol) 1–2 µg orally or IV Calcijex 1–2 µg along with IV calcium supplements may be necessary. Once the patient is stable, any oral vitamin D should be started as indicated (Table 18.5).

Chronic Hypocalcemia

- Treatment is aimed at correcting the cause, if possible.
- Oral calcium supplementation (500–1,500 mg elemental Ca^{2+}) and calcitriol 0.5–1 µg/day are generally used for patients with hypoparathyroidism or PTH resistance, chronic kidney disease, and osteomalacia.
- A few patients with hypoparathyroidism may benefit from thiazide diuretics.

- For patients with nutritional vitamin D deficiency, either cholecalciferol (effective dose 400–1,000 U/day) or ergocalciferol (effective dose 25,000–50,000 U three times/week) can be used. For many patients, lower doses may be sufficient.
- Maintain serum $[Ca^{2+}]$ slightly below normal to avoid hypercalciuria and subsequent nephrolithiasis.

Study Questions

Case 1 A 46-year-old hemodialysis-dependent woman is admitted for parathyroidectomy. She has been on maintenance hemodialysis for 6 years. She is noncompliant to diet and medications. She is normotensive. Her only complaint is bone pain. Pertinent laboratory results: serum $[Ca^{2+}]$ 12.4 mg/dL, phosphate 8.2 mg/dL, and PTH 3,940 pg/mL. She could not tolerate cinacalcet because of gastrointestinal problems. A sestamibi scan of parathyroid glands shows bilateral adenoma. She had a total parathyroidectomy. Postoperative serum $[Ca^{2+}]$ was 4.2 mg/dL with ionized Ca^{2+} 1.9 mg/dL. She complained of tingling and paresthesia of lower extremities. She had positive Trousseau's and Chvostek's signs.

Question 1 How would you manage her acute hypocalcemia?

Answer She developed hungry bone syndrome because of Ca^{2+} uptake by bones. Also, osteoclastic activity is suppressed. As a result, she developed symptomatic hypocalcemia, which requires urgent treatment. The drug of choice is IV calcium gluconate (10%) dissolved in 5% dextrose over a period of 10–15 min, followed by 1 mg/kg/h of elemental Ca^{2+} orally until symptoms improve.

Question 2 Does this patient require calcitriol administration?

Answer Yes. She required Calcijex 1 μg infusion in 20–30 min, followed by oral calcitriol of 1 μg in a period of 24 h.

Question 3 How would you manage her chronic hypocalcemia?

Answer She required oral calcium supplementation and vitamin D. Since she was on hemodialysis, she was asked to take two to three tablets of calcium carbonate (elemental Ca^{2+} 1,000–1,500 mg) per day with 2 μg of IV Zemplar on dialysis days (three times/week).

Case 2 You are asked to see a 70-year-old woman, a nursing home resident, for a serum Ca^{2+} level of 7.2 mg/dL and phosphate level of 1.9 mg/dL. Serum albumin and Mg^{2+} levels are normal. Renal and liver functions, except for alkaline phosphatase, are normal. She has a history of type 2 diabetes, and her diabetes is controlled with diet. Other than bone pain, she does not have any complaints.

On physical examination, she appears tired. Blood pressure is 146/84 mmHg with a pulse rate of 82 beats/min. Trousseau's and Chvostek's signs are negative, but calf and thigh muscle tenderness is significant.

Question 1 What other laboratory tests are helpful in making appropriate diagnosis?

Answer Serum ionized Ca^{2+}, PTH, $25(OH)D_3$, and $1,25(OH)_2D_3$. Alkaline phosphatase is also helpful in this patient. The following values were obtained:

Test	Value	Range
Ionized Ca^{2+}	3.5 mg/dL	4.5–5.0 mg/dL
PTH	74 pg/mL	10–65 pg/mL
$25(OH)D_3$	10 ng/mL	>30 ng/mL
$1,25(OH)_2D_3$	80 pg/mL	20–75 pg/mL
Alkaline phosphatase	300 U/L	30–120 U/L

Question 2 Which one of the following is the MOST likely diagnosis?

(A) Hyperparathyroidism
(B) Pseudohypothyroidism
(C) Vitamin D deficiency
(D) Low Ca^{2+} intake
(E) Type 2 diabetes

The answer is C Elevated PTH, $1,25(OH)_2D_3$, and alkaline phosphatase levels are observed in hyperparathyroidism; however, hypercalcemia is frequently associated with this disease. Pseudohypoparathyroidism is characterized by elevated phosphate and PTH levels, normal $25(OH)D_3$, and reduced $1,25(OH)_2D_3$ levels (Table 18.2). Low Ca^{2+} intake does not cause hypocalcemia, as Ca^{2+} levels are maintained by bone resorption. Type 2 diabetes is associated with vitamin D deficiency, but other biochemical abnormalities observed in this patient are very unlikely caused by diabetes. Thus, options A, B, D, and E are incorrect.

Vitamin D deficiency is the diagnosis in this patient, because of low $25(OH)D_3$. Active vitamin D_3 ($1,25(OH)_2D_3$) levels may be normal, slightly elevated, or reduced. Normal levels may be seen when all $25(OH)D_3$ is metabolized to $1,25(OH)_2D_3$; low levels are seen in the elderly as 1,α-hydroxylase enzyme activity is reduced. High levels are seen in some patients secondary to hypophosphatemia-enhanced 1,α-hydroxylase enzyme activity.

In this patient, vitamin D deficiency is related to decreased sun exposure, age, and lack of sufficient intake of milk and milk products. Vitamin D deficiency has been reported in 50% of nursing home residents. Lack of vitamin D leads to decreased gut absorption of Ca^{2+} and phosphate. The resultant hypocalcemia stimulates PTH secretion, which in turn promotes phosphate excretion and hypophosphatemia. Elevated PTH also increases bone turnover, resulting in high alkaline phosphatase activity and bone pain.

Question 3 How would you treat her vitamin D deficiency?

Answer Since the patient is not symptomatic from hypocalcemia, she should receive oral calcium and vitamin D preparations. Calcium carbonate 1250 mg tablet twice daily (elemental Ca^{2+} 1,000 mg) and cholecalciferol 1000 U/day should be sufficient initially. The patient should be followed frequently (every 2 weeks) with Ca^{2+} and phosphate measurements and adjustment of medications as needed. PTH, $25(OH)D_3$, and $1,25\ (OH)_2D_3$ should be determined in 2–3 months.

Case 3 A 70-year-old man is admitted for a suspicious lung mass. His blood pressure (BP), physical examination, and laboratory data are normal except for a creatinine of 1.2 mg/dL (estimate glomerular filtration rate (eGFR) 60 mL/min). An electrocardiogram (EKG) is also normal. He has an MRI of his chest, which shows a well-demarcated mass. The next morning, you are called by the laboratory for serum Ca^{2+} level of 6.5 mg/dL with normal phosphate and albumin. The patient is asymptomatic.

Which one of the following choices is CORRECT regarding the evaluation of his hypocalcemia?

(A) Obtain an EKG.
(B) Call either an endocrinologist or nephrologist for evaluation of Ca^{2+}.
(C) Order ionized Ca^{2+}.
(D) Repeat Ca^{2+} immediately.
(E) None of the above.

The answer is C This is pseudohypocalcemia secondary to MRI contrast agents. Serum Ca^{2+} is usually measured by the colorimetric assay, which uses a color-producing agent. This agent binds to Ca^{2+} and changes color in relation to the Ca^{2+} concentration. Of the four MRI contrast agents, gadodiamide (Omniscan) and gadoversetamide (OptiMARK) compete with Ca^{2+} for the colorimetric reagent and chelate Ca^{2+}, leading to falsely low Ca^{2+} concentration. Hypocalcemia persists as long as the contrast agent is in the blood. This pseudohypocalcemia does not occur with the remaining contrast agents, namely, gadopentetate dimeglumine (Magnevist) or gadoteridol (ProHance). Once pseudohypocalcemia is recognized, an EKG and a consult to either an endocrinologist or nephrologist are not necessary. To clarify pseudohypocalcemia, one can order ionized Ca^{2+}, which is usually measured by ion-specific electrode method. Thus, option C is correct.

Case 4 A 71-year-old alcoholic man is admitted for profuse lower gastrointestinal (GI) bleed, requiring 12 units of packed red blood cells (RBCs) in 6 h. Hemoglobin improved, but BP is slightly low. Although he is alert and oriented, he complains of oral tingling. His serum Ca^{2+} dropped from 9.2 to 6.0 mg/dL with normal Mg^{2+} level. His ionized Ca^{2+} is at the lower limit of normal. His liver function tests are slightly elevated.

Which one of the following is the MOST possible cause of his hypocalcemia?

(A) Hypokalemia-induced hypocalcemia due to blood transfusion
(B) Hypocalcemia due to liver disease
(C) Hypocalcemia due to blood transfusion
(D) Hypocalcemia due to transfusion-related coagulopathy
(E) None of the above

The answer is C Except for C, other answers are incorrect. Stored blood is usually anticoagulated with citrate (3 g of citrate per unit). Although the healthy liver metabolizes 3 g of citrate every 5 min, he has a heavy load of citrate from packed RBCs. He has a mild liver disease, which may impair citrate metabolism and result in citrate toxicity. Although total Ca^{2+} determination may not be that helpful because of hemodilution related to massive transfusion, ionized Ca^{2+} is helpful.

Citrate toxicity causes tetany, prolonged QT interval, hypotension due to decreased peripheral vascular resistance, decreased myocardial contractility, and muscle tremors. Intravenous Ca^{2+} is the appropriate treatment of transfusion-induced hypocalcemia.

Generally hyperkalemia is the common abnormality with blood transfusion; however, hypokalemia is infrequently observed once metabolic alkalosis ensues because of conversion of citrate into HCO_3^-. Mild liver disease may not cause symptomatic hypocalcemia. Coagulopathy is also a complication of massive blood transfusion, but has no relationship to hypocalcemia.

Case 5 A 50-year-old man is admitted for impending alcohol withdrawal. He complains of tingling around his lips and generalized weakness. His BP is 150/88 mmHg with a pulse rate of 96 beats/min. Abnormal laboratory results include K^+ 2.8 mEq/L, Ca^{2+} 6.8 mg/dL, Mg^{2+} 1.4 mg/dL, phosphate 2.1 mg/dL, and albumin 3.2 g/dL. EKG shows prolonged QT interval.

Which one of the following treatments will relieve his oral tingling?

(A) Administration of KCl
(B) Administration of calcium gluconate
(C) Administration of magnesium sulfate ($MgSO_4$)
(D) Administration of 5% dextrose in water (D5W) with KCl
(E) Administration of KCl, calcium gluconate, and $MgSO_4$

The answer is C Hypokalemia, hypocalcemia, hypomagnesemia, and hypophosphatemia are typical electrolyte abnormalities in a patient with either acute or chronic alcoholism. There are several mechanisms for hypomagnesemia in an alcoholic patient, which in turn can cause hypokalemia and hypocalcemia.

Hypokalemia in an alcoholic patient may be due to poor dietary intake, respiratory alkalosis, diarrhea, β-adrenergic stimulation during alcohol withdrawal, and Mg^{2+} deficiency.

Hypocalcemia is caused by hypomagnesemia by two mechanisms. First, hypomagnesemia impairs PTH secretion, and second, hypomagnesemia causes skeletal resistance to PTH action. Both mechanisms result in low PTH and Ca^{2+} levels. Also, levels of $1,25(OH)_2D_3$ were found to be low in hypomagnesemia because of decreased conversion from $25(OH)D_3$.

Alcoholism causes hypophosphatemia by poor dietary intake, transcellular distribution due to respiratory alkalosis and glucose intake, and hypomagnesemia. Since hypomagnesemia is responsible for other electrolyte abnormalities, it is the Mg^{2+} administration that corrects hypokalemia, hypocalcemia, and hypophosphatemia. Thus, option C is correct.

Unlike hypocalcemia induced by Mg^{2+} deficiency, hypocalcemia that is associated with gentamicin-induced hypomagnesemia may not improve with Mg^{2+} alone.

Suggested Reading

1. Dumitru C, Wysolmerski J. Disorders of calcium metabolism. In: Alpern RJ, Moe OW, Caplan M, editors. Seldin and Giebisch's the kidney. Physiology and pathophysiology. 5th ed. San Diego: Academic Press (Elsevier); 2013. p. 2273–309.
2. Hariri A, Mount DB, Rastegar A. Disorders of calcium, phosphorus, and magnesium metabolism. In: Mount DB, Sayegh MH, Singh AJ, editors. Core concepts in the disorders of fluid, electrolytes and acid-base balance. New York: Springer; 2013. p. 103–46.
3. Hoorn EJ, Zietse R. Disorders of calcium and magnesium balance: a physiology-based approach. Pediatr Nephrol. 2013;28:1195–206. doi:10.1007/s00467-012-2350-2.
4. Smogorzewski MJ, Stubbs JR, Yu ASL. Disorders of calcium, magnesium, and phosphate balance. In: Skorecki K, et al., editors. Brenner & Rector's the kidney. 10th ed. Philadelphia: Elsevier; 2016. p. 601–35.

Disorders of Calcium: Hypercalcemia

19

Hypercalcemia is defined as serum $[Ca^{2+}]$ >10.2 mg/dL in an individual with normal serum albumin concentration. Generally severe hypercalcemia is considered when serum $[Ca^{2+}]$ is above 14 mg/dL. It is a common electrolyte disorder that is frequently encountered by the primary care physicians. Hypercalcemia affects multiple organs in the body, including the kidney, heart, brain, peripheral nerves, and gut. Although causes of hypercalcemia are varied, they fall into four major categories (Table 19.1): (1) hypercalcemia secondary to increased Ca^{2+} mobilization from the bone, (2) hypercalcemia due to increased absorption of Ca^{2+} from the gastrointestinal (GI) tract, (3) hypercalcemia due to decreased urinary excretion of Ca^{2+}, and (4) hypercalcemia due to medications.

Table 19.1 Causes of hypercalcemia

Cause	Mechanism
Hypercalcemia secondary to increased Ca^{2+} mobilization from the bone	
Primary hyperparathyroidism	Increased bone resorption
Multiple endocrine neoplasia I and 2A	
Pseudohyperparathyroidism	
Renal failure	
Secondary hyperparathyroidism	
Tertiary hyperparathyroidism	
During recovery phase of acute kidney injury	
Malignancy	
Hyperthyroidism	
Immobilization	
Addison disease	Hemoconcentration, ↑ albumin, bone resorption

(continued)

© Springer Science+Business Media LLC 2018
A.S. Reddi, *Fluid, Electrolyte and Acid-Base Disorders*,
DOI 10.1007/978-3-319-60167-0_19

Table 19.1 (continued)

Cause	Mechanism
Hypercalcemia due to increased absorption of Ca²⁺ from the GI tract	
Granulomatous diseases (sarcoidosis, tuberculosis, histoplasmosis, coccidioidomycosis, berylliosis, leprosy, silicone)	Increased production of calcitriol by elevated 1,α-hydroxylase activity and increased GI and renal absorption of Ca²⁺
Vitamin D intoxication	
Milk (calcium)-alkali syndrome	
Hypercalcemia due to decreased urinary excretion of Ca²⁺	
Thiazide diuretics	Increased Ca²⁺ reabsorption by the proximal tubule
Familial hypercalcemic hypocalciuria	Inactivating mutations of Ca²⁺-sensing receptor (CaSR)
Medications (other than thiazide diuretics)	
Lithium	Increased PTH secretion
Vitamin D	Increased GI absorption of Ca²⁺
Vitamin A	Increased bone resorption
Growth hormone	Unknown
Estrogens/antiestrogens	Increased bone resorption
	↓ sensitivity of parathyroids to Ca²⁺
Theophylline	β₂-agonist mediation

GI gastrointestinal tract, *PTH* parathyroid hormone

Some Specific Causes of Hypercalcemia

Primary Hyperparathyroidism

- Primary hyperparathyroidism (PHPT) is the most underlying and leading cause of hypercalcemia in the general population.
- More common in elderly women than men. Postmenopausal women are at increased risk for hypercalcemia.
- PHPT is due to a single adenoma in 80–85% and hyperplasia of four glands in 15–20%.
- Clinically, PHPT presents as mild hypercalcemia (see Clinical manifestations for definition) with minimal or no symptoms, moderate hypercalcemia (20–25%) with nephrolithiasis and recurrent stones, or severe hypercalcemia (5–19%) with symptoms such as renal disease, bone disease, or GI tract problems.
- Diagnosis is made by measuring serum PTH levels and electrolytes. PTH is at times normal but commonly elevated. Hypercalcemia, hypophosphatemia, hyperchloremic metabolic acidosis, elevated alkaline phosphatase, and occasionally elevated uric acid are observed. Elevated levels of creatinine and blood urea nitrogen (BUN) are common in untreated patients for many years. Hypercalciuria, hyperphosphaturia, and elevated urinary cyclic adenosine monophosphate (cAMP) levels are characteristics of PHPT.
- Bone disease, called osteitis fibrosa cystica, is due to generalized increase in osteoclastic activity with mobilization of Ca²⁺ and phosphate from the bone (bone resorption). Pathologic fractures of bones are frequently seen.

Table 19.2 Indications for surgery in asymptomatic primary hyperparathyroidism

Serum Ca^{2+} level >1 mg/dL above normal
GFR <60 mL/min
Reduced bone mineral density (T-score <−2.5 at any site)
History of fracture
Age <50 years

GFR glomerular filtration rate

- Standard therapy for severe and symptomatic (renal stones, bone disease, and severe hypercalcemia) PHPT is still surgery. However, surgery versus medical therapy for asymptomatic patients remains unclear.
- Preoperative localization of parathyroid glands is usually done with sestamibi scan, which has a specificity of 90%. Ultrasonography of the neck is also useful in some patients.
- Some asymptomatic patients with PHPT may have evidence of reduced bone mass and masked neurocognitive abnormalities. Such patients may benefit from surgery. The indications for surgery in asymptomatic patients have been revised and published [1]. Table 19.2 shows these indications.
- Hypercalciuria is deleted from previous indications because it is not considered a risk factor for stone formation.
- Asymptomatic patients older than 50 years of age should get bone density measurements for 1–2 years with follow-up of renal function and serum Ca^{2+} levels. Their 25-hydroxyvitamin D level should be maintained >25 ng/mL.
- For those who are not surgical candidates or refuse surgery, medical therapy is indicated. Four classes of medications are available:
  1. Ca^{2+}-sensing receptor (CaSR) agonist—cinacalcet. Activation of CaSR inhibits PTH secretion.
  2. Bisphosphonates. Many drugs are available, which do not influence PTH secretion, but maintain bone mineral density by inhibiting osteoclast activity.
  3. Estrogens and progestins. Many drugs are available, which reduce serum and urinary Ca^{2+} levels and bone resorption. Adverse effects are major concern for their infrequent use.
  4. Selective estrogen modulator—raloxifene. It reduces serum Ca^{2+} level and bone turnover, but side effects may limit its use.
- Determination of PTH by appropriate assay is extremely important in patients with PHPT and chronic kidney disease (see Study Questions).

Multiple Endocrine Neoplasia Type 1 and Type 2a

- Multiple endocrine neoplasia (MEN) Type 1
  - Includes tumors of the parathyroid, anterior pituitary, and pancreas.
  - Of these tumors, parathyroid tumors are more prevalent.
  - It is caused by mutations in the tumor suppressor gene encoding menin.
  - Hypercalcemia due to hyperparathyroidism develops in the second and third decades of life. Parathyroidectomy improves hypercalcemia.

- MEN Type 2a
  - Includes medullary carcinoma of the thyroid, pheochromocytoma, and hyperparathyroidism due to hyperplasia and adenoma of parathyroid glands.
  - It is caused by mutations in the RET proto-oncogene.
  - Clinically, patients with MEN type 2a-associated hyperparathyroidism behave similarly as patients with PHPT.
  - Removal of the thyroid and/or parathyroid glands improves hyperparathyroidism.

Jansen's Disease

- A rare hereditary disorder caused by activating mutations of the gene for PTH receptor. The disease is characterized by dwarfism, hypercalcemia, hypophosphatemia, and metaphyseal chondrodysplasia. It is also called pseudohyperparathyroidism.

Familial Hypocalciuric Hypercalcemia

- Familial hypocalciuric hypercalcemia (FHH) is characterized by mild hypercalcemia, hypermagnesemia, hypocalciuria (calcium/creatinine clearance ratio <0.01), hypophosphatemia, and normal to slightly elevated PTH levels.
- Higher Ca^{2+} levels are needed to inhibit PTH secretion.
- Patients are always asymptomatic even from childhood to adulthood.
- FHH is caused by inactivating mutations of CaSR and is inherited as an autosomal dominant disease.
- No treatment is necessary for asymptomatic patients with FHH. However, possible parathyroidectomy is considered in adult patients with relapsing pancreatitis and serum $[Ca^{2+}]$ >14 mg/dL.

Neonatal Severe Hyperparathyroidism

A homozygous form of FHH (born to both parents with FHH) is a disease of life-threatening hypercalcemia with massive hyperplasia of the parathyroid glands. It is a lethal disease unless total parathyroidectomy is done.

Renal Failure

Secondary Hyperparathyroidism
Appropriate increase in PTH secretion in response to hypocalcemia is called secondary hyperparathyroidism. It usually occurs in chronic kidney disease (CKD) stages 4–5. Mechanisms include hyperparathyroidism due to hyperplastic parathyroid glands, bone disease, calcium supplements, and vitamin D administration.

Tertiary Hyperparathyroidism
- Occurs in a subset of CKD (CKD 5 and dialysis) patients and following renal transplantation. Hyperparathyroidism persists despite adequate treatment with calcium salts and active vitamin D compounds.
- Polyclonal parathyroid cell proliferation and monoclonal hypertrophy of adenomatous-like tissue, leading to an increase in parathyroid mass and continuous secretion of PTH, seem to be the underlying mechanism for hyperparathyroidism.
- Following renal transplantation, serum Ca^{2+} levels follow a biphasic pattern with hypocalcemia during the postoperative period followed by hypercalcemia.
- Hypercalcemia persists due to slow regression of hyperplastic parathyroid gland and generation of calcitriol by the transplanted kidney. It improves slowly in 6 months.
- Medical management of tertiary hyperparathyroidism includes calcimimetics such as cinacalcet.
- Parathyroidectomy for this condition is indicated in those dialysis patients with refractory hypercalcemia, severe bone disease, refractory pruritis, calciphylaxis, and progressive extraskeletal calcification.

Acute Kidney Injury
- Hypercalcemia is seen during the diuretic phase of acute kidney injury (AKI).
- Although hypercalcemia is common with rhabdomyolysis, other causes of AKI may also be associated with its development.
- Mechanisms of hypercalcemia include release of Ca^{2+} from myonecrosis, improved renal function, synthesis of calcitriol, and bone resorption due to decreased PTH resistance.

Milk (Calcium)-Alkali Syndrome

- This syndrome was initially described in patients with peptic ulcer disease who consumed calcium salts and milk for many years. With the introduction of new drugs for peptic ulcer disease, the use of calcium salts and milk has decreased substantially. However, calcium salts alone or in combination with vitamin D are being used to prevent and/or treat osteoporosis. Thus, the incidence of milk-alkali syndrome is increasing recently.
- Since milk is not consumed to prevent peptic ulcer or bone disease, and calcium supplements are recommended, the preferable term may be *calcium-alkali* syndrome.
- Calcium-alkali syndrome is characterized by the triad of hypercalcemia, metabolic alkalosis, and some degree of renal insufficiency.
- The generation and maintenance of hypercalcemia is dependent on several factors: (1) sufficient intake of Ca^{2+} over several days to weeks with increase in intestinal absorption; (2) decreased glomerular filtration rate (GFR) with decreased filtered load of Ca^{2+}, resulting in hypercalcemia and hypocalciuria; (3) hypercalcemia-induced nephrogenic diabetes insipidus (DI) and volume

depletion; and (4) increased renal reabsorption of Ca^{2+} in the proximal tubule due to volume depletion. The latter two factors with metabolic alkalosis tend to maintain hypercalcemia.
- It is of interest to note that hypercalcemia develops even in the presence of suppressed PTH and $1,25(OH)_2D_3$.
- Hydration with normal saline initially will improve both calcium and metabolic alkalosis, but elevated creatinine may persist.

Malignancy

- Malignancy is the second leading cause of hypercalcemia, which occurs in 20–30% of patients. The most common malignancy associated with hypercalcemia is the lung (35%), followed by the breast (25%), hematologic (14%), and other organs (3–7%). The mechanisms for malignancy-induced hypercalcemia are classified into four types (Table 19.3).

PTH-Related Protein (or Peptide) and Hypercalcemia
- A major factor that is responsible for hypercalcemia in >80% of tumors.
- PTH-related protein (PTH_rP) is similar to PTH because the initial eight amino acids at the N-terminus are identical. In the bone, PTH_rP interacts with PTH–PTH_rP receptor and activates bone resorption. In renal tubules, PTH_rP occupies the PTH–PTH_rP receptor as well and increases Ca^{2+} reabsorption. Both of these mechanisms maintain hypercalcemia.
- PTH_rP also causes hypophosphatemia and an increase in urinary excretions of phosphate and cAMP.

Table 19.3 Types of hypercalcemia associated with malignancy

Type	Occurrence (%)	Bone metastases	Causative factors	Associated tumors
Humoral hypercalcemia of malignancy	80	Minimal or absent	PTH-related protein (PTH_rP)	Squamous cell cancers (lung, head and neck, esophagus, and cervix), breast cancer, renal cell cancer, ovarian and endometrial cancers, HTLV-associated lymphoma
Local osteolytic hypercalcemia	20	Extensive	Cytokines, PTH_rP, chemokines	Breast cancer, multiple myeloma, lymphoma
$1,25(OH)_2D_3$ (calcitriol)-secreting lymphomas	<1	Variable	$1,25(OH)_2D_3$	Lymphomas (all types)
Ectopic hyperparathyroidism	<1	Variable	PTH	Variable

PTH parathyroid hormone, *HTLV* human T-lymphotropic virus

- Circulating levels of PTH$_r$P are negligible in normal individuals, and they are high in hyperornithinemia–hyperammonemia–homocitrullinuria syndrome (HHH).
- Unlike PTH, PTH$_r$P reduces 1,25(OH)$_2$D$_3$ production so that GI absorption of Ca^{2+} is decreased.

Cytokines and Hypercalcemia

Many tumors such as breast and prostate cancers as well as hematologic malignancies (multiple myeloma) cause hypercalcemia by generating osteoclast-activating cytokines such as IL-1, IL-6, IL-8, tumor necrosis factor-α (TNF-α), macrophage inflammatory-peptide (chemokine), and PTH$_r$P. These cause bone resorption. PTH$_r$P and the other cytokines induce receptor activator of nuclear factor κB (RANK) ligand, which mediates osteoclast bone resorption with resultant hypercalcemia.

1,25(OH)$_2$D$_3$ and Hypercalcemia

All types of lymphoma cells increase 1,α-hydroxylase and then conversion of 25-hydroxyvitamin D$_3$ to 1,25(OH)$_2$D$_3$ (calcitriol). As a result, intestinal Ca^{2+} absorption is increased. Hypercalcemia results from intestinal and bone resorption of Ca^{2+}.

Granulomatous Diseases

- Sarcoidosis and other granulomatous diseases, including silicone-induced granulomas, secrete 1,25(OH)$_2$D$_3$ with resultant hypercalcemia.
- Note that 1,25(OH)$_2$D$_3$ may be normal in certain granulomatous diseases.
- 1,α-hydroxylase is elevated in those with high 1,25(OH)$_2$D$_3.$
- Steroids improve hypercalcemia by decreasing 1,25(OH)$_2$D$_3$ levels.
- Chloroquine and ketoconazole also decrease 1,25(OH)$_2$D$_3$ by inhibiting 1,α-hydroxylase activity.

Vitamin D Overdose

- Doses >100,000 units/day of 25-hydroxyvitamin D are required to cause hypercalcemia, which is due to intestinal absorption of Ca^{2+} and 1,25(OH)$_2$D$_3$-induced bone resorption.
- Thus, most of the cases of vitamin D overdose are iatrogenic.
- PTH levels are low and 25(OH)D$_3$ levels are elevated. However, 1,25(OH)$_2$D$_3$ levels may be slightly elevated, low, or normal. Low levels may be due to suppressed 1,α-hydroxylase by low PTH and high levels may be related to displacement of calcitriol by weaker vitamin D metabolites from the vitamin D receptors.
- Discontinuation of vitamin D, hydration, bisphosphonates, and low-calcium diet improve hypercalcemia.

Table 19.4 Clinical manifestations of hypercalcemia

General	Weakness, malaise, and tiredness
Neuromuscular (psychiatric)	Confusion, impaired memory, lethargy, stupor, coma, muscle weakness, and hypotonia
Cardiac	Short QT interval, arrhythmias, bundle branch blocks, and hypertension
Renal	Dehydration, polyuria, polydipsia, nocturia (nephrogenic DI), nephrocalcinosis, nephrolithiasis, tubulointerstitial disease, and acute and chronic kidney disease
Gastrointestinal	Nausea, vomiting, poor appetite, weight loss, constipation, abdominal pain, and pancreatitis
Skeletal	Bone pain, arthritis, osteoporosis, osteitis fibrosa cystica
Calcifications	Band keratopathy, red eye syndrome, and conjunctival and vascular calcifications

DI diabetes insipidus

Clinical Manifestations

As Ca^{2+} is needed for functions of all organs, hypercalcemia affects all organ systems. The signs and symptoms of hypercalcemia depend on the severity and rate of rise of Ca^{2+} levels. Depending on serum Ca^{2+} levels, hypercalcemia is classified into mild (10.3–11.9 mg/dL), moderate (12–13.9 mg/dL), and severe (>14 mg/dL) hypercalcemia. Renal and neurologic manifestations worsen with increasing severity of hypercalcemia. Also, a rapid development of mild to moderate hypercalcemia results in severe neurologic dysfunction. In contrast, chronic hypercalcemia may cause minimal neurologic signs and symptoms. Mild hypercalcemia may be asymptomatic in younger individuals but may have profound effect in the elderly because of preexisting neurologic and cognitive dysfunctions. Table 19.4 lists signs and symptoms of hypercalcemia.

Diagnosis

Step 1 Confirm true hypercalcemia by measuring serum and ionized Ca^{2+} after hemoconcentration, Ca^{2+}-binding paraproteinemia, or thrombocythemia-associated hypercalcemia (Ca^{2+} is released from platelets) have been ruled out.

Step 2 Obtain electrolytes, creatinine, BUN, albumin, phosphate, and alkaline phosphatase, as well as complete blood count.

Take a good history regarding signs and symptoms of hypercalcemia and medications. Inquire about shortness of breath, and evaluate the most recent chest X-ray as well as electrocardiography (EKG). Also, inquire about frequent urination, abdominal pain, and/or constipation. History of low back pain, bone pain, ulcer

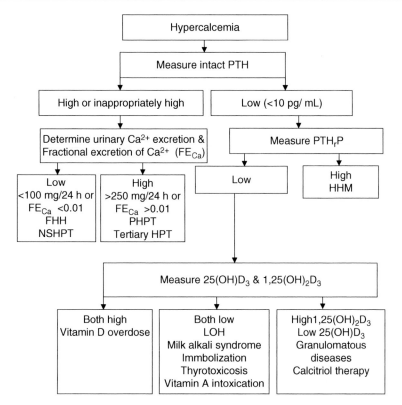

Fig. 19.1 Approach to the patient with hypercalcemia. *FHH* familial hypocalciuric hypercalcemia, *HHM* humoral hypercalcemia of malignancy, *LOH* local osteolytic hypercalcemia, *NSHPT* neonatal severe hyperparathyroidism, *PHPT* primary hyperparathyroidism, *PTH$_r$P* parathyroid hormone-related protein

disease, and kidney stones suggests chronic hypercalcemia. Establish acute onset or chronicity of hypercalcemia.

Step 3 Physical examination should include evaluation of blood pressure and pulse, volume status, eye examination for calcification, and neurologic status.

Step 4 Intact PTH determination is the single most important test in the differential diagnosis of hypercalcemia (Fig. 19.1). In addition, PTH$_r$P and vitamin D levels are usually ordered (Table 19.5).

Step 5 Also, 24 h urinary Ca^{2+} excretion (Table 19.5) or fractional excretion of Ca^{2+} can be useful in the differential diagnosis of hypercalcemia.

Step 6 If parathyroidectomy is indicated, sestamibi scan can be ordered. If malignancy is suspected, urine and serum immunoelectrophoresis, computed tomography (CT) of chest and abdomen, and a mammogram should be obtained.

Table 19.5 Biochemical abnormalities in various conditions of hypercalcemia

Condition	PO_4	PTH	PTH_rP	$25(OH)D_3$	$1,25(OH)_2D_3$	U_{Ca}	U_{cAMP}
Primary hyperparathyroidism	↓	↑	UD	N	↑	↑	↑
Secondary hyperparathyroidism	↑	↑	N	N	↓	NS	NS
FHH	↑	N/↑	UD	N	N	↓	N
Tumor-induced bone resorption	N/↑	↓	N/↑	N	N/↓	N/↑	N/↓
Humoral hypercalcemia of malignancy	N/↓	↓	↑	N	N/↓	↑	↑
Granulomatous diseases	N/↑	↓	UD	N	↑	↑	N
Vitamin D toxicity	N/↑	↓	UD	↑	N/↑/↓	↑	↓
Milk-alkali syndrome	N/↓	↓	UD	↑	↓	↓	N/↓

PTH parathyroid hormone, *PTHrP* PTH-related protein, U_{Ca} urinary calcium, U_{cAMP} urinary cyclic adenosine monophosphate, *FHH* familial hypocalciuric hypercalcemia, *(arrow sign)* decrease/increase, *UD* undetectable, *N* normal, *NS* not significant

Treatment

The primary goal of treatment of hypercalcemia is correction of the underlying cause. For example, parathyroidectomy is the definitive treatment for PHPT. Similarly, chemotherapy for malignant disease improves hypercalcemia. However, acute treatment is indicated in patients with signs and symptoms of hypercalcemia. In general, these signs and symptoms are mostly related to neuropsychiatric and GI systems.

Acute Treatment

The treatment of acute hypercalcemia includes:

1. Hydration with normal saline and then judicious administration of furosemide for volume overload. Note that furosemide-induced volume depletion may increase reabsorption of Ca^{2+} by the proximal tubule; therefore the use of furosemide in the management of acute hypercalcemia is questioned by many clinicians.
2. Inhibition of bone resorption of Ca^{2+}.
3. Decrease intestinal absorption of Ca^{2+}.
4. Removal of Ca^{2+} by hemodialysis using a dialysate bath containing low Ca^{2+}.

These treatment modalities are shown in Table 19.6. Following acute correction, chronic management of hypercalcemia includes removal of the cause.

Table 19.6 Treatment modalities of acute hypercalcemia

Treatment	Dosage	Route	Duration of effect	Mechanism
Promote Ca²⁺ excretion				
Normal saline	1–2 L every 6 h	IV	4–6 h	Improves GFR and promotes Ca²⁺ excretion
Furosemide	40–120 mg every 2–4 h	IV	2–4 h	Inhibits Ca²⁺ reabsorption in TALH
Decrease bone resorption				
Calcitonin	2–4 MRC units/kg every 4–8 h	IV	4–12 h	Inhibits bone resorption
Pamidronate[a]	30–90 mg in 100–200 mL saline or D5W once	IV over 4–24 h	2–3 weeks	Inhibits bone resorption. Clinical response takes 2–3 days
Zoledronate[a]	4 mg in 50 mL of saline or D5W once	IV over 15–20 min	2–3 weeks	Inhibits bone resorption. Clinical response takes 2–3 days
Gallium citrate	200 mg/m²/day in 1 L of saline for 5 days	IV	1–2 weeks	Inhibits bone resorption
Decrease intestinal absorption				
Prednisone	20–30 mg every 12 h	Oral	2–4 days	Inhibits gut absorption
Decrease plasma [Ca²⁺]				
Hemodialysis	Use dialysate bath containing low Ca²⁺		Few hours	Removal from blood

IV intravenous, *MRC* Medical Research Council, *TALH* thick ascending limb of Henle's loop, *GFR* glomerular filtration rate, *D5W* 5% dextrose in water

[a]Dose reduction or discontinuation in acute kidney injury or dialysis patients

Chronic Treatment

The goals of therapy include:

1. Correction of the underlying cause: parathyroidectomy and chemotherapy. Use cinacalcet (30–120 mg/day) for secondary hyperparathyroidism. Judicious use of cinacalcet in some patients with PHPT is recommended.
2. Maintenance of euvolemia: prescribe adequate amount of water that should be equal or slightly more than urine output and insensible loss.
3. Decrease the production of $1,25(OH)_2D_3$: low-calcium diet, avoid vitamin D intake, steroids, chloroquine (250 mg/day), hydroxychloroquine (400–600 mg/day), and ketoconazole (100–200 mg/day).
4. Decrease intestinal absorption of Ca²⁺: low-calcium diet, steroids, and avoidance of vitamin D preparations.
5. Decrease bone resorption: steroids, lower PTH levels, avoid vitamin D use, bisphosphonates, and receptor activator of nuclear factor-kB ligand (RANKL) inhibitor, and denosumab.

6. Bisphosphonates are used to treat hypercalcemia in patients with malignancy. They inhibit osteoclast-induced bone resorption. Of the available bisphosphonates, only pamidronate and zoledronate are approved for acute hypercalcemia management of malignancy in the USA. Ibandronate is approved in Europe. All are renally excreted. Reduction in dose and slow infusion are recommended in patients with renal failure. Zoledronate is more potent than pamidronate. The effect of bisphosphonates is seen in 48–72 h and lasts for 2–3 weeks. Repeat the dose, if necessary.
7. Denosumab is a humanized monoclonal antibody that inhibits osteoclastic activity and thereby bone resorption. It was initially approved for postmenopausal women with osteoporosis. It reduces serum Ca^{2+} level. Subsequently, it was approved for use in skeletal-related events such as hypercalcemia in patients with bone metastasis due to a solid tumor. Thus, denosumab is recommended for tumor-induced hypercalcemia when bisphosphonates do not work or failed to work.

Study Questions

Case 1 A 47-year-old man from New Guinea (immigrated to the USA 24 years ago) is admitted for complaints of productive cough with blood-tinged sputum, dyspnea for 1 week, and abdominal pain for 4 months. He also complained of nausea, vomiting, and dizziness for 1 week. The family noticed gradual weight loss and change in mental status. No history of kidney stones; however, he was diagnosed with tuberculosis at the age of 14 and was treated adequately. He is not on any prescription medications. He drinks milk and takes antacid for "heartburn." Chest X-ray shows bilateral infiltrates. EKG shows left bundle branch block. His blood pressure is 130/62 mmHg with a pulse rate of 84 beats per minute (sitting) and 100/50 mmHg with a pulse rate of 102 beats per minute (standing). There is no evidence of vascular calcifications. His laboratory results are as follows:

Na^+	140 mEq/L
K^+	4.1 mEq/L
Cl^-	96 mEq/L
HCO_3^-	28 mEq/L
Creatinine	2.7 mg/dL
BUN	52 mg/dL
Glucose	82 mg/dL
Ca^{2+}	21.6 mg/dL
Phosphate	5.3 mg/dL
Mg^{2+}	2.2 mg/dL
Total protein	7.2 g/dL
Albumin	4.0 g/dL
Alkaline phosphatase	105 IU/L
White blood cell count	15,000
Hemoglobin	13.8%
Platelets	327,000

Question 1 What is the appropriate differential diagnosis for hypercalcemia in this patient?

Answer Malignancy, PHPT, and granulomatous disease (reactivation of tuberculosis) are to be considered initially.

Question 2 What laboratory tests exclude PHPT?

Answer Normal Cl^-, slightly elevated HCO_3^- and phosphate, and normal alkaline phosphatase exclude the diagnosis of PHPT.

Question 3 What other pertinent laboratory tests you order at this time?

Answer Determinations of intact PTH, PTH_rP, $25(OH)D_3$, $1,25(OH)_2D_3$, and serum protein immunoelectrophoresis (SPEP) are appropriate tests to make the diagnosis.

The above tests were available 2 days later, which showed PTH, <10 pg/mL; PTH_rP, 20 pmol/L (reference <2 pmol/L); $25(OH)D_3$, normal; $1,25(OH)_2D_3$, low normal; and SPEP, normal.

Question 4 What is your diagnosis of his hypercalcemia?

Answer Humoral hypercalcemia of malignancy.

A CT scan of the lungs, abdomen, and brain showed enlarged lymph nodes in his abdomen. There were no malignant lesions either in lungs or brain. Serum creatinine increased from 2.7 to 5.7 mg/dL in 4 days despite adequate hydration and other appropriate therapeutic treatment modalities. A renal biopsy was performed for diagnostic and therapeutic considerations. The renal pathologist suggested HIV and human T-lymphotropic virus-1 (HTLV-1) testing. HIV test was negative, but HTLV-1 testing was positive in both serum and the renal tissue. The patient had acute tubular necrosis on renal biopsy.

The final diagnosis was hypercalcemia associated with HTLV-1-induced adult T-cell lymphoma/leukemia. Although chemotherapy improved hypercalcemia, the patient died.

Question 5 Explain the pathophysiology of hypercalcemia-associated volume depletion.

Answer Hypercalcemia induces nephrogenic DI with salt and water loss. Also, the patient had nausea and vomiting, thus limiting his fluid intake. Both mechanisms induce volume depletion. Hypercalcemia is perpetuated because of low GFR and enhanced Ca^{2+} reabsorption by the renal tubules.

Question 6 Discuss the epidemiology and clinical features of HTLV-1-induced T-cell lymphoma/leukemia.

Answer Adult T-cell lymphoma/leukemia is a rare and aggressive tumor that is linked to infection by the HTLV-1, a retrovirus that belongs to the HIV/AIDS virus. HTLV-1 infection is endemic in Japan, the Caribbean, South and Central America, parts of Africa, and the southeastern USA. The infection is acquired from sexual contact, virus-contaminated blood transfusion, and breast feeding from infected mother. There are no standardized protocols for treatment of HTLV-1-induced lymphoma. In general, the prognosis is poor.

Hypercalcemia is the significant electrolyte abnormality in these patients. PTH is suppressed, but PTH$_r$P levels are elevated.

Case 2 A 62-year-old man was brought to the emergency department with altered mental status. Physical examination showed a confused well-developed male with labored breathing. He was intubated to protect the airways. His blood pressure was 132/78 mmHg with a pulse rate of 100 beats per minute. Except for lower extremity ulcer, which was rapped with a bandage containing white powder, the rest of the examination was otherwise normal. His laboratory results were as follows:

Na$^+$	148 mEq/L
K$^+$	1.8 mEq/L
Cl$^-$	73 mEq/L
HCO$_3^-$	54 mEq/L
Creatinine	3.4 mg/dL
BUN	22 mg/dL
Glucose	110 mg/dL
Ca^{2+}	9.2 mg/dL
Phosphate	5.6 mg/dL
Total protein	7.1 g/dL
Albumin	2.7 g/dL
EKG	Normal sinus rhythm with prolonged QT interval
Arterial blood gas (ABG)	pH = 7.69, PO$_2$ = 45, PCO$_2$ = 48, HCO$_3^-$ = 53
Urine	pH = 5.8, Na$^+$ = 81 mEq/L, K$^+$ = 58 mEq/L, Cl$^-$ <10 mEq/L, Ca^{2+} = 150 mg/L
Urine toxicology	Negative
Chest X-ray	Normal

After vigorous hydration with normal saline and K$^+$ supplementation, electrolytes, creatinine, and pH improved. Blood pressure rose to 160/90 mmHg. The patient was successfully extubated. His intact parathyroid hormone (iPTH) and 1,25(OH)$_2$D$_3$ were low normal.

Which one of the following is the MOST likely diagnosis of his hypercalcemia?

(A) Sarcoidosis
(B) Hypercalcemia related to calcium-containing medications (milk-alkali syndrome)
(C) Familial hypocalciuric hypercalcemia (FHH)
(D) Occult malignancy
(E) Thiazide treatment

The answer is B Sarcoidosis is excluded based on normal $1,25(OH)_2D_3$ level, although normal values in some cases were observed. Also, FHH is unlikely because of normal Ca^{2+} excretion. Hypercalcemia is almost asymptomatic in FHH. Occult malignancy is possible; however, the patient does not have any evidence of malignancy. His chest X-ray and total protein concentration are normal. Further testing is necessary to completely rule out occult malignancy. Urine Cl^-<10 and urine Ca^{2+} 150 mg exclude the diagnosis of thiazide use. Based on the white powder that was covering the leg ulcer, the patient may be using a substance that contains Ca^{2+}. Indeed, the patient admitted to using baking soda ($CaHCO_3$) for the last 6 months as a remedy for leg ulcers. Thus, option B is correct.

Baking soda has been used as a home remedy for a number of conditions, including peptic ulcer disease and wound healing. Excessive ingestion or skin application of baking soda causes metabolic alkalosis, hypokalemia, hypercalcemia, volume contraction, and AKI. Hypercalcemia impairs HCO_3^- excretion, leading to metabolic alkalosis, volume contraction, and renal insufficiency, resulting in milk (calcium)-alkali syndrome.

Calcium-alkali syndrome can also develop without renal insufficiency. PTH and $1,25(OH)_2D_3$ are usually suppressed, but normal values also have been reported. Hydration and electrolyte replacements, as required, are generally sufficient to treat calcium-alkali syndrome. At times, renal insufficiency and hypercalcemia may slowly resolve. The definitive long-term treatment is withdrawal of the offending agent.

Case 3 A 45-year-old female patient was referred to the renal clinic for evaluation of hematuria and frequent urinary tract infections; she was found to have renal stones. During the workup of her renal stones, she was found to have a PTH level of 96 pg/mL (elevated).

Regarding the PTH assay, which one of the following statements is FALSE?

(A) The first-generation radioimmunoassay (RIA) measure either C-terminal (53–84) or midregion (48–68) of the PTH molecule
(B) The second-generation immunoradiometric assays (IRMA) measure intact (1–84) and other degradation fragments (7–84)
(C) The actions of intact PTH (1–84) are different than that of 7–84 fragment.
(D) The ratio of 1–84:7–84 discriminates low-turnover from high-turnover bone disease in dialysis patients
(E) The third-generation IRMA measures the biointact (1–84) and not 7–84 fragment of the PTH

The answer is D The intact PTH is a single-chain 84 amino acid peptide hormone. The Kidney Disease Outcomes Quality Initiative (K/DOQI) guidelines recommend that serum PTH levels of patients with CKD should be measured regularly and maintained within target ranges. For this reason, the methodology for PTH should be accurate because treatment decisions are made on the levels of PTH.

The first-generation RIA used polyclonal antibodies directed toward C-terminal or midregion of the PTH molecule. In addition, PTH fragments were also measured. Therefore, the PTH levels were greatly elevated. Thus, the first-generation assays became obsolete.

The second-generation PTH assays were introduced in mid-1980s as first- and second-generation assays. The first- and second-generation IRMA used two different antibodies, one directed toward the 39–84 portion and the second toward the 15–20 portion of the PTH molecule. These second-generation assays were called "INTACT PTH" assays as they were thought to measure only the full length 1–84 of the PTH. Soon it was realized that these assays had certain limitations, in particular, their values were high and overestimated (in the range of 400–500 pg/mL) because of recognition of another fragment with amino acids from 7 to 84 of the PTH molecule. The high intact PTH values in dialysis patients led the physician to take steps for suppression by either medical or surgical interventions, leading to low-turnover bone disease.

Further studies have shown that the newly measured 7–84 fragment has effects that are opposite to the intact 1–84 of the PTH, such as a decrease in serum Ca^{2+} and urine phosphate excretion and inhibition of bone resorption. These inhibitory effects of the 7–84 fragment seem to be mediated through a receptor called PTHR1, which is different from PTH–PTHrP receptor.

The third-generation PTH assay was first developed in 1999. It also used two antibodies, one directed toward C-terminal amino acids and the second toward the first amino acids (1–4). Thus, the third-generation IRMA does not recognize the 7–84 fragment and, therefore, measures the biointact PTH (1–84).

Subsequently, some authors suggested that the ratio 1–84:7–84 of the PTH (measured by the third- and second-generation assays, respectively) can discriminate between low- and high-turnover bone disease better than either one of the assays. However, it was later proven that the ratio has little discriminatory effect on bone disease. Thus, option D is false.

Case 4 A 20-year-old man is found to have a serum Ca^{2+} level of 10.9 mg/dL, which was confirmed by determining ionized Ca^{2+} on a routine physical examination. His Mg^{2+} is also slightly elevated and phosphate is low. His intact PTH level is 70 pg/mL, and vitamin D levels are normal. All other labs are normal. He is not on any medications. Physical examination is normal. He also had elevated serum Ca^{2+} levels 10 years ago when he was admitted to hospital for cough and sputum production.

Which one of the following is the MOST likely diagnosis in this subject?

(A) Primary hyperparathyroidism (PHPT)
(B) Secondary hyperparathyroidism
(C) Familial hypocalciuric hypercalcemia (FHH)
(D) Milk (calcium)-alkali syndrome
(E) Subclinical granulomatous disease

The answer is C The laboratory findings are consistent with asymptomatic PHPT and FHH. The distinction between PHPT and FHH in adults can be difficult. Parathyroidectomy is the cure for PHPT, whereas all the earlier biochemical abnormalities persist even after parathyroidectomy in patients with FHH. One way to distinguish between PHPT and FHH is to calculate the fractional excretion of Ca^{2+}, which is <0.01% in FHH and >0.01% in PHPT. Renal function is normal; therefore, secondary hyperparathyroidism is unlikely. Also, normal calcitriol and elevated PTH levels exclude the diagnoses of milk (calcium)-alkali syndrome and granulomatous diseases.

A 24-h urinary excretion of Ca^{2+} and creatinine were done, which showed Ca^{2+} levels of 54 mg and <0.01% fractional excretion of Ca^{2+}. Thus, this adult subject carries the diagnosis of FHH. Thus, option C is correct.

Case 5 A 30-year-old man with HIV/AIDS is found to have hypercalcemia, which is thought to be medication-induced.

Which one of the following drugs is NOT associated with hypercalcemia?

(A) Vitamin A
(B) Omeprazole
(C) Silicone
(D) Lithium
(E) Chloroquine

The answer is E Except for chloroquine, all other medications have been shown to cause hypercalcemia. Vitamin A intoxication causes bone resorption and elevates serum $[Ca^{2+}]$. Also, vitamin A analogs used in dermatologic and malignant conditions cause hypercalcemia.

Omeprazole, a proton pump inhibitor (PPI), has been shown to cause acute tubulointerstitial granulomatous disease and hypercalcemia with normal PTH levels. PPIs may also cause hypocalcemia.

The use of liquid silicone for soft tissue augmentation (breast and hip) has been shown to induce granulomas and hypercalcemia. Renal stones and renal failure due to obstruction and hypercalcemia do occur in some patients. Hypercalcemia improves with steroids. TNF-α inhibitors have also been used to prevent granuloma formation, as TNF-α induces granuloma formation. Chloroquine and denosumab can be used to treat hypercalcemia.

Lithium has been known for years to cause hypercalcemia by stimulating PTH secretion. This effect occurs probably through interaction with CaSR to alter the set point for PTH secretion in relation to plasma $[Ca^{2+}]$.

Chloroquine causes hypocalcemia by decreasing the production of $1,25(OH)_2D_3$. Thus, option E is correct.

Reference

1. Bilezikian JP, Khan AA, Potts JT Jr, on behalf of the Third International Workshop on the Management of Asymptomatic Primary Hyperthyroidism. Guidelines for the management of asymptomatic primary hyperparathyroidism: summary statement from the third international workshop. J Clin Endocrinol Metab. 2009;94:335–9.

Suggested Reading

2. Dumitru C, Wysolmerski J. Disorders of calcium metabolism. In: Alpern RJ, Moe OW, Caplan M, editors. Seldin and Giebisch's the kidney. Physiology and pathophysiology. 5th ed. San Diego: Academic Press (Elsevier); 2013. p. 2273–309.
3. Hariri A, Mount DB, Rastegar A. Disorders of calcium, phosphorus, and magnesium metabolism. In: Mount DB, Sayegh MH, Singh AJ, editors. Core concepts in the disorders of fluid, electrolytes and acid-base balance. New York: Springer; 2013. p. 103–46.
4. Hoorn EJ, Zietse R. Disorders of calcium and magnesium balance: a physiology-based approach. Pediatr Nephrol. 2013;28:1195–206. doi:10.1007/s00467-012-2350-2.
5. Rosner MH, Dalkin AC. Onco-nephrology: the pathophysiology and treatment of malignancy-associated hypercalcemia. Clin J Am Soc Nephrol. 2012;7:1722–9.
6. Smogorzewski MJ, Stubbs JR, Yu ASL. Disorders of calcium, magnesium, and phosphate balance. In: Skorecki K, et al., editors. Brenner and Rector's the kidney. 10th ed. Philadelphia: Elsevier; 2016. p. 601–35.
7. Stewart AF. Hypercalcemia associated with cancer. N Engl J Med. 2005;352:373–8.
8. Wysolmerski JJ. Parathyroid hormone-related protein: an update. J Clin Endocrinol Metab. 2012;97:2947–56.

Disorders of Phosphate: Physiology

20

General Features

Phosphate and phosphorus are generally used interchangeably. Phosphate, although not as abundant as Ca^{2+}, is an important constituent of the body. It plays a significant role in mitochondrial respiration and oxidative phosphorylation. Phosphate constitutes approximately 1% of the body weight. A 70 kg man contains about 700 g of phosphate. Of this amount, 85% is present in the bones and teeth, 14% in soft tissues, and the remaining 1% in the extracellular fluid.

In biologic fluids, phosphate is measured as elemental phosphorus. However, the latter participates in biologic functions as phosphate. For example, it is phosphate that is filtered at the glomerulus or transported across the renal tubules. In plasma, the concentration of phosphorus is expressed as mg/dL, and in transport and other processes, it is generally expressed as mEq or mmol/L.

In plasma, phosphate exists as *organic* (70%) and *inorganic* (30%) forms. The inorganic form is physiologically active. Only 10% of inorganic phosphate is bound to albumin. However, unlike Ca^{2+}, phosphate concentration is not influenced by changes in plasma albumin concentration. At a pH of 7.40, inorganic phosphate exists predominantly as divalent phosphate (HPO_4^{2-}) and monovalent phosphate ($H_2PO_4^-$) in the ratio of 4:1. However, at a pH of 6.8, which is the pK_a of this buffer pair, the ratio falls to 1:1.

The concentration of intracellular phosphate is several-fold higher than the plasma concentration. Inside the cell, 75% of phosphate exists as organic phosphate compounds such as adenosine triphosphate (ATP), creatine phosphate, and adenosine monophosphate. In red blood cells, it occurs predominantly as 2,3-diphosphoglycerate. Free phosphate in the cytosol accounts for 25% of the intracellular concentration of phosphate, and only this fraction is available for transport mechanisms.

© Springer Science+Business Media LLC 2018
A.S. Reddi, *Fluid, Electrolyte and Acid-Base Disorders*,
DOI 10.1007/978-3-319-60167-0_20

Phosphate Homeostasis

As in Ca^{2+} homeostasis, three main organs are involved in phosphate homeostasis: the intestine, the kidney, and the bone (Fig. 20.1). The dietary intake of phosphate varies from 1,000 to 1,400 mg daily. Of this amount, 300–500 mg are excreted in the feces and 700–900 mg in the urine to maintain a plasma phosphate concentration (abbreviated as [Pi]) between 2.5 and 4.5 mg/dL. Although phosphate exchange occurs between the extracellular fluid and bone, it is the balance between gut absorption and renal excretion that maintains phosphate homeostasis. For example, when gut absorption of phosphate increases, a transient increase in plasma [Pi] occurs. The kidneys excrete this excess amount in order to maintain the normal plasma [Pi].

In the intestine, both absorption and secretion of phosphate occur. Most of the dietary phosphate is absorbed in the duodenum and jejunum. Approximately 200 mg of phosphate is secreted into the gastrointestinal tract, mainly into saliva and bile. The net result is that about 65% of phosphate is absorbed in the gastrointestinal tract. Two important mechanisms seem to participate in this process. One, localized in the duodenum, is a Na$^+$-dependent secondary active transport system. The transporter involved in phosphate transport is called Na/Pi-type II$_b$ cotransporter. It is influenced by a number of factors. Arsenate, mercury, and calcitonin inhibit, whereas 1,25(OH)$_2$D$_3$ and low phosphate diet stimulate this cotransporter. The second mechanism is phosphate-dependent and is located in the jejunum and ileum. Phosphate absorption in these segments of the intestine depends on the luminal phosphate concentration. Absorption seems to be predominantly passive under

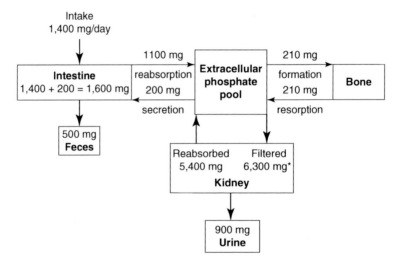

Fig. 20.1 Phosphate homeostasis in an adult subject. (The filtered load of phosphate equals the free plasma concentration of 3.5 mg/dL multiplied by the GFR of 180 L per day, i.e., 180 L×35 mg/L = 6,300 mg/day) (Modified from Nordin [5], with permission)

normal circumstances and occurs through the paracellular pathway. As stated above, active transport becomes prominent when dietary phosphate is extremely low. Ca^{2+}, Mg^{2+}, and aluminum are important elements that complex with phosphate and decrease its intestinal absorption. These compounds are thus used to treat increased plasma [Pi] in clinical practice.

Under normal conditions, the exchange of phosphate between the bone and the extracellular pool is rather small (see Fig. 20.1), and the release of phosphate is always accompanied by the release of Ca^{2+}. Thus, the release of phosphate is stimulated by the same hormones that stimulate the release of Ca^{2+}.

The kidneys play a significant role in the maintenance of phosphate homeostasis. Since the dietary intake of phosphate varies daily, the total body phosphate concentration would also vary were it not for the kidneys. The kidneys vary their excretion of phosphate to the varying amounts of phosphate absorption by the intestine to maintain normal serum [Pi].

Renal Handling of Phosphate

Renal handling of phosphate involves filtration and reabsorption. No secretion of phosphate probably occurs in humans. Plasma phosphate is filtered freely at the glomerulus. Of the filtered amount, about 80–90% is reabsorbed by the proximal tubule. Approximately 10% is reabsorbed by the distal convoluted tubule. Little or no phosphate transport occurs in the Henle's loop and collecting ducts. Therefore, the urine contains only 10% of the filtered phosphate. In conditions of high phosphate intake, urinary excretion may approach 20%.

Proximal Tubule

Transport of phosphate across the luminal membrane of the proximal tubule is transcellular and active (Fig. 20.2). The transport is unidirectional. There is no passive diffusion. The transport mechanisms of phosphate have been clearly demonstrated. Three types of Na/Pi cotransporters have been described: type I, type II, and type III. Type II cotransporter comprises three isoforms: type II_a, type II_b, and type II_c. Only types II_a and II_c are expressed in the apical membrane and thus involved in the transport of phosphate in the kidney. On the other hand, type II_b is involved in phosphate transport in the intestine and other organs. In the proximal tubule, 2 or 3 Na^+ ions are transported with one phosphate ion (Fig. 20.2). This cotransport system is driven by the energy supplied by the Na/K-ATPase located in the basolateral membrane.

Phosphate exit across the basolateral membrane occurs both by Na^+-dependent and Na^+-independent phosphate mechanisms (see Fig. 20.2). The Na^+-independent mechanism may involve an anion (Cl^-, lactate, etc.) exchange. Phosphate may also enter the blood by simple diffusion based on the electrochemical gradient.

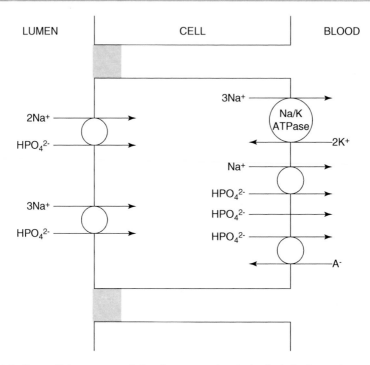

Fig. 20.2 Transcellular transport of phosphate across the proximal tubule. A^- = anion

Regulation of Renal Phosphate Handling

The proximal tubule has an intrinsic ability to modulate the reabsorption of phosphate depending on the need and the availability of phosphate. A number of factors and hormones influence the reabsorption and excretion of phosphate (Table 20.1). Of these, PTH and fibroblast growth factor (FGF)-23 are important regulators of phosphate homeostasis and deserve special mention here.

PTH: PTH decreases Na/Pi cotransport by decreasing the number of phosphate cotransporters, while parathyroidectomy increases the Na/Pi-II_a and II_b protein content of brush border vesicles by two- to threefold. Regulation of Na/Pi-II_a protein occurs via cAMP/PKA pathway.

PTH has opposing effects on phosphate excretion. First, it is phosphaturic; and second, it stimulates the synthesis of $1,25(OH)_2D_3$, which increases intestinal and renal reabsorption of phosphate. This results in reduced excretion of phosphate.

FGF-23: Like PTH, FGF-23 is also an important regulator. It was originally identified as one of the phosphatonins that was responsible for hypophosphatemia, renal phosphate wasting, and reduced $1,25(OH)_2D_3$ or calcitriol in patients with tumor-induced osteomalacia. This hormone is secreted by osteoblasts and osteocytes of the bone. FGF-23 has three important functions on phosphate

Table 20.1 Factors that regulate phosphate reabsorption and excretion in the proximal tubule

Factor	Mechanism
Factors that inhibit phosphate reabsorption and increase excretion	
PTH	Inhibition of Na/Pi-II$_a$ and IIc cotransports and Na/K-ATPase
FGF-23	Inhibition of type II$_a$ and decreased formation of calcitriol by 1,α-hydroxylase inhibition
Calcitriol	Inhibition of type II$_a$ cotransporter
Dopamine	Inhibition of type II$_a$ cotransporter and Na/K-ATPase
Glucocorticoids	Inhibition of type II$_a$ cotransporter
Volume expansion	Increase GFR and reduced Na$^+$ reabsorption
Chronic metabolic acidosis	Inhibition of type II$_a$ cotransporter and resorption of phosphate from bone
High phosphate intake	Inhibition of type II$_a$ and IIc cotransporters
Diuretics	Probably related to decreased Na$^+$ reabsorptions. Also, carbonic anhydrase inhibitors decrease type IIa cotransporter
Chronic hypercalcemia	Unknown
Hypokalemia	Inhibition of type IIc cotransporter
Factors that promote phosphate reabsorption and decrease excretion	
Parathyroidectomy	Increased type II$_a$ cotransporter activity
Insulin	Increased type II$_a$ cotransporter activity
Growth hormone	Increased type II$_a$ cotransporter activity
Volume contraction	Decreased GFR associated with increased Na$^+$ reabsorption
Metabolic alkalosis	Increased type II$_a$ cotransporter activity
Low phosphate intake	Increased type II$_a$ and type II$_c$ cotransporter activity
Hypocalcemia	Unknown
Hypermagnesemia	Increased type II$_a$ and type II$_c$ cotransporter activity

metabolism. First, FGF-23 inhibits Na$^+$-dependent phosphate cotransporter in the proximal tubule and promotes phosphate excretion. Second, FGF-23 inhibits 1,α-hydroxylase activity, leading to reduced levels of 1,25(OH)$_2$D$_3$. Since 1,25(OH)$_2$D$_3$ promotes intestinal and renal phosphate reabsorption, reduced level of this active vitamin D can cause reduced phosphate excretion, and, finally, FGF-23 inhibits the synthesis and secretion of PTH from the parathyroid glands and indirectly causes hypocalcemia. Thus, by direct and indirect means, FGF-23 lowers serum phosphate and Ca^{2+} levels by its coordinated effects on the kidney and parathyroid glands.

Most of the FGF family members exert their effects through interaction with FGF receptors (FGFRs). At least four FGFRs with various subtypes have been identified. Studies have shown that FGF-23 can interact with FGFR1c, 3c, and 4c. However, FGF-23-mediated receptor activation requires a cofactor called Klotho. The Klotho gene is an aging-suppressor gene, and its deficiency causes premature aging. Overexpression of this gene extends life span in animals. FGF-23 fails to exert its effects in the absence of Klotho. Thus, Klotho is required for phosphaturic and other effects of FGF-23. Klotho also has an independent phosphaturic effect in the kidney, and its deficiency plays a significant role in hyperphosphatemia in CKD and its progression.

FGF-23 is regulated by phosphate, vitamin D_3, and PTH. Studies have shown that high phosphate diet induces FGF-23 secretion, whereas low phosphate diet suppresses FGF-23 secretion. Exogenous administration of $1,25(OH)_2D_3$ is shown to increase FGF-23 expression and secretion due to a direct effect of this vitamin D on FGF-23 via a vitamin D response element located upstream of the FGF-23 promotor. PTH also seems to increase FGF-23 levels by stimulating the skeletal release of FGF-23, but the mechanism is unclear.

Klotho has two forms: a transmembrane form and a secreted form. Transmembrane form acts as a cofactor for FGF-23, whereas the secreted form promotes phosphate excretion independent of FGF-23. It also promotes Ca^{2+} reabsorption in the distal tubule. Thus, Klotho is involved in phosphate homeostasis.

Dietary phosphate: Serum phosphate levels are maintained between 2.5 and 4.5 mg/dL despite changes in dietary phosphate intake. When serum phosphate levels are low due to poor dietary intake, certain physiological changes occur to maintain normal phosphate levels. Low phosphate level causes two physiologic changes. First, it increases ionized Ca^{2+}, which inhibits PTH with resultant decrease in proximal tubular reabsorption of phosphate; and second, hypophosphatemia stimulates the production of $1,25(OH)_2D_3$ which increases the intestinal and renal reabsorption of phosphate. Both these processes maintain normal serum phosphate level (Fig. 20.3).

When serum phosphate level is high due to high dietary phosphate intake, changes, as shown in Fig. 20.4, occur, and normal serum phosphate level is maintained.

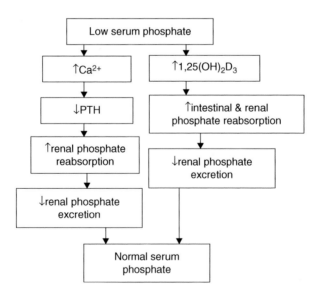

Fig. 20.3 Physiologic changes in response to low serum phosphate level

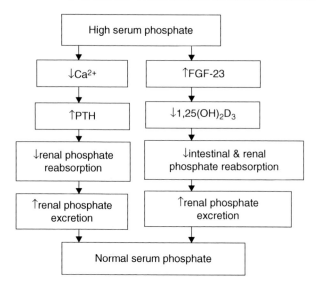

Fig. 20.4 Physiologic changes in response to high serum phosphate level

Suggested Reading

1. Bergwitz CJ, Jüppner H. Regulation of phosphate homeostasis by PTH, vitamin D, and FGF23. Annu Rev Med. 2010;61:91–104.

2. Berndt TJ, Thompson JR, Kumar R. The regulation of calcium, magnesium, and phosphate excretion by the kidney. In: Skorecki K, et al., editors. Brenner and Rector's the kidney. 10th ed. Philadelphia: Elsevier; 2016. p. 185–203.

3. Bindels RJM, Hoenderop GJ, Biber J. Transport of calcium, magnesium, and phosphate. In: Taal MW, Chertow GM, Marsden PA, et al., editors. Herausgeber. Brenner and Rector's the kidney. 9th ed. Philadelphia: Saunders; 2012. p. 226–51.

4. Hruska KA, Levi M, Slatopolsky E. Disorders of phosphorus, calcium, and magnesium metabolism. In: Coffman TM, Falk RJ, Molitoris BA, et al., editors. Herausgeber. Schrier's diseases of the kidney. 9th ed. Philadelphia: Lippincott Williams & Wilkins; 2013. p. 2116–81.

5. Nordin BEC, editor. Calcium, phosphate, and magnesium metabolism. Edinburgh: Churchill Livingstone; 1976.

Disorders of Phosphate: Hypophosphatemia

21

Hypophosphatemia is defined as serum [Pi] <2.5 mg/dL. Patients receiving mannitol develop *pseudohypophosphatemia*, which is caused by the binding of mannitol to the molybdate used to determine the serum [Pi]. Hypophosphatemia can be severe (serum [Pi] <1.0 mg/dL), moderate (serum [Pi] 1.0–1.9 mg/dL), or mild (serum [Pi] 2.0–2.5 mg/dL). Severe hypophosphatemia can occur in patients with prolonged use of antacids, such as aluminum hydroxide, magnesium hydroxide, or calcium carbonate or acetate. Moderate hypophosphatemia may be symptomatic or asymptomatic.

Hypophosphatemia is rather uncommon in the general population. However, the incidence of hypophosphatemia in hospitalized patients with sepsis, chronic alcoholism, and chronic obstructive pulmonary disease (COPD) is high. Patients with trauma also have high incidence of hypophosphatemia. The causes are varied but can be conveniently grouped under four categories (Table 21.1).

Table 21.1 Causes of hypophosphatemia

Cause	Mechanism
Shift from extracellular to intracellular compartment	
Glucose	Transcellular distribution
Insulin	Transcellular distribution
Catecholamines	Transcellular distribution
Hyperalimentation	Glucose-induced cellular uptake
Respiratory alkalosis	Transcellular distribution
Refeeding syndrome	Glucose and insulin-induced transcellular distribution, consumption during glucose metabolism, and ATP production
Rapid cellular proliferation	Cellular uptake

(continued)

© Springer Science+Business Media LLC 2018
A.S. Reddi, *Fluid, Electrolyte and Acid-Base Disorders*,
DOI 10.1007/978-3-319-60167-0_21

Table 21.1 (continued)

Cause	Mechanism
Decreased intestinal absorption	
Poor dietary intake/starvation	↓ intestinal absorption
Malabsorption	Disorders of duodenum and jejunum (celiac disease, tropical and nontropical sprue, regional enteritis), ↓ intestinal absorption
Phosphate binders	Calcium acetate or bicarbonate, aluminum hydroxide, and magnesium salts bind phosphate in the gut
Vitamin deficiency	↓ intestinal absorption
Vitamin D-dependent (VDD) rickets	
Typ e I VDD rickets	Low or deficiency of $1,25(OH)_2D_3$
Type 2 VDD rickets	Resistance to $1,25(OH)_2D_3$ action
Increased renal loss	
Primary and secondary hyperparathyroidism	↓ renal absorption
Increased fibroblast growth factor (FGF)-23 production or activity	↓ renal absorption
Inherited disorders	
X-linked hypophosphatemia	Mutations in PHEX gene
Autosomal dominant hypophosphatemia	Mutations in FGF-23 gene
Autosomal recessive hypophosphatemia	Mutations in DMP1 and ENPP1 genes
Acquired disorders	
Tumor-induced osteomalacia	Increased FGF-23 secretion and activity
Proximal tubule defect in phosphate reabsorption	↓ renal absorption
Hereditary hypophosphatemic rickets with hypercalciuria	Mutations in the gene-encoding Na/Pi-IIc cotransporter
Autosomal recessive renal phosphate wasting	Mutations in the gene-encoding Na/Pi-IIa cotransporter
Fanconi syndrome	A disorder causing decreased reabsorption of glucose, phosphate, amino acids, uric acid, bicarbonate, calcium, and potassium. Can be genetic or acquired
Renal transplantation	Tertiary hyperparathyroidism, excess FGF-23, immunosuppressive drugs, low $25(OH)D_3$ and $1,25(OH)_2D_3$ levels
Volume expansion, postobstructive diuresis, hepatectomy	↓ renal reabsorption and phosphaturia

Table 21.1 (continued)

Cause	Mechanism
Drugs	
Osmotic diuretics	↓ renal reabsorption and phosphaturia
Carbonic anhydrase inhibitor	↓ renal reabsorption and phosphaturia
Loop diuretics	↓ renal reabsorption and phosphaturia
Metolazone	↓ renal reabsorption and phosphaturia
Acyclovir	Inhibition of Na/Pi-IIa cotransporter
Acetaminophen poisoning	↓ renal reabsorption and phosphaturia
Intravenous iron administration	Increase in FGF-23 secretion and activity by inhibiting 1,α-hydroxylase
Tyrosine kinase inhibitors (imatinib, sorafenib)	↓Ca^{2+} and phosphate reabsorption and secondary hyperparathyroidism
Corticosteroids	↓ intestinal phosphate absorption and phosphaturia
Bisphosphonates	Inhibition of bone resorption
Cyclophosphamide, cisplatin	↑ phosphaturia
Ifosfamide, streptozotocin, suramin	Induction of Fanconi syndrome
Aminoglycosides, tetracyclines	Induction of Fanconi syndrome
Valproic acid	Induction of Fanconi syndrome
Tenofovir, cidofovir, adefovir	Induction of Fanconi syndrome
Miscellaneous causes	
Alcoholism	Poor intake, frequent use of phosphate binders, vitamin D deficiency, respiratory alkalosis, proximal tubule defect, ↓ intestinal absorption
Diabetic ketoacidosis	↓ total body phosphate due to osmotic diuresis at onset and hypophosphatemia after insulin administration
Toxic shock syndrome	Cellular uptake probably due to respiratory alkalosis

↑ increased, ↓ decreased

Some Specific Causes of Hypophosphatemia

X-Linked Hypophosphatemia

- It is the most common disorder inherited as an autosomal dominant disease, caused by inactivating mutations in the PHEX (phosphate-regulating gene with homologies to endopeptidases on the X chromosome) gene.
- Presents within 2 years of life.
- Characterized by hypophosphatemia, phosphaturia, short stature, rickets and osteomalacia, and dental abscesses. Decreased intestinal Ca^{2+} and phosphate absorption and decreased renal phosphate absorption have been described.
- Increased fibroblast growth factor (FGF)-23 levels are characteristic of this disorder. Serum Ca^{2+} and parathyroid hormone (PTH) levels are normal, but $1,25(OH)_2D_3$ levels are low owing to high FGF-23 activity.
- Treatment with oral calcitriol and phosphate improves growth retardation.

Autosomal Dominant Hypophosphatemic Rickets (ADHR)

- ADHR is a rare disorder caused by activating mutations in the FGF-23 gene, and these mutations prevent proteolytic cleavage of FGF-23 with the resultant increase in circulating levels of this hormone.
- The phenotype is similar to that of X-linked hypophosphatemia.
- Treatment includes calcitriol and phosphate.

Autosomal Recessive Hypophosphatemic Rickets (ARHR)

- ARHR is caused by inactivating mutations in the DMP (dentin matrix protein) 1 gene. DMP 1 is derived from osteoblasts and osteocytes and participates in bone mineralization of extracellular matrix.
- The deficiency of DMP 1 results in increased FGF-23 expression and levels and clinical manifestation similar to that of ADHR.
- Another inactivating mutation in the ENPPI (endonucleotide pyrophosphatase/ phosphodiesterase I) gene has been shown to cause ARHR.
- Treatment is calcitriol and phosphate.

Tumor-Induced Osteomalacia (TIO)

- TIO or oncogenic osteomalacia is an acquired paraneoplastic (usually mesenchymal tumor) syndrome that occurs during the sixth decade of life.
- In addition to FGF-23, three other phosphaturic factors, namely, sFRP-4 (frizzled-related protein-4), MEPE (matrix extracellular phosphoglycoprotein), and FGF-7 have been identified with the tumor.
- Biochemical findings are similar to ADHR (phosphaturia, elevated FGF-23, and normal Ca^{2+}, as well as PTH levels).
- Treatment includes identification of the tumor followed by resection or chemotherapy, calcitriol, and phosphate.

Hereditary Hypophosphatemic Rickets with Hypercalciuria (HHRH) Due to Type IIc Mutation

- It is a rare autosomal recessive disorder caused by mutations in the gene that encodes Na/Pi-type IIc cotransporter.
- It is characterized by growth retardation, rickets, and increased renal phosphate and Ca^{2+} excretion.
- Unlike other hypophosphatemic rickets, HHRH is characterized by elevated levels of $1,25(OH)_2D_3$, which cause hypercalciuria and hypercalcemia.
- Choice of treatment is only phosphate supplementation.
- Note that calcitriol is *not* recommended, as it further causes hypercalcemia and renal stone formation.

Hereditary Hypophosphatemic Rickets with Hypercalciuria (HHRH) Due to Type IIa Mutation

- This is another recessive disorder, similar to the above disease, due to mutations in the gene that encode Na/Pi-type IIa cotransporter.
- Unlike type IIc disease, type IIa disease is associated with Fanconi syndrome.

Refeeding Syndrome (RFS)

- RFS occurs in malnourished individuals following administration of oral, enteral, or parenteral nutrition.
- Commonly seen in hospitalized patients, who are malnourished because of poor oral intake, starvation, anorexia nervosa, or systemic illness such as malignancy.
- Hypophosphatemia is the most commonly observed electrolyte abnormality induced by RFS.
- Many mechanisms contribute to hypophosphatemia: (1) a high carbohydrate meal causing intracellular shift of phosphate, (2) increased consumption of phosphate during glycolysis, (3) depleted body stores of phosphate during poor oral intake, and (4) consumption of phosphate for formation of ATP and increased production of products such as creatine kinase and 2,3-diphosphoglycerate.
- Sudden deaths also have been reported following RFS with high-caloric diet owing to hypophosphatemia. Almost all organ systems fail.
- To prevent hypophosphatemia, the feeding should consist of low calories with gradual increase to maintain the target caloric intake.
- Along with hypophosphatemia, other electrolyte abnormalities such as hypokalemia and hypomagnesemia also occur due to high glucose.
- Supplementation of K^+, Mg^{2+}, and phosphate along with nutrition will prevent RFS.

Hypophosphatemia in Critical Care Units

- Electrolyte disorders are common in critically ill patients during their stay in the intensive care unit.
- Hypophosphatemia is a frequently observed electrolyte disorder.
- Common causes include glucose-containing solutions, insulin administration, starvation, refeeding, sepsis, shock, trauma, postoperative state, respiratory alkalosis, metabolic acidosis, medications such as catecholamines and diuretics, and renal replacement therapies.

Clinical Manifestations

The clinical manifestations of hypophosphatemia depend on its onset and severity. Two biochemical abnormalities underlie the manifestations of phosphate deficiency. One is depletion of ATP, and the second is a reduction in erythrocyte 2,3-diphosphoglycerate. Both depletions lead to altered cellular function and hypoxia. Table 21.2 shows clinical and biochemical manifestations of severe hypophosphatemia.

Table 21.2 Clinical and biochemical abnormalities of hypophosphatemia

Neurologic	Confusion
	Irritability
	Anorexia
	Ataxia, dysarthria, paresthesia
	Seizures, coma
Cardiovascular	Cardiomyopathy
	Decreased cardiac output
	Altered membrane potential
Skeletal muscle	Muscle weakness
	Rhabdomyolysis
Bone	Bone pain
	Rickets
	Osteomalacia
	Pseudofractures
	Osteopenia
Hematologic	*Red blood cells*
	Decreased 2,3-diphosphoglycerate content
	Decreased ATP production
	Increased oxygen affinity
	Hemolysis
	Decreased life span
	Leukocytes
	Impaired phagocytosis
	Impaired bactericidal activity
	Impaired chemotaxis
	Platelets
	Thrombocytopenia
	Decreased life span
	Megakaryocytosis
Carbohydrate metabolism	Decreased glucose metabolism
	Insulin resistance
Biochemical	Increased creatine kinase
	Increased aldolase
	Decreased parathyroid hormone (PTH)
	Hypomagnesemia
Renal	Decreased glomerular filtration rate (GFR)
	Hypercalciuria
	Hypermagnesuria
	Hypophosphaturia
	Increased $1,25(OH)_2D_3$
	Decreased renal gluconeogenesis
	Decreased renal HCO_3^- threshold
	Decreased net titratable acidity

Table 21.2 (continued)

Respiratory	Respiratory muscle weakness
	Impaired diaphragmatic contractility
	Respiratory failure
	Difficulty in weaning
	Hypoxia

Diagnosis

Step 1
- First, the cause of hypophosphatemia should be established from the history, physical examination, and the clinical setting in which it occurs.
- History: Inquire about signs and symptoms, as listed in Table 21.2. History of alcoholism and medications is important. In hospitalized patients, review of dietary intake, IV fluids, and diagnosis is also important.

Step 2
- Physical examination should focus on musculoskeletal system.
- Muscle tenderness and pain—rhabdomyolysis.
- Pathologic or pseudofractures and skeletal deformities—rickets in children.
- Rachitic features in adults—chronic hypophosphatemia.
- Short stature with increased upper to lower body ratio—previous childhood rickets.
- Sinus tumors—TIO.
- Hepatomegaly—chronic alcoholism, tumors.
- Limited spine, joint, and hip motion in adults—X-linked hypophosphatemia.

Step 3
- Serum electrolytes, Ca^{2+}, phosphate, Mg^{2+}, alkaline phosphatase, and GFR
- Measure urine phosphate and creatinine.
- Calculate fractional excretion of phosphate (FE_{PO4}), which suggests renal or non-renal loss of phosphate.
- If FE_{PO4} is <5%, hypophosphatemia is nonrenal, suggesting transcellular distribution or decreased gastrointestinal absorption.
- If FE_{PO4} is >5%, hypophosphatemia is renal in origin.

Step 4
- Serum and urine Ca^{2+}, PTH, $25(OH)D_3$, and $1,25(OH)_2D_3$ levels are usually helpful in the differential diagnosis of various causes of hypophosphatemia.

Step 5
- Increased alkaline phosphatase and PTH levels suggest primary and secondary hyperparathyroidism as well as FGF-23-mediated hypophosphatemia.
- Serum FGF-23 levels are elevated in X-linked hypophosphatemia, ADHR, ARHR, TIO, and after transplantation.

Step 6
- Imaging studies for chronic hypophosphatemia:
  - Plain radiographs—fractures and skeletal abnormalities
  - Dual-energy X-ray absorptiometry scan—bone density and osteomalacia
  - Bone scan—increased uptake of ^{99}technitium at multiple sites in osteomalacia
  - Computed tomography (CT), magnetic resonance imaging (MRI), positron-emission tomography (PET)—TIO

Treatment

Treatment of hypophosphatemia depends on the onset and severity of symptoms and is aimed at removing the causes such as medications or dietary deficiency whenever possible (Fig. 21.1).

Acute Severe Symptomatic Hypophosphatemia

- It usually occurs in hospitalized patients and carries high morbidity and mortality.
- Although oral route is the safest, IV administration of either sodium or potassium phosphate with frequent monitoring of serum [Pi] is warranted.
- Table 21.3 shows IV and oral phosphate preparations.
- In hyperalimentation-induced hypophosphatemic (< 1.5 mg/dL) patients in an intensive care setting, infusion of 1 mmol/kg (1 mmol = 3.1 mg/dL) phosphorus diluted in 100 or 250 mL of either normal saline or 5% dextrose in water (D5W) at a rate not exceeding 7.5 mmol/h is sufficient to normalize serum phosphate in 48 h.
- In surgical intensive care patients, Taylor et al. [1] used a weight-based and serum phosphate-based protocol for IV phosphate repletion (Table 21.4). Either sodium or potassium phosphate, depending on serum K^+ levels, was dissolved in

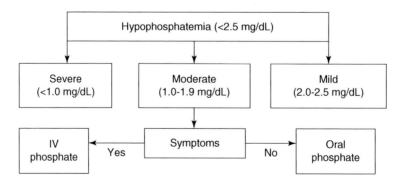

Fig. 21.1 Treatment algorithm for hypophosphatemia

Table 21.3 Intravenous and oral phosphate preparations

Preparation	Phosphate (PO_4)	Na^+ (mEq/L)	K^+ (mEq/L)
Intravenous			
Neutral Na/K PO_4	1.1 mmol/mL	0.2	0.02
Neutral $NaPO_4$	0.09 mmol/mL	0.2	0
Sodium PO_4	3 mmol/mL	4	0
Potassium PO_4	3 mmol/mL	0	4.4
Oral			
Skim milk	1 g/L	28	38
Neutra-phos	250 mg/packet	7.1/packet	7.1/packet
Neutra-phos K	250 mg/capsule	0	14.25/capsule
Phospho soda	150 mg/mL	4.8	0
K-Phos Original	150 mg/capsule	0	3.65/capsule
K-Phos Neutral	250 mg/tablet	13	1.1

Phosphate: 1 mmol/L = 3.1 mg/dL

Table 21.4 Intravenous phosphorus (mmol) repletion protocol

Serum phosphate	Weight (40–60 kg)	Weight (61–80 kg)	Weight (81–120 kg)
<0.32 mmol/L (<1 mg/dL)	30	40	50
0.32–0.54 mmol/L (1–1.7 mg/dL)	20	30	40
0.58–0.7 mmol/L (1.8–2.2 mg/dL)	10	15	20

250 mL of D5W and infused over 6 h as a single dose to severely hypophosphatemic (<1 mg/dL) or moderately hypophosphatemic (1.5–1.8 mg/dL) patients. Successful repletion occurred in 63% of severe and 78% of moderate hypophosphatemic patients. Thus, severe hypophosphatemic patients may benefit from more aggressive and tailored IV phosphorous regimens.

- Note that IV phosphate administration is associated with hypocalcemia and hyperphosphatemia. Fluid overload in congestive heart failure patients is a problem. In general, moderate hypophosphatemia does not require IV phosphate administration, except when symptoms warrant IV therapy.
- Parental calcium is needed in those with combined hypophosphatemia and hypocalcemia. In such cases, *do not* add either bicarbonate or phosphate to calcium-containing solutions.

Chronic Hypophosphatemia

- Management depends on the underlying cause.
- Oral therapy is indicated.
- Note that long-term oral therapy may suppress $1,25(OH)_2D_3$ levels and raise PTH and FGF-23 levels. To suppress PTH levels, concomitant administration of calcitriol is suggested.

- In renal transplant patients, an increase in dietary phosphate may improve hypophosphatemia. Oral phosphate therapy may be indicated in severe hypophosphatemia; however, hyperphosphatemia is a major concern. Therefore, cinacalcet may be indicated in some patients with close monitoring. Figure 21.1 summarizes the treatment modalities of hypophosphatemia.

Study Questions

Question 1 In hospitalized patients and clinical practice, hypophosphatemia is a common electrolyte disorder. Which one of the following drugs does NOT cause hypophosphatemia?

(A) Imatinib
(B) Tenofovir
(C) Corticosteroids
(D) Glucose
(E) Calcitriol

The answer is E Except for calcitriol, all other drugs cause hypophosphatemia. Imatinib, a tyrosine kinase inhibitor, is used in many malignant diseases. Long-term use of imatinib causes hypophosphatemia and secondary hyperparathyroidism. Tenofovir, a nucleotide that reverses transcriptase inhibitor, causes transient hypophosphatemia owing to Fanconi syndrome.

Corticosteroids cause a decrease in intestinal absorption of phosphate, and they also promote renal excretion of phosphate. Both these processes account for hypophosphatemia. Intravenous glucose or carbohydrate intake transports phosphate into the cell, causing hypophosphatemia.

Calcitriol increases gastrointestinal absorption of phosphate and causes relative hyperphosphatemia. Therefore, option E is correct.

Question 2 Which one of the following metabolic abnormalities is NOT related to severe hypophosphatemia (<1.0 mg/dL)?

(A) Rhabdomyolysis
(B) Metabolic acidosis
(C) Increased susceptibility to infection
(D) Decreased cardiac output
(E) Metabolic alkalosis

The answer is E Moderate hypophosphatemia is defined as serum phosphate level between 1.2 and 1.8 mg/dL, whereas severe hypophosphatemia constitutes serum phosphate level <1.0 mg/dL. Metabolic complications are clearly evident with severe hypophosphatemia. Muscle requires adequate amounts of ATP and creatine phosphate for its actions. Phosphate depletion leads to low intracellular phosphate and an increase in Na^+, Cl^-, and water, resulting in myopathy, weakness, and muscle injury. Rhabdomyolysis is a complication of low serum phosphate, which may present with acute kidney injury.

Metabolic acidosis due to severe hypophosphatemia is related to a decrease in net acid excretion (titratable acid and ammonium), resulting in retention of H^+. Also, hypophosphatemia decreases renal tubular reabsorption of HCO_3^-. Thus, metabolic acidosis in severe hypophosphatemia is due to the above mechanisms.

Increased susceptibility to infection is related to leukocyte dysfunction caused by decreased ATP production.

Severe hypophosphatemia is associated with cardiomyopathy and low cardiac output, which are due to low myocyte concentration of phosphate, ATP, and creatine phosphate. Metabolic alkalosis is not a complication of severe hypophosphatemia, and thus option E is correct.

Question 3 Regarding treatment of hypophosphatemia, which one of the following statements is FALSE?

(A) In asymptomatic ambulatory patient, moderate hypophosphatemia (1.2–1.8 mg/dL) can be corrected by oral phosphate repletion
(B) Hyperalimentation-induced severe hypophosphatemia (<1 mg/dL) requires aggressive intravenous (IV) treatment with 1 mmol/kg over 10 h
(C) Intravenous phosphate repletion depends on the severity of phosphate deficiency and body weight
(D) Moderate degree of hypophosphatemia after heavy carbohydrate meal does not require phosphate repletion
(E) Moderate hypophosphatemia (>1 mg/dL) generally causes severe metabolic complications and requires vigorous IV replacement of phosphate

The answer is E The treatment of hypophosphatemia depends on its signs and symptoms and the degree (severity) of phosphate deficiency. Asymptomatic patients should be treated with oral preparations (Table 21.3). Serum phosphate levels can rise by as much as 1.5 mg/dL 60–120 min after oral intake of 1 g of elemental phosphate. In children and malnourished individuals, skim milk is an adequate repletion of phosphate because each liter contains 1 g of elemental phosphate and is better tolerated than regular milk.

Intravenous administration of phosphate is reserved for patients with severe hypophosphatemia (<1 mg/dL) with symptoms and those receiving hyperalimentation and critically ill patients. In surgical intensive care patients, Taylor et al. [1] used a weight-based and serum phosphate-based protocol for IV phosphate repletion (see Table 21.4).

Transcellular distribution of phosphate from extracellular fluid (ECF) to intracellular fluid (ICF) occurs after a carbohydrate load or glucose infusion, which does not require immediate treatment. Serum phosphate level >1 mg/dL may not cause

Table 21.5 Serum chemistry in disorders of hypophosphatemia

Disorder	Phosphate	Ca^{2+}	1,25(OH)$_2$D3	PTH	FGF-23
ADHR	↓	N	↓	N	↑
ARHR	↓	N	N	N	↑
XLH	↓	N	↓/N	N	↑
TIO	↓	N	↓/N	N	↑
Primary Hyperparathyroidism	↓	↑	↑	↑	↑/N

↑ increased, ↓ decreased, *N* normal, ↓/*N* low/normal, *ADHR* autosomal dominant hypophosphatemic rickets, *ARHR* Autosomal recessive hypophosphatemic rickets, *XLH* X-linked hypophosphatemia, *TIO* tumor-induced osteomalacia, *PTH* parathyroid hormone, *FGF-23* fibroblast growth factor-23

severe metabolic complications, and vigorous IV treatment is not necessary. Thus, option E is false.

Question 4 Which one of the following human phosphate wasting diseases is *ASSOCIATED* with high levels of active vitamin D (1,25 (OH)$_2$D3)?

(A) Autosomal dominant hypophosphatemic rickets (ADHR)
(B) Autosomal recessive hypophosphatemic rickets (ARHR)
(C) X-linked hypophosphatemia (XLH)
(D) Tumor-induced osteomalacia (TIO)
(E) Primary hyperparathyroidism

The answer is E The etiology for hypophosphatemia in the above disorders other than primary hyperparathyroidism is elevated levels of FGF-23. In these disorders, the active vitamin D levels are generally low to normal, but in hyperparathyroidism, they are elevated. Thus, option E is correct. Table 21.5 shows the levels of phosphate, Ca^{2+}, vitamin D, PTH, and FGF-23 in all of the above disorders.

Question 5 Match the following serum values with the patient history.

Option	Phosphate	Ca^{2+}	1,25(OH)$_2$D$_3$	PTH	FGF-23
A	↓	↑	↑	↑	N↑
B	↓	↑	↓	N↓	↑
C	N	↑	↑	↓	↑
D	↓	↓	N↓	↑	↑ (?)
E	↑	↓	↓	↑	↑

↑ increased, ↓ decreased, *N* normal, *PTH* parathyroid hormone, *FGF-23* fibroblast growth factor-23

1. A 45-year-old African-American woman with hilar adenopathy on chest X-ray (CXR) and decreased diffusing lung capacity on pulmonary function tests
2. A 30-year-old obese female with short-bowl resection and subsequent fat malabsorption

3. A 60-year-old man with long history of smoking and a lung mass on CXR
4. A 24-year-old female with bilateral flank pain, frequent urinary tract infections (UTIs) with hematuria, and envelope-like crystals on urine microscopy
5. A 50-year-old housewife with joint pain, headache, hypertension, and nocturia, and a urinalysis revealing dysmorphic RBCs and 1 + proteinuria

Answers: A = 4; B = 3; C = 1; D = 2, E = 5 The patient described in A seems to have sarcoidosis. The patient with sarcoidosis usually has hypercalcemia due to elevated calcitriol secreted by the granuloma. PTH is generally low because of its inhibition by high levels of calcitriol and hypercalcemia. Phosphate levels are normal. FGF-23 may be elevated or remains normal. Labs shown in option C are consistent with sarcoidosis.

Subjects with short-bowl syndrome develop vitamin D deficiency, which causes low calcitriol, hypocalcemia, and hypophosphatemia. Hypocalcemia and low calcitriol stimulate PTH secretion, resulting in elevated PTH levels. Low calcitriol stimulates FGF-23, which in turn causes phosphaturia and hypophosphatemia. High PTH may also contribute to hypophosphatemia. Laboratory results shown in D are suggestive of vitamin D deficiency.

The patient with lung mass seems to have lung cancer that secretes PTH$_r$P (PTH-related protein), which causes hypercalcemia. Patients with humoral hypercalcemia also demonstrate hypophosphatemia, inappropriately low calcitriol, and low calcitriol-induced high FGF-23 levels, the latter causing hypophosphatemia. PTH may be either normal or slightly low. Laboratory results shown in B are consistent with lung malignancy.

The description of a young female with UTIs and envelope-like crystals (calcium oxalate) is suggestive of primary hyperparathyroidism, causing elevated PTH, hypercalcemia, and hypophosphatemia. FGF-23 levels have been shown to be either normal or elevated in primary hyperparathyroidism. Laboratory results given in A are consistent with primary hyperthyroidism.

The clinical manifestations of the housewife (choice 5) are suggestive of stage 3–4 chronic kidney disease (CKD) probably related to analgesic use. Hypocalcemia, hyperphosphatemia, hyperparathyroidism, and elevated FGF-23 levels are related to declining renal function. Values shown in E are suggestive of CKD.

Case 1 A 67-year-old thin woman with colon cancer and colostomy is admitted for poor oral intake, weakness, dizziness, and weight loss. She is receiving chemotherapy. The oncologist starts her on total parenteral nutrition with 2,000 calories a day. Serum chemistry is normal, including Ca^{2+}, Mg^{2+}, and phosphate. Two days later, the patient complains of worsening weakness. Repeat laboratory results show K^+ 3.1 mEq/L, Ca^{2+} 7.8 mg/dL, Mg^{2+} 1.6 mEq/L, and phosphate 1.1 mg/dL.

Which one of the following describes the BEST for the above abnormalities in laboratory results?

(A) Metabolic acidosis
(B) Respiratory alkalosis
(C) Refeeding syndrome
(D) Chemotherapy
(E) None of the above

The answer is C Refeeding syndrome (RFS) occurs in malnourished individuals following administration of oral, enteral, or parenteral nutrition. Hypophosphatemia is the most commonly observed electrolyte abnormality induced by RFS. Along with hypophosphatemia, other electrolyte abnormalities such as hypokalemia and hypomagnesemia also occur because of high glucose. Supplementation of K^+, Mg^{2+}, and phosphate along with nutrition will prevent RFS. Other options do not describe adequately the clinical picture of the patient.

Reference

1. Taylor BE, Huey WY, Buchman TG, et al. Treatment of hypophosphatemia using a protocol based on patient weight and serum phosphorus level in a surgical intensive care unit (see comment). J Am Coll Surg. 2004;198:198–204.

Suggested Reading

2. Amanjadeh J, Reilly RF Jr. Hypophosphatemia: an evidence-based approach to its clinical consequences and management. Nat Clin Pract Nephrol. 2006;2:136–48.
3. Bacchetta I, Salusky I. Evaluation of hypophosphatemia: lesions from patients with genetic disorders. Am J Kidney Dis. 2012;59:152–9.
4. Brunelli SM, Goldfarb S. Hypophosphatemia: clinical consequences and management. J Am Soc Nephrol. 2007;18:1999–2003.
5. Felsenfeld AJ, Levine BS. Approach to treatment of hypophosphatemia. Am J Kidney Dis. 2012;60:655–61.
6. Geerse DA, Bindels AJ, Kuiper MA, et al. Treatment of hypophosphatemia in the intensive care unit: a review. Crit Care. 2010;14:R147.
7. Hruska KA, Levi M, Slatopolsky E. Disorders of phosphorus, calcium, and magnesium metabolism. In: Coffman TM, Falk RJ, Molitoris BA, et al., editors. Schrier's diseases of the kidney. 9th ed. Philadelphia: Lippincott Williams & Wilkins; 2013. p. 2116–81.
8. Imel EA, Econs MJ. Approach to the hypophosphatemic patient. J Clin Endocrinol Metab. 2012;97:696–706.
9. Liams G, Milionis HJ, Elisaf M. Medication-induced hypophosphatemia: a review. Q J Med. 2010;103:449–59.
10. Smogorzewski MJ, Stubbs JR, Yu ASL. Disorders of calcium, magnesium, and phosphate balance. In: Skorecki K, et al., editors. Brenner and Rector's the kidney. 10th ed. Philadelphia: Elsevier; 2016. p. 601–35.
11. Subramanian R, Khardori R. Severe hypophosphatemia. Pathophysiologic implications, clinical presentations, and treatment. Medicine. 2000;79:1–8.
12. Tennenhouse HS, Murer H. Disorders of renal tubular phosphate transport. J Am Soc Nephrol. 2003;14:240–7.

Disorders of Phosphate: Hyperphosphatemia

22

Hyperphosphatemia is defined as serum [Pi] >4.5 mg/dL. Spurious increase in serum [Pi] is called *pseudohyperphosphatemia*. It is rather rare but has been described in conditions of hyperglobulinemia, hypertriglyceridemia, and hyperbilirubinemia. This spurious increase has been attributed to the interference of proteins and triglycerides in the colorimetric assay of phosphate. The causes of true hyperphosphatemia can be discussed under three major categories: (1) addition of phosphate from the intracellular fluid (ICF) to extracellular fluid (ECF) compartment, (2) a decrease in renal excretion of phosphate, and (3) drugs (Table 22.1). In clinical practice, acute and chronic kidney diseases are probably the most significant causes of hyperphosphatemia.

Table 22.1 Major causes of hyperphosphatemia

Cause	Mechanism
Addition of phosphate to ECF compartment	
Endogenous	
Hemolysis	Release from hemolyzed red blood cells
Rhabdomyolysis	Release from muscle cells
Tumor lysis syndrome	Release from tumor cells due to chemotherapy or cell turnover
High catabolic state	Release from cells
Exogenous	
Oral intake or through IV route	Ingestion of sodium phosphate solution for bowl preparation or IV Na/K phosphate in hospitalized patients
Phosphate-containing enemas	Phosphate absorption from enemas (fleet enema)
Respiratory acidosis	Release from cells
Lactic acidosis	Phosphate utilization during glycolysis, leading to its depletion and subsequent release from cells
Diabetic ketoacidosis	Shift of phosphate from ICF to ECF due to insulin deficiency and metabolic acidosis

(continued)

© Springer Science+Business Media LLC 2018
A.S. Reddi, *Fluid, Electrolyte and Acid-Base Disorders*,
DOI 10.1007/978-3-319-60167-0_22

Table 22.1 (continued)

Cause	Mechanism
Decreased renal excretion	
Chronic kidney disease stages 4 and 5	Inability of the kidneys to excrete phosphate load
Acute kidney injury	Inability to excrete phosphate and release from muscle during rhabdomyolysis
Hypoparathyroidism	Increased renal phosphate reabsorption
Pseudohypoparathyroidism	Renal and skeletal resistance to PTH
Familial tumor calcinosis	Mutations in GALNT3, FGF-23, and KLOTHO genes
Drugs	
Excess vitamin D	Increased gastrointestinal (GI) absorption of phosphate
Bisphosphonates	Decreased phosphate excretion, cellular shift
Growth hormone	Increased proximal tubule reabsorption
Liposomal amphotericin B	Contains phosphatidyl choline and phosphatidyl serine
Sodium phosphate (oral)	GI absorption of phosphate

Some Specific Causes of Hyperphosphatemia

Acute Kidney Injury (AKI)

Serum phosphate levels between 5 and 10 mg/dL are common in patients with AKI. However, when AKI is caused by rhabdomyolysis, tumor lysis syndrome, hemolysis, or severe burns, serum levels may be as high as 20 mg/dL. The mechanisms for hyperphosphatemia in AKI include (1) decreased $1,25(OH)_2D_3$ production, (2) skeletal resistance to parathyroid hormone (PTH) action, and (3) metastatic deposition as calcium phosphate in soft tissues.

Chronic Kidney Disease (CKD)

In early stages of CKD (glomerular filteration rate (GFR) 30–60 mL/min), phosphate homeostasis is maintained by progressive increase in phosphate excretion by the surviving nephrons. As a result, FE_{PO4} increases to >35% (normal 5–7%).

This increased phosphate excretion is due to elevated FGF-23 levels, which subsequently inhibit $1,25(OH)_2D_3$ production. The low production of $1,25(OH)_2D_3$ stimulates the secretion of PTH causing secondary hyperparathyroidism. Both FGF-23 and PTH inhibit reabsorption of phosphate in the proximal tubule and enhance its urinary excretion. Thus, FE_{PO4} increases by >35% to maintain normal serum phosphate level at the cost of high FGF-23 and PTH.

In CKD stages 4 and 5, the GFR is <30 mL/min. In these stages of CKD, hyperphosphatemia develops due to decreased excretion and release of phosphate from the bone. At the same time, deficiency of Klotho occurs with the development of CKD. This deficiency in Klotho's expression causes an increase in FGF-23 secretion, which lowers $1,25(OH)_2D_3$. This reduction in active vitamin D stimulates PTH secretion. Increased PTH induces more FGF-23 levels, which reduce the levels of $1,25(OH)_2D_3$ even further. Deficiency of Klotho causes resistance to FGF-23 action on phosphate excretion, as Klotho is a cofactor for FGF-23.

This cycle—of Klotho's deficiency with resistance of FGF-23 and decreased phosphate excretion—leads to hyperphosphatemia in CKD stages 4 and 5.

Deficiency of Klotho can also cause secondary hyperparathyroidism via FGF-23. In normal subjects, Klotho is expressed not only in the kidney but parathyroid glands as well. In CKD 4 and 5, there is deficiency of Klotho in parathyroid glands. This deficiency of Klotho causes FGF-23 resistance and prevents suppression of PTH, causing secondary hyperparathyroidism. Thus, secondary hyperparathyroidism occurs by reduced levels of $1,25(OH)_2D_3$ and nonsuppressability of PTH by FGF-23. Also, the independent phosphaturic effect of Klotho is lost by its deficiency, causing hyperphosphatemia in CKD. Figure 22.1 summarizes the pathogenesis of hyperphosphatemia and secondary hyperparathyroidism in CKD 4 and 5 patients.

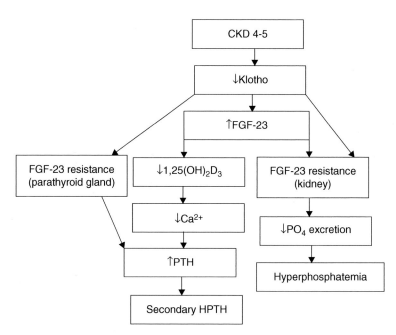

Fig. 22.1 Pathogenesis of hyperphosphatemia and secondary hyperparathyroidism in CKD 4 and 5. *HPTH* hyperparathyroidism

Sodium Phosphate Use and Hyperphosphatemia

Oral sodium phosphate (OSP) solution is the most commonly used agent for bowl preparation for colonoscopy. It is given as two 45 mL doses, 9–12 h apart. The 90 mL solution contains 43.2 g of monobasic and 16.2 g of dibasic sodium phosphate. Because of its high phosphate content, hyperphosphatemia is an early observed electrolyte abnormality. Death due to severe hyperphosphatemia had been reported.

Hypocalcemia develops because of hyperphosphatemia. Hyponatremia is also a common electrolyte abnormality because of excessive water intake, particularly in elderly women who are on thiazide diuretics, antidepressants, or angiotensin-converting enzyme inhibitors. Hypokalemia has also been observed because of K^+ loss in the GI tract and kidneys. In some patients, hypernatremia has been observed, which is due to high Na^+ content in OSP solutions.

About 1–4% of subjects develop acute phosphate nephropathy with normal or near-normal renal function. Besides electrolyte abnormalities, AKI also develops after OSP administration.

Familial Tumor Calcinosis (FTC)

- Familial tumor calcinosis (FTC) is a rare autosomal recessive disorder.
- This disease has been described in families from Africa and Mediterranean areas.
- Hyperphosphatemia is related to increased proximal tubular reabsorption of phosphate.
- The disease is caused by loss-of-function mutations in three genes:
  1. GALNT3 (the uridine-diphosphate-N-acetyl-α-D-galactosamine), which causes aberrant FGF-23 glycosylation
  2. FGF-23, a missense mutation in the gene inhibiting FGF-23 secretion
  3. KLOTHO, causing resistance to FGF-23 action
- Clinically, the patients present with deposition of calcium phosphate crystals in the hip, elbow, or shoulder.
- Serum Ca^{2+}, PTH, and alkaline phosphatase levels are normal, but $1,25(OH)_2D_3$ levels are slightly elevated.
- Treatment includes low phosphate diet, phosphate binders, and acetazolamide. Surgery may occasionally be needed.

Clinical Manifestations

Clinical manifestations are related to hyperphosphatemia-induced hypocalcemia (paresthesia, tetany). In patients with CKD stage 5 and patients on dialysis, hyper-phosphatemia is common, and precipitation of calcium phosphate occurs in vascular and muscular systems. Skin deposition is also common. Hyperphosphatemia is an independent risk factor for all-cause or cardiovascular mortality in CKD stages 4 and 5 (see Question 1).

Diagnosis

Step 1 Following the history and physical examination, obtain complete metabolic panel, hemoglobin, and iron indices. Obtain PTH and $1,25(OH)_2D_3$ levels.
Step 2 Confirm true hyperphosphatemia after ruling out pseudohyperphosphatemia.
Step 3 Establish the severity and onset of hyperphosphatemia.
Step 4 Check blood urea nitrogen (BUN) and creatinine. If normal, look for causes (exogenous or endogenous) of acute phosphate load and those that promote renal reabsorption of phosphate. If BUN and creatinine are elevated, differentiate between AKI and CKD.

Treatment

Hyperphosphatemia is a risk factor for cardiovascular morbidity and mortality, vascular classification, and secondary hyperparathyroidism. Therefore, control of hyperphosphatemia is extremely important. The treatment strategies include control of dietary phosphate, phosphate binders, and dialysis.

Diet

The best practice of hyperphosphatemia management in CKD stages 4 and 5 or dialysis patients are restriction of dietary protein and avoidance of phosphate-containing foods. Dietician's consultation is needed for prescription of an appropriate diet to prevent malnutrition. Processed foods and beverages that contain phosphate should be minimized in planning a diet for CKD patients. However, the patients do not adhere to the diet because of low palatability. Therefore, control of hyperphosphatemia with intestinal phosphate-binding agents is necessary.

Phosphate Binders

Table 22.2 shows the classification of available phosphate binders.

- Historically *aluminum hydroxide* was used as a phosphate binder. However, it caused adynamic bone disease with bone pain and fractures, microcytic anemia, and dementia in a substantial number of patients. Therefore, its use has been abandoned.
- Subsequently, calcium (Ca)-containing binders, such as Ca carbonate (Caltrate, Os-Cal) and *Ca acetate* (PhosLo) became available. Although they reduce serum phosphate level, it became apparent that they cause hypercalcemia and vascular calcification. These complications prompted the nephrologists to use non-Ca-containing binders such as sevelamer HCl.

Table 22.2 Phosphate binders

Binder	Common name	How supplied	Starting dose
Ca-containing binders			
Ca carbonate	Caltrate, Tums, Os-Cal, Calcichew	Variable	500–2,000 mg/day
Ca acetate	PhosLo, Phoslyra	667 mg or 667 mg/5 mL	1–2 tabs or 5–10 mL with meals
Non-Ca-containing binders			
Sevelamer HCl	Renagel	400–800 mg	400 or 800 mg Tables 1–2 with meals
Sevelamer carbonate	Renvela	800 mg tab or powder	1–2 with meals
Metal-based binders			
Lanthanum carbonate	Fosrenol	500, 750, 1,000 mg chewable tab or 750 or 100 mg powder	500 mg with meals
Aluminum hydroxide (not used chronically)	Amphogel (other names available)	Variable	30–50 mL in between or with meals
Iron-containing binders			
Sucroferric oxyhydroxide	Velphoro	500 mg chewable tab	500 mg with meals
Ferric citrate	Auryxia	100 mg tab	2 tabs with meals
Newer binders			
Colestilan[a]	BindRen	1,000 mg tab	1 tab with meals

[a]Available in the UK

- *Sevelamer HCl (Renagel)* has been shown to control phosphate as much as Ca-containing binders without causing hypercalcemia. Studies also have shown that sevelamer slowed the progression of coronary artery calcification, as compared with a Ca-containing binder. In addition, sevelamer lowered low-density lipoprotein (LDL) cholesterol levels in dialysis patients, and survival benefit has also been reported. However, it is expensive and causes hyperchloremic metabolic acidosis. To improve metabolic acidosis, the next-generation sevelamer compound has been introduced. It is called sevelamer carbonate (Renvela). It was shown that sevelamer carbonate has the physiologic and biochemical profile as sevelamer HCl except for an increase of serum HCO_3^- level of approximately 2 mEq/L.
- Another non-Ca-containing phosphate binder is *lanthanum carbonate* (Fosrenol), which binds phosphate ionically. Unlike other binders, the potency of lanthanum carbonate as a binder is so great that the pill burden is reduced which may aid the patient's adherence to therapy. Several concerns have been raised about its long-term safety as it belongs to the family of aluminum in the periodic table. However, studies have shown no adverse effects in dialysis patients who were followed for a period of 6 years. In one study, the incidence of hypercalcemia was 0.4% in the lanthanum group compared to 20.2% in the Ca-treated group.
- Two iron-binding agents (sucroferric oxyhydroxid or Velphoro and ferric citrate or Auryxia) have been introduced in recent years. Both drugs seem to lower phosphate as efficiently as sevelamer.

Table 22.3 Effects of some commonly used phosphate (PO$_4$) binders for hyperphosphatemia on biochemical parameters relevant to mineral bone disorder

Binder	Ca^{2+}	PO$_4$	PTH	LDL-C	Vascular calcification	Comment
Ca carbonate	↑↑	↓↓	↓↓	↔	↑	Hypercalcemia, ↑vascular complications, low cost
Ca acetate	↑↑	↓↓	↓↓	↔	↑	Hypercalcemia, increased vascular complications, low cost (US$ 1,000–2,000/year)
Sevelamer HCl	↔	↓	↓	↓	↓	Metabolic acidosis, higher pill burden, abdominal pain and bloating, N/V, expensive (US$ 4,400–8,800/year)
Sevelamer carbonate	↔	↓	↓	↓	↓	Metabolic acidosis, higher pill burden, abdominal pain and bloating, N/V, expensive (US$ 5,500–11,000/year)
Lanthanum carbonate	↔	↓↓	↓	↔	↔	N/V, diarrhea, constipation, hypercalcemia, long-term safety (?), expensive (US$ 7,000–14,000/year)

↔ No significant change, ↑ mild increase, ↑↑ moderate increase, ↓ mild decrease, ↓↓ moderate decrease, *PTH* Parathyroid hormone, *LDL-C* low-density lipoprotein cholesterol, *N/V* nausea/vomiting

- *Magnesium (Mg) carbonate* is less effective than Ca-containing binder, but it is less often used in dialysis patients because of the fear of diarrhea and aggravation of hypermagnesemia. However, Mg carbonate may improve vascular calcification. Despite this beneficial effect, the use of Mg carbonate is not preferred at this time. Table 22.3 summarizes the effects of phosphate binders on various biochemical parameters relevant to mineral bone disorder in CKD stage 5 (on dialysis) patients.

Acute Hyperphosphatemia

Eliminate the cause. Use phosphate binders as needed. Aluminum hydroxide, although not recommended for chronic use, has been found to be useful in controlling moderate hyperphosphatemia in hospitalized patients with normal renal function. At times, hemodialysis is necessary when hyperphosphatemia is due to rhabdomyolysis or tumor lysis syndrome.

Chronic Hyperphosphatemia

- Mostly seen in patients with CKD stage 5 and on dialysis.
- Dietary restriction of phosphate is extremely important.

- Restricted intake of milk, milk products, meat, grains, and processed foods is to be recommended in consultation with a dietician.
- Phosphate binders are needed in almost all patients on dialysis in addition to dietary restriction.
- Select a phosphate binder that is easy to take and low in cost, provides maximum benefit, and has low adverse effects. Unfortunately, none of the phosphate binders (Table 22.2) fulfils all of these criteria.
- Selection between a Ca-containing binder and non-Ca-containing binder is difficult.
- Advantages of sevelamer HCl or carbonate are prevention and improvement in vascular calcification (Table 22.2).
- Advantage of lanthanum is a decrease in pill burden (3–4 tablets/day). Good as a second-on drug addition.
- Cinacalcet, a calcimimetic, lowers both Ca^{2+} and phosphate in dialysis patients with secondary hyperparathyroidism.

Study Questions

Question 1 High serum phosphate (PO_4) level is an independent risk factor for cardiovascular morbidity and mortality in CKD 4 and dialysis patients. Which one of the following factors regarding hyperphosphatemia is FALSE?

(A) Hyperphosphatemia stimulates PTH secretion independent of Ca^{2+} levels
(B) Hyperphosphatemia may increase cell proliferation and growth of parathyroid through transforming growth factor-α (TGF-α)
(C) Hyperphosphatemia reduces the expression of the calcium-sensing receptor (CaSR) and the ability of the parathyroid gland to respond to changes in ionized Ca^{2+}
(D) Hyperphosphatemia indirectly increases PTH by inhibiting 1α-hydroxylase activity, thereby reducing the production of active vitamin D_3
(E) Hyperphosphatemia alone is not sufficient to cause vascular calcification in the absence of hypercalcemia

The answer is E Studies have shown that hyperphosphatemia can stimulate PTH secretion directly and indirectly. Regulation of PTH secretion by PO_4 alone was demonstrated in CKD animals with PO_4-restricted diet. In these studies, low PO_4 diet reduced PTH secretion independent of serum Ca^{2+} and $1,25(OH)_2D_3$ levels. These results were reproduced in CKD patients. It appears that the parathyroid gland responds to changes in serum PO_4 at the level of secretion, gene expression, and cell proliferation through phospholipase A_2-activated signal transduction mechanism. It was also shown that hyperphosphatemia may promote cell proliferation and growth of parathyroid via TGF-α and epidermal growth factor.

Hyperphosphatemia has also been shown to reduce the expression of CaSR, thereby decreasing the ability of the parathyroid gland to respond to changes in ionized Ca^{2+}. Restriction of PO_4 in diet restores the expression and sensitivity of the receptor.

Hyperphosphatemia stimulates PTH secretion indirectly by lowering Ca^{2+} via inhibition of 1α-hydroxylase in the kidney, thereby reducing the conversion of $25(OH)_2$ to $1,25(OH)_2D_3$. Also, several studies have shown that hyperphosphatemia alone can cause vascular calcification in CKD patients without the combination of hypercalcemia and vitamin D. Thus, option E is false.

Question 2 With regard to PO_4 binders and vascular calcification (VC), which one of the following statements is FALSE?

(A) The Renagel in New Dialysis (RIND) study showed that the absolute median increase was 11-fold greater in coronary artery calcification (CAC) score with Ca-containing binders than with sevelamer in hemodialysis (HD) patients
(B) The treat-to-goal (TTG) study reported that Ca binder suppressed iPTH below target range of 150–300 pg/mL than sevelamer in HD patients
(C) The Calcium Acetate Renagel Evaluation 2 (CARE-2) study concluded that sevelamer is noninferior to Ca acetate with respect to CAC score in HD patients
(D) The phosphate binder impact on bone remodeling and coronary calcification (BRiC) showed no significant difference on CAC score between Ca acetate and sevelamer-treated HD patients
(E) In predialysis patients, treatment with either Ca carbonate or sevelamer had no beneficial effect on CAC score

The answer is E There are several studies that evaluated the effects of Ca-based and non-Ca-based binders on VC: six on HD and one on predialysis patients. Table 22.4 summarizes the results of these studies.

Question 3 With regard to phosphate (PO_4) binders and mortality, which one of the following statements is FALSE?

(A) A prospective study showed that mortality was higher in HD patients with Ca-based binder compared to non-Ca-based binder
(B) A retrospective study reported improved survival in HD patients treated with sevelamer compared to those HD patients on Ca-based binder
(C) Non-Ca-based binder increases both PO_4 and Ca^{2+} in HD patients and improves survival
(D) Non-Ca-based binder decreases PO_4 and Ca × PO_4 product without any effect on Ca in HD patients and improves survival
(E) The Dialysis Clinical Outcomes Revisited (DCOR) trial showed no difference in all-cause mortality between Ca-based binder and non-Ca-based binder in HD patients

Table 22.4 Effects of Ca-based and non-Ca-based binders on vascular calcification

Study (reference)	Study patients	Study duration (months)	No. randomized	Results
TTG (Chertow et al. [1])	HD	12	101 Ca[a]/99 S[b]	Increase in coronary artery and aorta calcification (CAC) with Ca vs S
Braun et al. [2]	HD	12	59 CaCO₃/55 S	Increase in CAC with Ca vs S
RIND (Block et al. [3])	HD	18	75 Ca[a]/73 S[b]	Rapid and severe increase in CAC with Ca vs S
Russo et al. [4]	Predialysis (no previous treatment with binders)	24	30 low-P diet; 30 low-P diet + CaCO₃; 30 low-P diet + S	Progression of CAC greatest with low-P diet followed by Ca and then S
BRiC (Barreto et al. [5])	HD	12	49 Ca acetate/52 S	No difference in CAC between Ca and S
CARE2 (Quniby et al. [6])	HD	12	103 Ca acetate + atorvastatin/100 S + atorvastatin	No difference in CAC between Ca and S
Takei et al. [7]	HD	6	20 CaCO₃/22 S	Greater progression of CAC with Ca vs S

HD Hemodialysis
[a]CaCO₃ or Ca acetate
[b]Sevelamer

The answer is C Several studies addressed the issue of PO_4 binders and mortality in HD patients, as reviewed by Molony and Stephens [8]. For example, the RIND study [3] showed that the all-cause mortality was higher in Ca-treated patients than sevelamer-treated patients over a 4-year period. A retrospective VA study also showed a survival advantage with sevelamer over Ca carbonate for up to 2 years. In contrast, the DCOR study [9] showed no overall mortality advantage with sevelamer compared to Ca acetate up to 2 years. However, there was a 20% reduction in mortality in patients over 65 years of age who were treated with sevelamer. Also, multiple all-cause hospitalization rate and hospital days were much lower in the sevelamer group. In general, these studies demonstrate a survival advantage with sevelamer.

It is the experience of many investigators that sevelamer lowers PO_4 similar to Ca-based binders without increasing serum Ca^{2+}. Thus, option C is false.

Case 1 A 68-year-old woman with diabetes mellitus is admitted for mucormycosis of the left ear. She is started on high doses of liposomal amphotericin B (L-AMP). One week later, her serum phosphate increased from 4.2 to 10.8 mg/dL, and repeat phosphate is 11.2 mg/dL. Her creatinine, Ca^{2+}, uric acid, and creatine kinase (CK) are normal.

Question 1 Which one of the following is the MOST likely cause of her hyperphosphatemia?

(A) Rhabdomyolysis
(B) Respiratory alkalosis
(C) Liposomal amphotericin B
(D) Tumor calcinosis
(E) None of the above

The answer is C The sudden increase in serum phosphate in a patient who is not on phosphate replacement could indicate laboratory error. Repeat analysis confirmed hyperphosphatemia. The patient was asymptomatic. Rhabdomyolysis can be ruled out based on normal creatinine, Ca^{2+}, uric acid, and CK levels. Arterial blood gas showed chronic respiratory alkalosis, which causes hypophosphatemia by transcellular distribution of phosphate. Tumor calcinosis is a rare genetic disorder that is characterized by hyperphosphatemia, elevated levels of $1,25(OH)_2D_3$, and decreased renal excretion of phosphate. Thus, options A, B, D, and E are incorrect.

L-AMP is an antifungal preparation that contains amphotericin B embedded in a phospholipid bilayer of unilamellar liposomes. Measurement of phosphate from L-AMP-treated patients with a specific autoanalyzer, Synchron LX20 (Beckman Coulter), gives a high level of serum phosphate with normal Ca^{2+} levels. This autoanalyzer measures the phosphate at low pH (<1.0). At this acid pH, organic phosphate contained in the lipid bilayer of the liposomes is hydrolyzed and gives falsely high levels of serum phosphate. Thus, high doses of L-AMP will give pseudohyperphosphatemia when measured with LX20 system. Other autoanalyzers measure the reaction at high pH and do not give pseudohyperphosphatemia. However, some authors believe that L-AMP adds phosphorus derived from phosphotidyl choline and phosphotidyl serine present in liposomes. Thus, option C is correct.

Case 2 A 56-year-old man with estimated GFR (eGFR) of 16 mL/min, on calcium acetate 667 mg (one tablet) with each meal, is found to have serum Ca^{2+} level of 10.8 mg/dL and a phosphate level of 7.2 mg/dL. He says that he follows the physician's and dietician's orders very strictly. A repeat eGFR is 16 mL/min.

Question 1 Explain the mechanisms for hyperphosphatemia in this patient.

Answer As stated under CKD stages 4 and 5, there are several mechanisms for hyperphosphatemia:

1. Decreased excretion of phosphate because of low GFR
2. Decreased expression of Klotho
3. Increased levels of FGF-23 with renal resistance
4. Increased PTH levels
5. Decreased synthesis and levels of $1,25(OH)_2D_3$

Question 2 Why is his serum Ca^{2+} level high?

Answer It is not uncommon to see hypercalcemia with calcium acetate treatment either in predialysis or dialysis patients. It is one of the adverse effects of calcium-containing phosphate binders.

Question 3 How is phosphate homeostasis maintained in CKD patients with eGFR 30–60 mL/min?

Answer FGF-23 is an important regulator of phosphate homeostasis in early stages of CKD. A small rise in serum phosphate stimulates FGF-23 synthesis in bone cells, and FGF-23 levels increase. FGF-23 inhibits renal reabsorption of phosphate. As a result, the surviving nephrons excrete a large amount of phosphate in the urine.

FGF-23 also decreases the production of $1,25(OH)_2D_3$ synthesis with resultant hypocalcemia. Hypocalcemia is a stimulant of PTH synthesis and secretion. High PTH levels also inhibit renal reabsorption of phosphate, promoting its urinary excretion. Thus, FGF-23 and PTH maintain normal phosphate homeostasis until GFR falls < 30 mL/min.

Question 4 How would you treat his hyperphosphatemia?

Answer First, calcium acetate should be discontinued. Based on serum HCO_3^- concentration, either sevelamer HCl or sevelamer carbonate should be started. Lowering phosphate level lowers Ca^{2+} as well. If the patient is on vitamin D, it should be discontinued. Also, if serum PTH level is >600 µg/mL, cinacalcet lowers PTH, Ca^{2+}, and phosphate, although cinacalcet is not recommended in CKD stages 3 and 4. However, our patient has eGFR of 16 mL/min, which is close to CKD stage 5.

References

1. Chertow GM, Burke SK, Raggi P. Treat to goal working group. Sevelamer attenuates the progression of coronary and aortic calcification in hemodialysis patients. Kidney Int. 2002;62:245–52.
2. Braun J, Asmus H-G, Holzer H, et al. Long term comparison of a calcium free phosphate binder and calcium carbonate-phosphorus metabolism and cardiovascular calcification. Clin Nephrol. 2004;62:104–15.
3. Block GA, Spiegel DM, Ehrlich J, et al. Effects of sevelamer and calcium on coronary artery calcification in patients new to dialysis. Kidney Int. 2005;68:1815–24.
4. Russo D, Miranda I, Ruocco C, et al. The progression of coronary artery calcification in predialysis patients on calcium calbonate or sevelamer. Kidney Int. 2007;72:1255–61.
5. Barreto DV, Barreto Fde C, de Carvalho AB, Cuppari L, Draibe SA, Dalboni MA, et al. Phosphate binder impact on bone remodeling and coronary calcification–results from the BRiC study. Nephron Clin Pract. 2008;110:273–83.
6. Qunibi W, Moustafa M, Muenz LR, et al. A 1-year randomized trial of calcium acetate versus sevelamer on progression of coronary artery calcification in hemodialysis patients with comparable lipid control: the calcium acetate renagel evaluation-2 (CARE-2) study. Am J Kidney Dis. 2008;51:952–65.

7. Takei T, Otsubo S, Uchida K, Matsugami K, Mimuro T, Kabaya T, et al. Effects of sevelamer on the progression of vascular calcification in patients on chronic haemodialysis. Nephron Clin Pract. 2008;108:c278–83.

8. Molony DA, Stephens BW. Derangements in phosphate metabolism in chronic kidney diseases/endstage renal disease: therapeutic considerations. Adv Chronic Kidney Dis. 2011;18:120–31.

9. St Peter WL, Liu J, Weinhandl E, Fan Q. A comparison of sevelamer and calcium-based phosphate binders on mortality, hospitalization, and morbidity in hemodialysis: a secondary analysis of the dialysis clinical outcomes revisited (DCOR) randomized trial using claims data. Am J Kidney Dis. 2008;51:445–54.

Suggested Reading

10. Hruska KA, Levi M, Slatopolsky E. Disorders of phosphorus, calcium, and magnesium metabolism. In: Coffman TM, Falk RJ, Molitoris BA, et al., editors. Schrier's diseases of the kidney. 9th ed. Philadelphia: Lippincott Williams & Wilkins; 2013. p. 2116–81.

11. Komaba H, Lanske B. Vitamin D and Klotho in chronic kidney disease. In: Ureña Torres PA, et al., editors. Vitamin D in chronic kidney disease. Switzerland: Springer; 2016. p. 179–94.

12. Kuro-O M. Phosphate and KLOTHO. Kidney Int. 2011;79(suppl 121):S20–3.

13. Razzaque MS. Bone-kidney axis in systemic phosphate turnover. Arch Biochem Biophys. 2014;561:154–8.

14. Smogorzewski MJ, Stubbs JR, Yu ASL. Disorders of calcium, magnesium, and phosphate balance. In: Skorecki K, et al., editors. Brenner and Rector's the kidney. 10th ed. Philadelphia: Elsevier; 2016. p. 601–35.

15. Tonelli M, Pannu N. Oral phosphate binders in patients with kidney failure. N Engl J Med. 2010;362:1312–24.

16. Gutiérrez OM. Fibroblast growth factor 23, Klotho, and phosphorus metabolism in kidney disease. Turner N et al. Oxford textbook of clinical nephrology. 4 Oxford. Oxford University Press; 2016. 947–56.

Disorders of Magnesium: Physiology

23

General Features

Magnesium (Mg^{2+}) is the second most common intracellular cation next to K^+ in the body. A 70 kg individual has approximately 25 g of Mg^{2+}. About 67% of this Mg^{2+} is present in the bone, about 20% in the muscle, and 12% in other tissues such as the liver. Only 1–2% is present in the extracellular space. In plasma, Mg^{2+} exists as free (60%) and bound (40%) forms. About 10% is bound to HCO_3^-, citrate, and phosphate and 30% to albumin. Only the free and nonprotein-bound Mg^{2+} is filtered at the glomerulus.

Mg^{2+} plays an essential role in cellular metabolism. It is involved in activation of enzymes such as phosphokinases and phosphatases. Mg-ATPase is also involved in the hydrolysis of ATP and thus the generation of energy that is utilized in several ion pump activities. In addition, Mg^{2+} plays a critical role in protein synthesis and cell volume regulation. Because of its pivotal role in cellular physiology, Mg^{2+} deficiency adversely affects many cellular functions.

Mg^{2+} Homeostasis

The daily intake of Mg^{2+} in the diet is approximately 300 mg (200–340 mg). However, the serum concentration of Mg^{2+} (abbreviated as $[Mg^{2+}]$) is maintained between 1.7 and 2.7 mg/dL (1.4–2.3 mEq/L). As in Ca^{2+} and phosphate homeostasis, Mg^{2+} homeostasis is regulated by the intestine, bone, and kidneys. Of ingested Mg^{2+}, 30–40% is absorbed by the jejunum and ileum (Fig. 23.1). About 30 mg/day is secreted into the gastrointestinal tract. The fecal excretion, which is calculated as the intake plus secretion minus absorption, amounts to 200 mg/day. Intestinal absorption of Mg^{2+} occurs by transcellular and paracellular pathways. Active Mg^{2+} transport occurs via TRPM6 (transient receptor potential melastatin6) channel, whereas the paracellular movement occurs via tight junctions and follows Na^+ and water absorption. Active vitamin D_3 ($1,25(OH)_2D_3$) increases the intestinal absorption of Mg^{2+}, whereas diets rich in Ca^{2+} and phosphate decrease its absorption.

© Springer Science+Business Media LLC 2018
A.S. Reddi, *Fluid, Electrolyte and Acid-Base Disorders*,
DOI 10.1007/978-3-319-60167-0_23

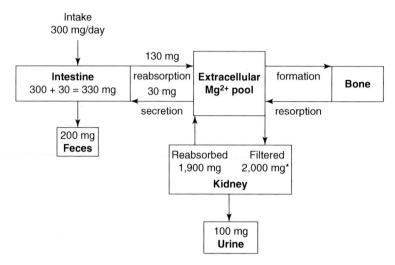

Fig. 23.1 Mg^{2+} homeostasis in an adult subject. (Filtered load of Mg^{2+} equals plasma-free Mg^{2+} concentration of 1.1 mg/dL times GFR of 180 L/day; i.e., 180 L × 11 mg/L = 1,980 mg/day). Note that the intake of 300 mg/day is excreted in the feces (200 mg) and urine (100 mg) to maintain Mg^{2+} homeostasis. (Modified from Nordin [6], with permission)

Mg^{2+} homeostasis is also dependent on the exchange between the extracellular pool and the bone. The Mg^{2+} available in the surface pool of the bone is involved in the homeostatic regulation of extracellular Mg^{2+}.

The kidney also maintains Mg^{2+} homeostasis because it regulates the rate of excretion depending on the Mg^{2+} concentration. Normally, the excretory fraction of Mg^{2+} is 5%. In states of Mg^{2+} deficiency, the excretion can be as low as 0.5%. In states of Mg^{2+} excess or in chronic kidney disease, excretion can be as high as 50%.

Renal Handling of Mg^{2+}

Free and nonprotein-bound Mg^{2+} is filtered at the glomerulus. Approximately 2000 mg of Mg^{2+} are filtered, and only 100 mg are excreted in the urine, which implies that 95% of the filtered Mg^{2+} is reabsorbed. The proximal tubule reabsorbs about 20% of the filtered Mg^{2+}. This amount is relatively low when compared to the reabsorption of Na^+, K^+, Ca^{2+}, or phosphate at the proximal tubule. The most important segment for Mg^{2+} reabsorption is the cortical thick ascending limb of Henle's loop. In this segment, about 40–70% of Mg^{2+} is reabsorbed. The distal convoluted tubule reabsorbs 5–10% of the filtered Mg^{2+}, and very little reabsorption occurs in the collecting duct. Under steady state conditions, the urinary excretion of Mg^{2+} is about 5% of the filtered load.

Proximal Tubule

The transport of Mg^{2+} in the proximal tubule is passive and unidirectional down an electrochemical gradient. It is dependent on the concentration of Mg^{2+} in the luminal fluid. Mg^{2+} reabsorption occurs in parallel with Na^+ reabsorption and thus is influenced by changes in extracellular fluid volume.

Thick Ascending Limb of Henle's Loop (TALH)

The transport of Mg^{2+} in the cortical TALH is both passive and active. Passive transport is dependent on the lumen-positive voltage difference secondary to Na/K/2Cl cotransporter activity and back-leak of K^+ into the lumen via ROMK (Fig. 23.2). This positive voltage difference facilitates paracellular movement of Mg^{2+}. Inhibition of the Na/K/2Cl cotransporter by a loop diuretic diminishes Mg^{2+} reabsorption. A similar decrease in Mg^{2+} reabsorption is also observed with volume expansion.

The paracellular movement of Mg^{2+} is thought to be mediated by proteins of the claudin family of tight junction proteins. The important protein of the claudin family is paracellin-1 or claudin-16. Mutations of the gene-encoding paracellin cause hypomagnesemia (discussed later).

Evidence also exists for active transport of Mg^{2+} in the cortical TALH. This mechanism has been suggested based on the observation that Mg^{2+} transport is stimulated by antidiuretic hormone (ADH) and glucagon without any change in the potential difference.

Mg^{2+} ions exit across the basolateral membrane by being actively extruded against their electrochemical gradient. Although the mechanisms have not been

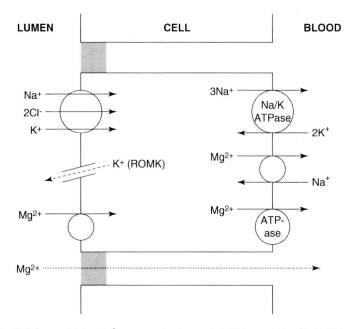

Fig. 23.2 Cellular model for Mg^{2+} transport in the cortical thick ascending limb of Henle's loop

Table 23.1 Effect of various factors on TRPM6 activity and urinary Mg^{2+}

Factor	Effect	Urinary Mg^{2+}
Epidermal growth factor	↑	↓
Estradiol	↑	↓
Hypomagnesemia	↑	↓
Hypermagnesemia	↓	↑
Chronic metabolic acidosis	↓	↑
Metabolic alkalosis	↑	↓
Cyclosporine	↓	↑
Tacrolimus	↓	↑
Thiazide diuretics	↓	↑

↑ increase; ↓ decrease

studied in epithelial cells, the existence of a Mg-ATPase that extrudes Mg^{2+} has been reported in other cells. Also, a Na/Mg exchanger has been demonstrated in erythrocytes (see Fig. 23.2).

Distal Convoluted Tubule (DCT)

As stated earlier, the DCT reabsorbs 5–10% of Mg^{2+}, and the transport is active and transcellular. Mg^{2+} transport from the lumen to the cell occurs via an epithelial Mg^{2+} channel called the TRPM6. The DCT determines the final urinary excretion of Mg^{2+}, as no or very little reabsorption occurs beyond this segment. Several factors influence TRMP6 expression and activity and thus influence urinary excretion of Mg^{2+} (Table 23.1).

Factors that Alter Renal Handling of Mg^{2+} in TALH and DCT

Several factors influence the tubular reabsorption of Mg^{2+} and are summarized in Table 23.2. Volume expansion decreases proximal tubular reabsorption of Na^+ and water. As a result, Mg^{2+} reabsorption is also decreased. Conversely, volume depletion causes an increase in Mg^{2+} reabsorption. Hypermagnesemia inhibits Mg^{2+} reabsorption, whereas hypomagnesemia causes renal retention of Mg^{2+}. Hypercalcemia markedly increases Mg^{2+} excretion by inhibiting reabsorption in the proximal tubule and TALH. Hypocalcemia has the opposite effect. Phosphate depletion enhances Mg^{2+} excretion by reducing its absorption in TALH and DCT. Acute acidosis seems to inhibit Mg^{2+} reabsorption in TALH and thus enhances its excretion. Chronic metabolic acidosis suppresses TRPM6 expression and activity in DCT and enhances Mg^{2+} excretion. On the other hand, metabolic alkalosis decreases urinary excretion of Mg^{2+} by enhancing its reabsorption in the proximal straight tubule and DCT. Cyclic AMP-mediated hormones such as parathyroid hormone and ADH enhance Mg^{2+} reabsorption in TALH and DCT and decrease its urinary excretion. Osmotic diuretics, such as mannitol and urea, promote Mg^{2+} excretion by predominantly inhibiting its reabsorption in TALH and to some extent in the proximal tubule. Loop diuretics, such as furosemide, inhibit Mg^{2+} reabsorption in TALH and

Table 23.2 Factors influencing Mg^{2+} reabsorption and excretion

Factor	TALH	DCT	Urinary excretion
Volume expansion	↓	↓	↑
Volume contraction	↑	↑	↓
Hypermagnesemia	↓	↓	↑
Hypomagnesemia	↑	↑	↓
Hypercalcemia	↓	↓	↑
Hypocalcemia	↑	↑	↓
Hypophosphatemia	↓	↓	↑
Metabolic acidosis	↓	↓	↑
Metabolic alkalosis	↑	↑	↓
PTH	↑	↑	↓
ADH	↑	↑	↓
Glucagon	↑	↑	↓
Osmotic diuretics	↓	↓	↑
Loop diuretics	↓	NC	↑
Thiazide diuretics	NC	↓	↑
Amiloride	NC	↑	↓

↑ increase; ↓ decrease; *NC* no change; *DCT* distal convoluted tubule; *TALH* thick ascending limb of Henle's loop

cause magnesuria. Thiazide diuretics (hydrochlorothiazide) act in DCT and may cause a mild increase in Mg^{2+} excretion.

Suggested Reading

1. Alexander RT, Hoenderop JG, Bindels RJ. Molecular determinants of magnesium homeostasis: insights from human disease. J am Soc Nephrol. 2008;19:1451–8.
2. Berndt TJ, Thompson JR, Kumar R. The regulation of calcium, magnesium, and phosphate excretion by the kidney. In: Skorecki K, et al., editors. Brenner & Rector's the kidney. 10th ed. Philadelphia: Elsevier; 2016. p. 185–203.
3. Houillier P. Magnesium homeostasis. Turner N et al. Oxford textbook of clinical nephrology. 4th ed. Oxford. Oxford University Press; 2016. 243–248.
4. Hruska KA, Levi M, Slatopolsky E. Disorders of phosphorus, calcium, and magnesium metabolism. In: Coffman TM, Falk RJ, Molitoris BA, et al., editors. Herausgeber. Schrier's diseases of the kidney. 9th ed. Philadelphia: Lippincott Williams & Wilkins; 2013. p. 2116–81.
5. Schlingmann KP, Quamme GA, Konrad M. Mechanisms and disorders of magnesium metabolism. In: Alpern RJ, Moe OW, Caplan M, editors. Seldin and Giebisch's the kidney. Physiology and pathophysiology. 5th ed. San Diego: Academic Press (Elsevier); 2013. p. 2139–65.
6. Nordin BEC, editor. Calcium, phosphate, and magnesium metabolism. Edinburgh: Churchill Livingstone; 1976.

Disorders of Magnesium: Hypomagnesemia

24

Hypomagnesemia is defined as serum $[Mg^{2+}] <1.7$ mg/dL. The prevalence of hypomagnesemia in outpatient and hospitalized patient population is 6–12%. The incidence of hypomagnesemia is approximately 65%. The causes of hypomagnesemia fall into four major categories: (1) decreased intake of Mg^{2+}, (2) decreased intestinal absorption, (3) increased urinary losses, and (4) drugs (Table 24.1). In addition to these causes, cellular uptake of Mg^{2+} is caused by infusion of glucose or epinephrine.

Table 24.1 Causes of hypomagnesemia

Cause	Mechanism
Decreased intake	
Protein-calorie malnutrition	Poor Mg^{2+} intake
Starvation	Poor Mg^{2+} intake
Prolonged IV therapy without Mg^{2+}	Poor Mg^{2+} intake
Chronic alcoholism	Possible mechanisms include (1) poor dietary intake, (2) alcohol-induced renal Mg^{2+} loss, (3) diarrhea, and (4) starvation ketosis-induced renal Mg^{2+} loss
Decreased intestinal absorption	
Prolonged nasogastric suction	Removal from saliva and gastric secretions
Malabsorption (nontropical sprue and steatorrhea)	Loss from the intestine
Diarrhea	Loss from the intestine
Intestinal and biliary fistulas	Loss from stool and urine
Excessive use of laxatives	Loss from stool due to diarrhea
Resection of the small intestine	Defective Mg^{2+} absorption
Familial hypomagnesemia with secondary hypocalcemia	Mutation in intestinal TRPM6 gene

(continued)

© Springer Science+Business Media LLC 2018
A.S. Reddi, *Fluid, Electrolyte and Acid-Base Disorders*,
DOI 10.1007/978-3-319-60167-0_24

Table 24.1 (continued)

Cause	Mechanism
Increased urinary loss	
Inherited disorders of TALH	
Familial hypomagnesemia with hypercalciuria and nephrocalcinosis	Mutations in CLDN 16 gene (claudin-16 or paracellin-1) of tight junction proteins
Familial hypomagnesemia with hypercalciuria and nephrocalcinosis with ocular manifestation	Mutations in CLDN19 gene (claudin-19) of tight junction protein
Disorders of Ca/Mg-sensing receptor	Inactivating mutations in TALH/DCT Ca/Mg-sensing receptor
Bartter syndrome	Mutations in Na/K/2Cl, ROMK, ClC-Ka/Kb-Barttin
Inherited disorders of DCT	
Familial hypomagnesemia with secondary hypocalcemia	Mutations in TRPM6 gene
Isolated recessive hypomagnesemia with normocalciuria	Mutations in epidermal growth factor (EGF) gene
Isolated dominant hypomagnesemia with hypocalciuria	Mutations in FXYD2 gene encoding γ-subunit of Na/K-ATPase
Acquired causes other than drugs	
Volume expansion	Increased GFR with increased Na^+, water, and Mg^{2+} excretion
Hypercalcemia	Increased Mg^{2+} excretion
Diabetic ketoacidosis	Increased Mg^{2+} excretion
Hyperaldosteronism	Increased Mg^{2+} excretion
Drugs	
Diuretics	
Osmotic, loop, and thiazide diuretics	Renal Mg^{2+} wasting, inhibition of TRPM6 by thiazides
Antibiotics	
Aminoglycosides	Activation of CaSR receptors and renal Mg^{2+} wasting
Amphotericin B	Renal Mg^{2+} wasting (unknown molecular mechanism)
Pentamidine	↓ Mg^{2+} reabsorption probably in DCT
Foscarnet	Complexes with Mg^{2+} and Ca^{2+}? Fanconi syndrome
Antineoplastics	
Cisplatin	Renal Mg^{2+} wasting
EGF receptor antagonist (Cetuximab)	Inhibits TRPM6 activity
Proton pump inhibitors	Possible mechanisms include (1) decreased intestinal absorption due to achlorhydria, (2) increased intestinal secretion and loss in feces, (3) decreased intestinal TRPM6 activity because of inhibition of H/K-ATPase, and (4) decreased transport via paracellular pathway

Table 24.1   (continued)

Cause	Mechanism
Immunosuppressives	
Cyclosporine and tacrolimus	Inhibit TRPM6 activity
Rapamycin	Renal Mg^{2+} wasting due to inhibition of Na/K/2Cl and TRPM6 activity
Miscellaneous	
Hyperthyroidism	Cellular shift
Hungry bone syndrome	Uptake by bones following parathyroidectomy
Neonatal hypomagnesemia	Renal loss in diabetic pregnant mothers, use of stool softeners by pregnant mothers, malabsorption/or hyperparathyroidism in mothers

Some Specific Causes of Hypomagnesemia

Familial Hypomagnesemia with Hypercalciuria and Nephrocalcinosis (FHHNC)

- Inherited as an autosomal recessive disorder.
- Caused by loss-of-function mutations in the CLAN16 gene that encodes claudin-16 (paracellin-1) tight junction protein.
- Clinically characterized by hypomagnesemia, renal wasting of Mg^{2+} and Ca^{2+}, nephrocalcinosis, and renal failure (30%).
- Polyuria, polydipsia, and urinary tract infections are common.
- Treatment includes oral citrates, thiazide diuretics, and enteral Mg^{2+} salts.

Familial Hypomagnesemia with Hypercalciuria and Nephrocalcinosis with Ocular Manifestation

- A subset of these patients demonstrates additionally ocular abnormalities, such as myopia, chorioretinitis, nystagmus, and hearing impairment. Such patients have been shown to have mutations in CLAN19 gene encoding claudin-19 protein.
- Treatment is similar to that of FHHNC.

Familial Hypomagnesemia with Secondary Hypocalcemia

- Inherited as an autosomal dominant disorder.
- Caused by mutations in TRPM6 gene encoding the Mg^{2+} channel in DCT and the intestine.
- Patients present with profound hypomagnesemia and generalized seizures during the first few months of life. Also, hypocalcemia is prominent.
- Treatment is IV Mg^{2+} infusion during seizure activity followed by life-long oral therapy.

Isolated Dominant Hypomagnesemia with Hypocalciuria

- Inherited as an autosomal dominant disorder.
- Caused by mutations in the FXYD2 gene that encodes γ-subunit of the Na/K-ATPase in DCT.
- Malfunction of Na/K-ATPase leads to intracellular accumulation of Na^+ and inhibition of Mg^{2+} transport, resulting in hypomagnesemia.
- Clinical manifestations include generalized seizures, mental retardation with severe hypomagnesemia, and hypocalciuria.
- Similar to Gitelman syndrome with respect to hypocalciuria, but hypokalemia and metabolic alkalosis are absent in this disorder.
- Occurs in infants and adults.

Isolated Recessive Hypomagnesemia (IRH) with Normocalciuria

- A rare disorder characterized by seizures and psychomotor retardation during childhood and mental retardation during adult life.
- Caused by the mutation in EGF gene encoding the pro-epidermal growth factor (pro-EGF), which is cleaved by proteases to EGF in the kidney. In normal DGT, EGF occupies its receptor and activates TRPM6 channel so that Mg^{2+} reabsorption is increased.
- Mutations in pro-EGF gene prevent full EGF synthesis, leading to low TRPM6 activity and decreased Mg^{2+} reabsorption.
- Only hypomagnesemia is present. Ca^{2+} excretion is normal.

Bartter and Gitelman Syndromes (see Chaps. 3 and 15)

- Clinical and biochemical characteristics of some inherited hypomagnesemic disorders are shown in Table 24.2.

Hypomagnesemia-Induced Hypocalcemia

- Common in hypomagnesemic subjects.
- Hypomagnesemia inhibits PTH release and also causes skeletal resistance to PTH action.
- Only Mg^{2+} repletion corrects hypocalcemia in a hypomagnesemia–hypocalcemia patient.

Table 24.2 Clinical and biochemical characteristics of inherited disorders of hypomagnesemia

Disorder	Onset	Serum Mg²⁺	Serum Ca²⁺	Serum K⁺	Urine Mg²⁺	Urine Ca²⁺	Blood pH	Nephrocalcinosis	Renal stones	Clinical characteristics
Familial hypomagnesemia with hypercalciuria and nephrocalcinosis	Childhood/adult	↓	N	N	↑↑	↑↑	N	Yes	Yes	Polyuria, renal failure
Familial hypomagnesemia with secondary hypocalcemia	Infancy	↓↓	↓	N	↑	N	N	No	No	Tetany, seizures
Isolated dominant hypomagnesemia with hypocalciuria	Childhood	↓	N	N	↑	↓	N	No	No	Seizures, chondrocalcinosis
Isolated recessive hypomagnesemia with normocalciuria	Childhood	↓	N	N	↑	N	N	No	No	Tetany, seizures
Gitelman syndrome	Variable	↓	N	↓↓	↑	↓↓	↑	No	No	Weakness, chondrocalcinosis, salt-craving
Classic Bartter syndrome	Infancy	↓	N	↓↓	↑/N	↑/↓/N	↑	Rare	No	Weakness

↑increase, ↓decrease, *N* normal

Hypomagnesemia-Induced Hypokalemia

- Hypokalemia is very common in hypomagnesemic patient.
- Increased kaliuresis and hypokalemia were observed in humans on Mg^{2+}-deficient diet.
- The mechanism of hypokalemia in Mg^{2+} deficiency remains unclear. It has been proposed that Mg^{2+} deficiency inhibits skeletal muscle Na/K-ATPase, causing efflux of K^+ and secondary kaliuresis.
- The currently proposed mechanism is that changes in intracellular Mg^{2+} concentration affect K^+ secretion through ROMK channel in the DCT. At the physiologic intracellular Mg^{2+} concentration (e.g., 1 mM), K^+ entry through ROMK is more than its exit, because the intracellular Mg^{2+} binds ROMK and blocks K^+ exit. It seems Mg^{2+} deficiency may lower intracellular Mg^{2+} concentration which relieves the binding and promotes K^+ secretion, causing hypokalemia.
- Hypokalemia is refractory to KCl administration unless hypomagnesemia is treated.

Clinical Manifestations

The clinical manifestations of hypomagnesemia are listed in (Table 24.3). These manifestations are often difficult to differentiate from those of hypocalcemia. This difficulty is due to hypomagnesemia-induced hypocalcemia and also hypokalemia. The manifestations are mostly related to neuromuscular and cardiovascular systems.

Table 24.3 Clinical manifestations of hypomagnesemia

Signs	Symptoms
Chvostek's sign	Nausea
Trousseau's sign	Vomiting
Tremors	Apathy
Muscle fasciculations	Weakness
Hyperreflexia	Anorexia
Seizures	Mental retardation
Depression	
Psychosis	
Prolonged QT interval	
Cardiac arrhythmias	
Decreased myocardial contractility	
Hypertension	
Sudden death	

Diagnosis

Step 1

- History: The two most common disorders of hypomagnesemia are GI and renal loss of Mg $^{2+}$. Therefore, inquire about diarrhea or malabsorption, or drugs that cause renal Mg^{2+} loss (Fig. 24.1).
- In children, family history is extremely important.

Step 2

- Physical examination is important. Elicit signs and symptoms of hypomagnesemia.

Step 3

- Obtain pertinent labs, including Ca^{2+}, phosphate, and albumin.
- If the cause is not obvious, obtain a 24 h urine Mg^{2+} and creatinine. If 24 h urine collection is not possible, calculate FE_{Mg} in a spot urine.
- If FE_{Mg} is <5%, consider GI losses or cellular uptake.
- If FE_{Mg} is >5%, consider renal losses.
- Serum [Mg^{2+}] may be normal despite total body deficit of Mg^{2+}. In such cases, some physicians recommend a Mg^{2+}-loading test (2.4 mg/kg of elemental Mg^{2+} in D5W to be infused over a 4 h period, and <70% urinary excretion indicates Mg^{2+} deficiency) to estimate total body deficit. Because of high false positives (diarrhea, malabsorption) and false negatives (renal Mg^{2+} wasting), this test is not routinely recommended. The following algorithm may help you evaluate hypomagnesemia (Fig. 24.1).

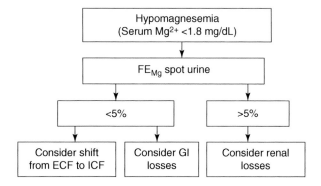

Fig. 24.1 Evaluation of hypomagnesemia

Table 24.4 Magnesium salts available for treatment of hypomagnesemia

Compound	Molecular wt[a]	Elemental Mg^{2+} (%)[a]
Oral		
Magnesium chloride ($MgCl_2$ $6H_2O$)	203	12
Magnesium oxide (MgO)	40	60
Magnesium hydroxide (Mg $(OH)_2$)	58	42
Magnesium carbonate ($MgCO_3$)	84	29
Magnesium acetate tetrahydrate (Mg $(C_2H_3O_2)_2$ $4H_2O$)	214	11
Magnesium gluconate ($MgC_{12}H_{22}O_{14}$)	415	17
Magnesium citrate ($MgC_6H_6O_7$)	214	11
Magnesium lactate ($MgC_6H_{10}O_6$)	202	10
Parenteral		
Magnesium sulfate ($MgSO_4$ $7H_2O$)[b]	247	10

Magnesium sulfate is also available as powder
[a]Rounded to the nearest number
[b]Available in 2 mL quantity as 50% solution, containing 8 Eq/L or 4 mmol

Treatment

Treatment of hypomagnesemia depends on the severity of symptoms. Symptoms usually develop once serum $[Mg^{2+}]$ is <1.0 mg/dL. Since hypocalcemia and hypokalemia coexist with hypomagnesemia, it is often difficult to distinguish the clinical manifestations related to hypomagnesemia. Therefore, it is advisable to treat hypomagnesemia first and then other electrolyte abnormalities. In some patients, both calcium gluconate and KCl administration are necessary to replenish the deficits of both electrolytes following Mg^{2+} administration. A variety of magnesium salts are available for oral therapy, and only magnesium sulfate is used parenterally (Table 24.4).

Acute Treatment

Severe Symptomatic Hypomagnesemia
- Intravenous magnesium sulfate (2 mL dissolved in 100 mL normal saline) over a 10 min period for patients with arrhythmias, seizures, or severe neuromuscular irritability and hemodynamically unstable patients.
- Continue IV therapy with 2 mL magnesium sulfate every 3–4 h until serum $[Mg^{2+}]$ reaches above 1.0 mg/dL.
- Note that most of the administered magnesium is excreted in patients with normal renal function. Therefore, serum creatinine levels should be followed to avoid hypermagnesemia.
- Dose reduction (50%) is required in patients with renal impairment.

Hemodynamically Stable Patients with Symptomatic Hypomagnesemia ($\geq$ 1.0 mg/dL)
- Intravenous magnesium sulfate (4–8 mL dissolved in 1 L of normal saline or D5W) over 12–24 h. This dose can be repeated as necessary until serum $[Mg^{2+}]$ reaches above 1.0 mg/dL.

Special Groups of Patients Requiring Intravenous Magnesium Sulfate

- Patients receiving total parenteral nutrition, post-op patients, and those with diarrheal disorders require IV magnesium to maintain near-normal serum [Mg^{2+}]. In addition, those patients with massive renal loss require IV therapy.

Chronic Treatment

- Encourage magnesium-rich foods, such as green leafy vegetables, meat, seafood, nuts, etc.
- If medication is needed, oral therapy is recommended.
- Several oral preparations are available (Table 24.4). All of them have adverse effects, such as diarrhea and abdominal cramping or pain.
- Selection of oral preparation is dependent both on the physician and patients.
- Dose and frequency depend on the patients' tolerability.
- Usual dose is 240–1,000 mg of elemental Mg^{2+} in divided doses per day for patients with normal renal function.
- Sustained release preparations (magnesium chloride, Mag Delay, Slow-Mag, or magnesium lactate, Mag-Tab SR) are preferred because of slow absorption and minimum renal Mg^{2+} excretion.
- Magnesium oxide (400–1,200 mg daily), if no slow release preparation is available.
- Amiloride can be used in those with renal Mg^{2+} wasting and normal renal function.
- Use with care with those drugs that promote Mg^{2+} excretion.

Study Questions

Case 1 A 62-year-old man is admitted for chemotherapy of small cell (oat cell) cancer of the lung with cisplatin. The patient is hydrated with 3 L of normal saline prior to the initiation of chemotherapy. He subsequently develops shortness of breath for which he receives furosemide 80 mg intravenously. He excreted 4 L of urine in 24 h. 7 days later, the patient started feeling weak. Physical examination reveals tetany, and Chvostek's and Trouasseau's signs could be elicited. The labs:

$$Na^+ = 135 \text{ mEq/L}$$
$$K^+ = 2.9 \text{ mEq/L}$$
$$Cl^- = 100 \text{ mEq/L}$$
$$HCO_3^- = 26 \text{ mEq/L}$$
$$BUN = 30 \text{ mg/dL}$$
$$Creatinine = 1.6 \text{ mg/dL}$$
$$Ca^{2+} = 7.0 \text{ mg/dL}$$
$$Phosphate = 3.0 \text{ mg/dL}$$
$$Albumin = 3.5 \text{ mg/dL}$$
$$Mg^{2+} = 0.7 \text{ mEq/dL}$$

Question 1 What is the most likely cause of Chvostek's and Trousseau's signs?

Answer Both hypocalcemia and hypomagnesemia cause tetany, carpopedal spasm, and positive Chvostek's and Trousseau's signs. However, in this patient, Mg^{2+} depletion is more severe than Ca^{2+} depletion.

Question 2 What precipitated this patient's hypomagnesemia?

Answer Although loop diuretics (furosemide) cause significant magnesuria, it is the cisplatin that caused profound hypomagnesemia secondary to excess urinary losses of Mg^{2+}. The mechanism seems to be cisplatin's inhibition of Mg^{2+} reabsorption by the loop of Henle or the destruction of loop of Henle due to interstitial nephritis caused by cisplatin. Hypokalemia and hypocalcemia also result from cisplatin therapy.

Question 3 How would you treat this patient?

Answer Replacement of K^+ and Ca^{2+} would not prevent tetany. The appropriate treatment is the IV administration of $MgSO_4$. 1 gram of $MgSO_4$ $7H_2O$ provides 97.6 mg of elemental or 8 mEq/L Mg^{2+}. It is available in 2 mL quantity as 50% solution, which can be added to 100 mL of normal saline and given in 30–60 min. This treatment can be continued until plasma $[Mg^{2+}]$ returns to normal. Normalization of plasma $[Mg^{2+}]$ corrects Ca^{2+} and K^+, and phosphate deficiency can be corrected by potassium phosphate.

Case 2 You are asked to see a 20-year-old woman for recurrent urinary tract infections (UTIs). An abdominal plain film showed nephrolithiasis. Upon questioning, she tells that she had renal stones since the age of 10. Her parents also had history of hypomagnesemia. There are no eye or ocular problems. Pertinent labs: K^+ 3.4 mEq/L; Ca^{2+} 7.2 mg/dL; Mg^{2+} 1.2 mEq/dL; phosphate 3.2 mg/dL; albumin 3.9 g/dL.

Question 1 Based on the above history and lab data, which one of the following gene defects is the *MOST* likely cause of her disorder?

(A) TRPM6
(B) CLDN-16
(C) CLDN-19
(D) FXYD2
(E) Pro-EGF

The answer is B This patient carries the diagnosis of familial hypomagnesemia with hypercalciuria and nephrocalcinosis. This disorder is caused by mutations in the gene CLDN-16, which encodes claudin-16, a protein of tight junctions. The remaining gene defects cause other hypomagnesemic disorders that are not associated with nephrolithiasis.

Question 2 How would you treat her electrolyte abnormalities?

Answer This patient requires life-long Mg^{2+} supplementation and K citrate with regular follow-up of her labs.

Question 3 What is her serious long-term complication other than renal colic and UTIs?

Answer About 30% of these patients develop CKD; therefore, regular follow-up of her renal function is indicated.

Study Question 1 With regard to Mg^{2+} handling by the nephron, which one of the following statements is *INCORRECT*?

(A) Mg^{2+} reabsorption is only 20% of the filtered load in the proximal tubule
(B) Both Na^+ and Mg^{2+} are equally reabsorbed in the proximal tubule
(C) About 70% of the filtered load of Mg^{2+} is reabsorbed in thick ascending limb of loop of Henle (TALH)
(D) Only 10% of filtered load of Mg^{2+} is reabsorbed in the distal convoluted tubule (DCT)
(E) Fractional excretion of Mg^{2+} is 5%, and it can be decreased to <0.5% in hypomagnesemia

The answer is B Mg^{2+} is the second most common intracellular cation next to K^+ in the body. A 70 kg individual has approximately 25 g of Mg^{2+}. About 67% of this Mg^{2+} is present in the bone, about 20% in the muscle, and 12% in other tissues such as the liver. Only 1–2% is present in the extracellular space. In plasma, Mg^{2+} exists in free (60%) and bound (40%) forms. About 10% is bound to HCO_3^-, citrate, and phosphate and 30% to albumin. Only the free and nonprotein-bound Mg^{2+} is filtered at the glomerulus.

Approximately 2,000 mg of Mg^{2+} are filtered, and only 100 mg are excreted in the urine, which implies that 95% of the filtered Mg^{2+} is reabsorbed. The proximal tubule reabsorbs about 20% of the filtered Mg. This amount is relatively low when compared to the reabsorption of Na^+, K^+, Ca^{2+}, or phosphate at the proximal tubule. Thus, option B is incorrect.

The most important segment for Mg^{2+} reabsorption is the cortical TALH. In this segment, about 70% of Mg^{2+} is reabsorbed. The transport of Mg in the TALH is both passive and active. Passive transport is dependent on the lumen-positive voltage difference secondary to Na/K/2Cl cotransport and back-leak of K^+ into the lumen via ROMK. This positive voltage difference facilitates paracellular movement of Mg^{2+}. Evidence also exists for active transport of Mg^{2+} in the cortical TALH. This mechanism has been suggested based on the observation that Mg^{2+} transport is stimulated by antidiuretic hormone and glucagon without any change in the potential difference.

The DCT reabsorbs about 5–10% of the filtered Mg^{2+}, and very little reabsorption occurs in the collecting duct. Thus, the DCT is the last site of Mg^{2+} reabsorption in the nephron. It occurs by an active transcellular mechanism. At the lumen, Mg^{2+} enters the cell via TRPM6 (transient receptor potential melastatin6). Under steady-state conditions, the urinary excretion of Mg^{2+} is about 5% of the filtered load and decreases to <0.5% in severe hypomagnesemia.

Study Question 2 Which one of the following drugs does *NOT* cause hypomagnesemia?

(A) Cisplatin
(B) Amphotericin B (Amp B)
(C) Proton pump inhibitor (PPI)
(D) Alcohol
(E) Vancomycin

The answer is E Except for vancomycin, all other drugs cause hypomagnesemia. Cisplatin and Amp B cause renal wasting of Mg^{2+}. Both drugs also cause hypocalciuria. PPIs have been shown to induce hypomagnesemia by various mechanisms. Not only hypomagnesemia but also hypokalemia and hypocalcemia have been reported with PPIs. Hypokalemia is due to renal wasting of K^+. Patients with chronic alcoholism may develop hypomagnesemia by several mechanisms, including inadequate dietary intake, steatorrhea, diarrhea, phosphate deficiency, fatty acid or ATP–Mg complex formation, and alcohol-induced magnesuria. To date, vancomycin has not been shown to cause hypomagnesemia, making choice E incorrect.

Study Question 3 Of the following, which one is the recently proposed mechanism for hypomagnesemia-induced hypokalemia?

(A) Inhibition of Na/K/2Cl cotransporter
(B) Inhibition of Na/Cl cotransporter
(C) Blockage of ROMK channel by Mg^{2+} in distal convoluted tubule (DCT)
(D) Inhibition of epithelial Na^+ channel (ENaC)
(E) None of the above mechanisms

The answer is C Combined Mg^{2+} and K^+ deficiency is seen in many conditions such as loop or thiazide diuretics, alcoholism, diarrhea, Bartter and Gitelman syndrome, aminoglycosides, amphotericin B, and cisplatin. Inhibition of Na/K/2Cl and Na/Cl cotransporters cause Bartter and Gitelman syndromes, respectively. However, hypokalemia can be to some extent corrected by administration of KCl. In contrast, hypokalemia induced by Mg^{2+} deficiency is not corrected by KCl alone. The mechanism of hypokalemia in Mg^{2+} deficiency remains unclear. However, several lines of evidence suggest that Mg^{2+} administration decreases K^+ secretion and Mg^{2+} deficiency promotes K^+ excretion. These effects occur independent of Na/K/2Cl, Na/Cl, and ENaC participation. It has been proposed that Mg^{2+} deficiency inhibits skeletal muscle Na/K-ATPase, causing efflux of K^+ and secondary kaliuresis.

The currently proposed mechanism is that changes in intracellular Mg^{2+} concentration affect K^+ secretion through ROMK channel in DCT. At the physiologic intracellular Mg^{2+} concentration (e.g., 1 mM), K^+ entry through ROMK exceeds its exit, because the intracellular Mg^{2+} binds ROMK and blocks K^+ exit. In Mg^{2+} deficiency, the intracellular Mg^{2+} concentration decreases. This relieves the binding of Mg^{2+} from ROMK, thus promoting K^+ secretion. Thus, option C is correct.

Suggested Reading

1. Alexander RT, Hoenderop JG, Bindels RJ. Molecular determinants of magnesium homeostasis: insights from human disease. J Am Soc Nephrol. 2008;19:1451–8.
2. Hruska KA, Levi M, Slatopolsky E. Disorders of phosphorus, calcium, and magnesium metabolism. In: Coffman TM, Falk RJ, Molitoris BA, et al., editors. Schrier's diseases of the kidney. 9th ed. Philadelphia: Lippincott Williams & Wilkins; 2013. p. 2116–81.
3. Knoers NVA. Inherited forms of renal hypomagnesemia: an update. Pediatr Nephrol. 2009;24:697–705.
4. Konrad M, Weber S. Recent advances in molecular genetics of hereditary magnesium-losing disorders. J am Soc Nephrol. 2003;14:249–60.
5. Lameris AL, Monnens LA, Bindels RJ, et al. Drug-induced alterations in Mg^{2+} homeostasis. Clin Sci. 2012;123:1–14.
6. Naderi ASA, Reilly RF Jr. Hereditary etiologies of hypomagnesemia. Nat Clin Pract Nephrol. 2008;4:80–9.
7. Schlingmann KP, Quamme GA, Konrad M. Mechanisms and disorders of magnesium metabolism. In: Alpern RJ, Moe OW, Caplan M, editors. Seldin and Giebisch's the kidney. Physiology and pathophysiology. 5th ed. San Diego: Academic Press (Elsevier); 2013. p. 2139–65.
8. Smogorzewski MJ, Stubbs JR, Yu ASL. Disorders of calcium, magnesium, and phosphate balance. In: Skorecki K, et al., editors. Brenner & Rector's the kidney. 10th ed. Philadelphia: Elsevier; 2016. p. 601–35.

Disorders of Magnesium: Hypermagnesemia

25

Hypermagnesemia, which is defined as serum $[Mg^{2+}]$ >2.7 mg/dL, is not a common electrolyte disorder in individuals with normal renal function. As stated in Chap. 23, the kidney is able to maintain serum $[Mg^{2+}]$ within normal range by enhancing its excretion in situations of excess Mg^{2+} intake. Therefore, a decrease in glomerular filtration rate (GFR), as seen in chronic kidney disease, seems to be the most common cause of hypermagnesemia. The other major cause is an exogenous load of Mg^{2+}. Excess intake of Mg^{2+} can occur when a patient with preeclampsia (a condition characterized by proteinuria and hypertension during third trimester of pregnancy) is treated with magnesium sulfate or when individuals take Mg^{2+}-containing antacids or enemas. Infants born to mothers who were treated with magnesium for preeclampsia/ eclampsia may develop hypermagnesemia. Elderly individuals are particularly susceptible to Mg^{2+} toxicity because of decreased renal function with aging and excessive use of Mg^{2+}-containing medications and vitamins. Subjects with familial hypocalciuric hypercalcemia may have elevated Mg^{2+} levels. Acromegalics and patients with adrenal insufficiency may have hypermagnesemia. The various causes of hypermagnesemia are summarized in Table 25.1.

Clinical Manifestations

The clinical manifestations of hypermagnesemia are related to serum $[Mg^{2+}]$, as shown in Table 25.2. Two organ systems are greatly affected by hypermagnesemia: the neuromuscular and cardiovascular systems.

© Springer Science+Business Media LLC 2018
A.S. Reddi, *Fluid, Electrolyte and Acid-Base Disorders*,
DOI 10.1007/978-3-319-60167-0_25

Table 25.1 Causes of hypermagnesemia

Cause	Mechanism
Systemic diseases	
Acute kidney injury	↓ Excretion
Chronic kidney disease stages 4–5	↓ Excretion
Familial hypocalciuric hypercalcemia	↓ Excretion
Adrenal insufficiency	↑Renal absorption
Acromegaly	↓ Excretion
Mg^{2+} load in patients with low GFR	
Administration of Mg^{2+} to treat hypomagnesemia	Exogenous load and ↓ excretion
Mg^{2+}-containing laxatives	Exogenous load and ↓ excretion
Mg^{2+}-containing antacids	Exogenous load and ↓ excretion
Epsom salts	Exogenous load and ↓ excretion
Mg^{2+} load in patients with normal GFR	
Treatment of preeclampsia/eclampsia	Exogenous load
Treatment of hypertension in pregnant women	Exogenous load and↓ excretion
Infants born to mothers treated with Mg^{2+} for preeclampsia/eclampsia	Transfer from mother to fetus
Sea water ingestion or drowning	Exogenous load (normal sea water 14 mg/dL; dead sea water 394 mg/dL)

Table 25.2 Clinical manifestations of hypermagnesemia

Signs/symptoms	Serum [Mg^{2+}] (mg/dL)
Nausea and vomiting	3.6–6.0
Sedation, hyporeflexia, muscle weakness	4.8–8.4
Bradycardia, hypotension	6.0–12.0
Absent reflexes, respiratory paralysis, coma	12.0–18.0
Cardiac arrest	>18.0

Treatment

Asymptomatic Patient

- Removal of the cause will normalize plasma [Mg^{2+}].
- If the plasma concentration does not return to normal, volume expansion and a loop diuretic promote Mg^{2+} excretion in a patient with normal GFR.

Symptomatic Patient

- Intravenous calcium gluconate (15 mg/kg) should be given over a 4-h period. Ca^{2+} antagonizes the neuromuscular and cardiovascular effects of hypermagnesemia.
- For a patient with renal insufficiency, hemodialysis using a Mg^{2+}-free dialysate is the treatment of choice. Since Mg^{2+} is removed by hemodialysis, this treatment provides an efficient means of lowering plasma [Mg^{2+}] within a short period of time.

Study Questions

Case 1 A 22-year-old pregnant woman in her third trimester was admitted for severe hypertension (180/110 mmHg) and proteinuria. She was started on magnesium sulfate ($MgSO_4$) and labetalol (an antihypertensive agent). Her blood pressure was controlled at 140/90 mmHg. Four days later, she developed nausea and vomiting and progressively became lethargic. Her blood pressure dropped to 100/70 mmHg. Deep tendon reflexes were decreased. Her serum creatinine was 2.0 mg/dL and Mg^{2+} was 6.2 mEq/dL.

Question 1 Why did the patient develop hypermagnesemia?

Answer The causes for this patient's elevated serum $[Mg^{2+}]$ were increased exogenous load and reduced excretion by the kidney. $MgSO_4$ is given to reduce blood pressure in a pregnant woman. A creatinine value of 2.0 mg/dL in this patient represents moderate renal failure, because the serum creatinine is usually <0.8 mg/dL in a normal pregnant woman.

Question 2 How would you recognize Mg^{2+} intoxication at the bed side?

Answer Besides hypotension and central nervous system depression, decreased deep tendon reflexes should alert the physician for Mg^{2+} intoxication.

Question 3 How would you treat this patient?

Answer First, $MgSO_4$ administration should be discontinued. Second, calcium gluconate (20 mL of 10% solution) should be given intravenously over a 10-min period to counteract the manifestations of hypermagnesemia. Third, if the symptoms persist, hemodialysis with a dialysate containing low-Mg^{2+} concentration should be done to remove Mg^{2+}.

Case 2 An 18-year-old male student is found to have a serum $[Mg^{2+}]$ of 3.1 mg/dL on a routine medical checkup. He has normal renal function. He denies any medication use, including illicit drugs. His blood pressure is normal. Pertinent labs: Ca^{2+} 11.1 mg/dL, phosphate normal, and parathyroid hormone (PTH) 84 pg/mL (normal 10–65 pg/mL). A 24-h urine Ca^{2+} excretion is 56 mg.
    Which one of the following is the MOST likely cause of his hypermagnesemia?

(A) Use of excess Epsom salt in mouthwash
(B) Excess use of antacids
(C) Excess use of laxatives
(D) Adrenal insufficiency
(E) Familial hypocalciuric hypercalcemia (FHH)

The answer is E Epsom salts (used in mouthwash), Mg^{2+}-containing antacids, and laxatives cause hypermagnesemia only in patients with GFR <30 mL/min. This student's renal function is normal. Therefore, options A, B, and C are incorrect. In patients with adrenal insufficiency due to lack of mineralocorticoid, renal reabsorption of Mg^{2+} is increased. This student has normal blood pressure and normal renal function. Thus, option D is incorrect.

This student carries the diagnosis of FHH, which is due to inactivating mutation in calcium-sensing receptor. The subjects with this mutation do not have any clinical manifestations of hyperparathyroidism. Hypermagnesemia is one of the lab abnormalities in these subjects.

Suggested Reading

1. Hruska KA, Levi M, Slatopolsky E. Disorders of phosphorus, calcium, and magnesium metabolism. In: Coffman TM, Falk RJ, Molitoris BA, et al., editors. Schrier's diseases of the kidney. 9th ed. Philadelphia: Lippincott Williams & Wilkins; 2013. p. 2116–81.
2. Smogorzewski MJ, Stubbs JR, Yu ASL. Disorders of calcium, magnesium, and phosphate balance. In: Skorecki K, et al., editors. Brenner & Rector's the kidney. 10th ed. Philadelphia: Elsevier; 2016. p. 601–35.
3. Topf JM, Murray PT. Hypomagnesemia and hypermagnesesemia. Rev Endocrinol Metab Disord. 2003;4:195–206.

Acid–base physiology deals with the maintenance of normal hydrogen ion concentration (abbreviated as [H⁺]) in body fluids. The normal [H⁺] in the extracellular fluid is about 40 nmol/L or 40 nEq/L (range 38–42 nmol/L), which is precisely regulated by an interplay between body buffers, lungs, and kidneys. Since many functions of the cell are dependent on the optimum [H⁺], it is extremely important to maintain [H⁺] in blood ~40 nmol/L. Any deviation from this [H⁺] results either in acidemia ([H⁺] >40 nmol/L) or alkalemia ([H⁺] <40 nmol/L). This chapter provides an overview of the role of buffers, lungs, and kidneys in regulating [H⁺] in body fluids. The [H⁺] in blood is so low that it is not measured routinely. However, the [H⁺] is measured as pH, which is expressed as:

$$pH = -\log\left[H^+\right]. \tag{26.1}$$

Thus, pH is defined as the negative logarithm of the [H⁺]. An inverse relationship exists between pH and [H⁺]. In other words, as the pH increases, the [H⁺] decreases and vice versa. Cells cannot function at a pH below 6.8 and above 7.8. The normal arterial pH ranges from 7.38 to 7.42, which translates to a [H⁺] of 38–42 nmol/L.

Blood pH is under constant threat by endogenous acid and base loads. If not removed, these loads can cause severe disturbances in blood pH and thus impair cellular function. However, three important regulatory systems prevent changes in pH and thus maintain blood pH in the normal range. These protective systems, as previously stated, are buffers, lungs, and kidneys.

Production of Endogenous Acids and Bases

An acid is a proton donor, whereas a base is a proton acceptor. Under physiological conditions, the diet is a major contributor to endogenous acid and base production.

© Springer Science+Business Media LLC 2018
A.S. Reddi, *Fluid, Electrolyte and Acid-Base Disorders*,
DOI 10.1007/978-3-319-60167-0_26

Endogenous Acids

The oxidation of dietary carbohydrates, fats, and amino acids yields CO_2. About 15,000 mmol of CO_2 are produced by cellular metabolism daily. This CO_2 combines with water in the blood to form carbonic acid (H_2CO_3):

$$CO_2 + H_2O \overset{CA}{\leftrightarrow} H_2CO_3 \leftrightarrow H^+ + HCO_3^-. \qquad (26.2)$$

This reaction is catalyzed by carbonic anhydrase (CA), an enzyme present in tissues and red blood cells but absent in plasma. When H_2CO_3 dissociates into CO_2 and H_2O (a process called dehydration), the CO_2 is eliminated by the lungs. For this reason, H_2CO_3 is called a *volatile acid*.

In addition to volatile acid, the body also generates *nonvolatile (fixed) acids* from cellular metabolism. These nonvolatile acids are produced from sulfur-containing amino acids (i.e., cysteine and methionine) and phosphoproteins. The acids produced are sulfuric acid and phosphoric acid, respectively. Other sources of endogenous nonvolatile acids include glucose, which yields lactic and pyruvic acids; triglycerides, which yield acetoacetic and β-hydroxybutyric acids; and nucleoproteins, which yield uric acid. Hydrochloric acid is also formed from the metabolism of cationic amino acids (i.e., lysine, arginine, and histidine). Sulfuric acid accounts for 50% of all acids produced. A typical North American diet produces 1 mmol/kg/day of endogenous nonvolatile acid.

Under certain conditions, acids are produced from sources other than the diet. For example, starvation produces ketoacids, which can accumulate in the blood. Similarly, strenuous exercise generates lactic acid. Drugs such as corticosteroids cause endogenous acid production by enhancing catabolism of muscle proteins.

Endogenous Bases

Endogenous base (HCO_3^-) is generated from anionic amino acids (glutamate and aspartate) in the diet. Also, citrate or lactate generated during metabolism of carbohydrate yields HCO_3^-. Vegetarian diets contain high amounts of anionic amino acids and small amounts of sulfur- and phosphate-containing proteins. Therefore, these diets generate more bases than acids. In general, the production of acid exceeds that of base in a person ingesting a typical North American diet.

Maintenance of Normal pH

Buffers

All acids that are produced must be removed from the body in order to maintain normal blood pH. Although the kidneys eliminate most of these acids, it takes hours to days to complete the process. Buffers (both cellular and extracellular) are the first line of defense against wide fluctuations in pH.

The most important buffer in blood is bicarbonate/carbon dioxide (HCO_3^-/CO_2). Other buffer systems are disodium phosphate/monosodium phosphate ($Na_2HPO_4^{2-}$/$NaH_2PO_4^-$) and plasma proteins. In addition, erythrocytes contain the important hemoglobin (Hb) system, reduced Hb (HHb^-), and oxyhemoglobin (HbO_2^{2-}). Bones also participate in buffering.

The HCO_3^-/CO_2 system provides the first line of defense in protecting pH. Its role as a buffer can be described by incorporating this system into the Henderson–Hasselbalch equation as follows:

$$pH = pKa + \log \frac{\left[HCO_3^- \right]}{\left[H_2CO_3 \right]}. \tag{26.3}$$

Although H_2CO_3 cannot be measured directly, its concentration can be estimated from the partial pressure of CO_2 (pCO_2) and the solubility coefficient (α) of CO_2 at known temperature and pH. At normal temperature of $37\,^\circ$C and pH of 7.4, the pCO_2 is 40 mmHg, α is 0.03, and pK_a is 6.1. The Henderson–Hasselbalch equation can be appropriately written as

$$pH = 6.1 + \log \frac{\left[HCO_3^- \right]}{0.03 \times pCO_2}. \tag{26.4}$$

Normal plasma [HCO_3^-] is 24 mEq/L. Therefore,

$$pH = 6.1 + \log \frac{24}{0.03 \times 40}$$
$$pH = 6.1 + \log \frac{24}{1.2} = 6.1 + \log \frac{20}{1} \tag{26.5}$$
$$pH = 6.1 + 1.3 = 7.4$$

It should be noted from the Henderson–Hasselbalch equation that the pH of a solution is determined by the pK_a and the ratio of [HCO_3^-] to pCO_2 and not by their absolute values. Thus, because the kidneys regulate the [HCO_3^-] and the lungs pCO_2, the kidneys and lungs determine the pH of extracellular fluids.

Phosphate buffers are effective in regulating intracellular pH more efficiently than extracellular pH. Their increased effectiveness intracellularly is due to their higher concentrations inside the cell. Also, the pK_a of this system is 6.8, which is close to the intracellular pH.

Plasma proteins contain several ionizable groups in their amino acids that buffer either acids or bases. For example, the imidazole groups of histidine and the N-terminal amino groups have pK_a that are close to extracellular pH and thus function as effective buffers. In blood, Hb is an important protein buffer because of its abundance in red blood cells.

Extracellular buffering to an acid load is complete within 30 min. Subsequent buffering occurs intracellularly and takes several hours to complete. Most of this intracellular buffering occurs in the bone. The bone becomes an important source of buffering acid load acutely by an uptake of H^+ in exchange for Na^+, K^+, and bone minerals. These bone minerals rescue the HCO_3^-/CO_2 system in severe acidosis.

It is apparent from the Henderson–Hasselbalch equation (Eq. 26.3) that any change either in [HCO_3^-] or pCO_2 can cause a change in blood pH. The acid–base disturbance that results from a change in plasma [HCO_3^-] is termed a *metabolic acid–base disorder* whereas that due to a change in pCO_2 is called a *respiratory acid–base disorder*.

Lungs

After buffers, the lungs are the second line of defense against pH disturbance. In a normal individual, pCO_2 is maintained around 40 mmHg. This pCO_2 is achieved by expelling the CO_2 that is produced by cellular metabolism through the lungs. Any disturbance in the elimination of CO_2 may cause a change in blood pH. Thus, alveolar ventilation maintains normal pCO_2 to prevent an acute change in pH. Alveolar ventilation is controlled by chemoreceptors located centrally in the medulla and peripherally in the carotid body and aortic arch. Blood [H^+] and pCO_2 are important regulators of alveolar ventilation. The chemoreceptors sense the changes in [H^+] or pCO_2 and alter alveolar ventilatory rate. For example, an increase in [H^+], i.e., a decrease in pH, stimulates ventilatory rate and decreases pCO_2. These responses, in turn, raise pH (see Eq. 26.4). Conversely, a decrease in [H^+] or an increase in pH depresses alveolar ventilation and causes retention of pCO_2 so that the pH is returned to near normal. An increase in pCO_2 stimulates ventilatory rate, whereas a decrease depresses the ventilatory rate. The respiratory response to changes in [H^+] takes several hours to complete.

Kidneys

As stated earlier, 1 mmol/kg/day of fixed acid is produced from the diet. If not removed, this acid is retained and plasma [HCO_3^-] decreases. The result is metabolic acidosis. In a healthy individual, metabolic acidosis does not occur because the kidneys excrete the acid load and maintain plasma [HCO_3^-] around 24 mEq/L. The maintenance of [HCO_3^-] is achieved by three renal mechanisms:

1. Reabsorption of filtered HCO_3^-
2. Generation of new HCO_3^- by titratable acid (TA) excretion
3. Formation of HCO_3^- from generation of NH_4^+

Reabsorption of Filtered HCO₃⁻

HCO_3^- is freely filtered at the glomerulus. The daily filtered load (plasma concentration × glomerular filtration rate) of HCO_3^- is 4,320 mEq (24 mEq/L × 180 L/day = 4,320 mEq/day). Almost all of this HCO_3^- is reabsorbed by the tubular segments of the nephron, and urinary excretion is negligible (<3 mEq). HCO_3^- reabsorption by various segments of the nephron can be summarized as follows:

- Proximal tubule, 80%
- Loop of Henle, 10%
- Distal tubule, 6%
- Collecting duct, 4%

Proximal Tubule

As stated earlier, the proximal tubule has a high capacity for HCO_3^- reabsorption. This reabsorption occurs because of H^+ secretion into the tubular lumen via the Na/H exchanger (Fig. 26.1). Another transporter, called H-ATPase, is also responsible for transport of some protons into the lumen (see Fig. 26.1). The H^+ combines with the filtered HCO_3^- to form H_2CO_3. The apical membrane is rich in carbonic anhydrase IV, which splits H_2CO_3 into H_2O and CO_2. The CO_2 diffuses into the cell where it is hydrated to form H_2CO_3 in the presence of carbonic anhydrase II. H_2CO_3 is dehydrated to form H^+ and HCO_3^-. H^+ are subsequently secreted into the lumen via the Na/H exchanger and H-ATPase to start the cycle again.

HCO_3^- exit across the basolateral membrane occurs via an Na/HCO_3 symporter, in which 2–3 HCO_3^- ions are transported for each Na^+ ion. Another mechanism occurs through the Cl/HCO_3 antiporter, in which one HCO_3^- is exchanged for one Cl^-. Both the energy and electrochemical gradient for H^+ secretion and HCO_3^- exit are provided by the Na/K-ATPase pump located in the basolateral membrane.

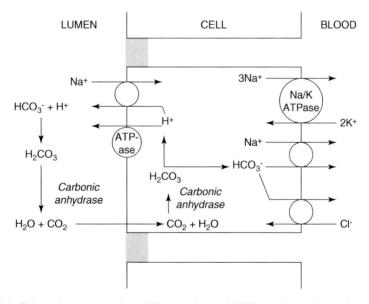

Fig. 26.1 Schematic representation of H^+ secretion and HCO_3^- reabsorption in the proximal tubule cell

Loop of Henle

Most HCO_3^- reabsorption occurs in the thick ascending Henle's loop. The mechanisms for H^+ secretion into the lumen and HCO_3^- exit across the basolateral membrane appear to be similar to those described for the proximal tubule.

Distal Tubule

For the purpose of understanding HCO_3^- reabsorption, it is helpful to divide the distal tubule into three distinct segments: (1) distal convoluted tubule, (2) connecting tubule, and (3) cortical collecting duct. Very little is known about H^+ secretion and HCO_3^- reabsorption by the distal convoluted tubule. This tubule consists of only one cell type, which contains H-ATPase in its apical membrane. The other two segments of the distal tubule consist of principal cells and intercalated cells. The latter cells are responsible for acid–base transport. The intercalated cells in the cortical collecting duct are of three types: Type A, Type B, and Type C cells. Type A intercalated cells contain H-ATPase and K/H exchanger in the apical membrane. H^+ that is formed inside the cell from dehydration of H_2CO_3 is secreted into the lumen by these transporters (Fig. 26.2). HCO_3^- exit is facilitated by the Cl/HCO_3 exchanger.

In contrast, Type B intercalated cells secrete HCO_3^- into the lumen (Fig. 26.3). These cells possess pendrin, a Cl/HCO_3 exchanger, in the apical membrane and H-ATPase in the basolateral membrane. HCO_3^- secretion is stimulated by alkali loading and inhibited by depletion of luminal Cl^-.

Type C (formerly non-A, non-B) cells express H-ATPase and pendrin (Cl/HCO_3 exchanger) in the apical membrane. These cells also participate in HCO_3^- handling.

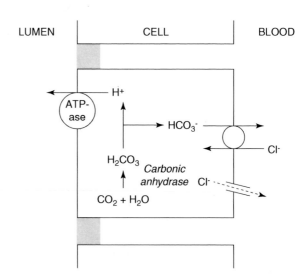

Fig. 26.2 Cellular model for H^+ secretion and HCO_3^- reabsorption by Type A intercalated cell of the cortical collecting duct. *Broken arrow* represents a conductance channel

Fig. 26.3 Cellular model for HCO$_3^-$ secretion and H$^+$ reabsorption by Type B intercalated cell of the cortical collecting duct. *CA* carbonic anhydrase. *Broken arrow* represents a conductance channel

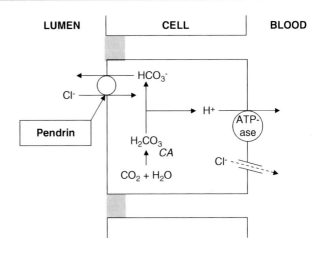

Collecting Duct

The collecting duct includes the cortical portion and outer and inner medullary portions. The cellular mechanisms of HCO$_3^-$ reabsorption in the cortical collecting duct have been discussed in the previous paragraph. The intercalated cells of the outer medullary and inner medullary collecting duct reabsorb HCO$_3^-$ and secrete protons similar to the Type A cell mechanisms (see Fig. 26.2). The cells of outer medullary and inner medullary collecting duct do not secrete HCO$_3^-$ into the lumen.

Regulation of HCO$_3^-$ Reabsorption

A number of factors influence HCO$_3^-$ reabsorption both in the proximal tubule and distal segments of the nephron. These factors are summarized in Tables 26.1 and 26.2. Since the Na/H antiporter is the major mechanism for H$^+$ secretion, any factor that enhances or inhibits this antiporter stimulates or decreases HCO$_3^-$ reabsorption.

Aldosterone plays an important role in HCO$_3^-$ reabsorption and H$^+$ secretion by the intercalated (Type A) cell. It also stimulates Na$^+$ reabsorption by the principal cell. As a result of this Na$^+$ reabsorption, the lumen becomes electrically negative, which promotes H$^+$ secretion. Aldosterone seems to have little effect on HCO$_3^-$ reabsorption in the proximal tubule.

Generation of New HCO$_3^-$ by Titratable Acid Excretion

Generally, one HCO$_3^-$ ion is reclaimed for each H$^+$ that is secreted into the lumen. This mechanism alone does not replenish the HCO$_3^-$ lost in buffering the daily acid load. Additional HCO$_3^-$ has to be generated. How does the new HCO$_3^-$ form? The answer is as follows: whenever an H$^+$ is secreted into the tubule, it combines with the filtered HCO$_3^-$ or with two important urinary buffers, namely, HPO$_4^{2-}$ and NH$_3$,

Table 26.1   Factors affecting HCO_3^- reabsorption (or H^+ secretion) by the proximal tubule

Factor	HCO_3^- reabsorption	Possible mechanism
Increase in filtered load of HCO_3^-	↑	Glomerulotubular balance (G-T) is maintained so that a constant fraction of filtered load of HCO_3^- is reabsorbed
Volume contraction	↑	Promotes HCO_3^- reabsorption by ↑ Na/H exchange
Hypokalemia	↑	↓ Intracellular pH increases $[H^+]$ and promotes proton secretion by stimulation of Na/H antiporter
↑ pCO_2	↑	↓ Intracellular pH and ↑ Na/H antiporter
↑Plasma $[H^+]$	↑	↓ Intracellular pH and ↑ Na/H antiporter
Cl^- depletion	↑	↓ Volume and GFR
Hypercalcemia	↑	Probable ↓ volume and GFR
Volume expansion	↓	↑ GFR. Although G-T balance is maintained, still some HCO_3^- escapes from reabsorption
PTH	↓	Probable ↑ in cytosolic Ca^{2+}. No effect on GFR
↓ pCO_2	↓	↑ Intracellular pH
Hypophosphatemia	↓	↑ Intracellular pH
Acetazolamide	↓	↓ Carbonic anhydrase activity

↑ increase, ↓ decrease

Table 26.2   Factors affecting HCO_3^- reabsorption by the distal tubule

Factor	HCO_3^- reabsorption	Possible mechanism
Aldosterone	↑	↑ H^+ secretion
↑ pCO_2	↑	↓ Intracellular pH
↑ Plasma $[H^+]$	↑	↓ Intracellular pH
Impermeant anions (sulfate, phosphate)	↑	↑ H^+ excretion
Hypokalemia (man and rat)	↑	↓ GFR
↓ pCO_2	↓	↑ Intracellular pH
↓ Plasma $[H^+]$	↓	↑ Intracellular pH
Adrenalectomy	↓	↓H^+ secretion

↑ increase, ↓ decrease

to form $H_2PO_4^-$ and NH_4^+, respectively. For each H^+ that combines with HPO_4^{2-}, one new HCO_3^- is formed and reabsorbed. The process is different when NH_3 is converted into NH_4^+. In this conversion, HCO_3^- is produced from glutamine metabolism. This process is discussed in the next section. In addition to the generation of new HCO_3^-, the urinary buffers also help to maintain acid urine pH (i.e., 4.5–6.0). If these buffers did not exist, the daily acid load would be excreted into the urine and its pH would be < 4.5. The amount of free H^+ in the urine is about 0.04 mmol/L. In the absence of urinary buffers, an individual has to excrete 1,750 L of urine to eliminate 70 mmol/L of acid load. Obviously, this amount of urine excretion is impossible. Let us now see how urinary buffers replenish the HCO_3^- load.

As mentioned previously, the two major urinary buffers are $HPO_4^{2-}/H_2PO_4^-$ and NH_3/NH_4^+. About 40% of H^+ is excreted as phosphate and the remaining 60% as

Fig. 26.4 Schematic representation for titratable acid formation in the collecting duct cell. *CA* carbonic anhydrase

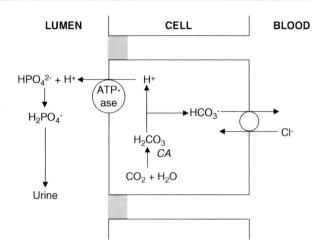

ammonium. The contribution of phosphate to urinary acid excretion is termed *titratable acidity*, which is defined as the number of equivalents of hydroxyl ions required to titrate a unit volume of acidic urine to the pH of the blood (i.e., pH of 7.4). Thus, the amount of hydroxyl ions used in the titration is equal to the amount of H ions that were buffered in the tubular lumen. If 30 mmol of hydroxyl ions are used to raise urine pH to 7.4, then 30 mmol of H ions are titrated, and 30 mmol of HCO_3^- are generated. Other organic substances, such as creatinine and urate, also contribute to TA excretion to a minor degree. Compared to creatinine and urate, the phosphate buffer pair has a pK_a of 6.8 and thus appears to be an ideal urinary buffer. Figure 26.4 shows the mechanisms by which TA excretion occurs in the collecting duct cell. The filtered phosphate (HPO_4^{2-}) combines with the H^+ secreted in the lumen via H-ATPase to form $H_2PO_4^-$. The H ions are formed inside the cell due to dehydration of H_2CO_3 by the catalytic action of carbonic anhydrase II. Note that one HCO_3^- ion is formed for each H^+ secreted.

Generation of HCO₃⁻ from NH₄⁺

Renal handling of NH_4^+ is summarized as follows:

1. NH_4^+ is formed from glutamine in the proximal tubule. It is secreted into the tubular lumen via the Na/H antiporter replacing H^+ in this transporter.
2. NH_4^+ is subsequently reabsorbed in the thick ascending Henle's loop via the Na/K/2Cl cotransporter by replacing K^+. In the medulla, NH_4^+ is split into NH_3 and H^+. As a result, NH_3 accumulates. NH_3 then diffuses into the collecting tubule where it combines with H^+ to form NH_4^+, which is excreted in the urine.
3. The excretion of NH_4^+ per se does not generate HCO_3^-. Instead, new HCO_3^- is formed from the metabolism of glutamine and its organic anions (α-ketoglutarate). Both NH_4^+ formation and excretion are necessary to prevent HCO_3^- loss. If all NH_4^+ formed in the proximal tubule were returned to the general circulation, it would be

used for urea synthesis in the liver. During urea synthesis, H ions are formed which would neutralize the HCO_3^- generated from glutamine. This neutralization would lower $[HCO_3^-]$ and thus negate the beneficial effect of NH_4^+ generation.

Formation of HCO_3^- from glutamine occurs by the following reaction:

$$\text{Glutamine} \overset{(1)}{\leftrightarrow} NH_4^+ + \text{Glutamate} \overset{(2)}{\leftrightarrow} NH_4^+ + \alpha\text{-Ketoglutarate} \leftrightarrow 2HCO_3^-$$

The first reaction is catalyzed by a phosphate-dependent glutaminase and the second reaction by glutamate dehydrogenase. The net result is the formation of two NH_4^+ and two HCO_3^- ions.

Net Acid Excretion (Urinary Acidification)

As stated previously, the H ions that are generated as fixed acids must be excreted daily in the urine to maintain normal acid–base balance. These H^+ are not excreted as free ions. Instead, they are excreted in the form of TA and NH_4^+. Only a small amount of H^+ is excreted as free ions. Each liter of urine contains approximately 0.04 mmol of free H^+. Because of this negligible amount of free H^+, the urine pH is maintained between 4.5 and 6.0. Another reason for the maintenance of acid urine pH is the relatively low concentration of HCO_3^- (<3 mEq/L of urine). Urinary loss of HCO_3^- greater than 5 mEq would generally raise the pH above 6.0 and make the urine alkaline. HCO_3^- loss in the urine is generally equated as a gain of H^+ to the body.

The excretion of H^+ as TA and NH_4^+ is quantified as *net acid excretion* (NAE). NAE is defined as the sum of TA and NH_4^+ minus any H^+ that is added to the body because of urinary loss of HCO_3^-. Therefore, NAE is calculated as follows:

$$NAE = TA + NH_4^+ - HCO_3^-.$$

Metabolic acidosis increases the NAE because the excretion of both TA and NH_4^+ increases. Thus, NAE reflects the amount of H^+ excretion in the form of urinary buffers.

Suggested Reading

1. DuBose TD. Disorders of acid-base balance. In: Skorecki K, et al., editors. Brenner & Rector's the kidney. 10th ed. Philadelphia: Elsevier; 2016. p. 511–58.
2. Hamm LL. Renal regulation of hydrogen ion balance. In: Gennari FJ, Adrogué HJ, Galla JH, Madias NE, editors. Acid–base disorders and their treatment. Boca Raton: Taylor & Francis; 2005. p. 79–117.
3. Hamm LL, Nakhoul N, Hering-Smith KS. Acid-base homeostasis. Clin J Am Soc Nephrol 2015;10:2232–42.
4. Palmer BF. Normal acid-base balance. In: Johnson RJ, Feehally J, Floege J, editors. Comprehensive clinical nephrology. 5th ed. Philadelphia: Mosby; 2015. p. 142–8.
5. Weiner ID, Verlander JW, Wingo CS. Renal acidification mechanisms. In: Mount DB, Sayegh MH, Singh AK, editors. Core concepts in the disorders of fluid, electrolytes and acid–base balance. New York: Springer; 2013. p. 203–33.

Evaluation of an Acid–Base Disorder

27

In Chap. 26, we stated that a change in plasma [HCO$_3^-$] results in a metabolic acid–base disturbance, whereas a change in arterial pCO$_2$ results in a respiratory acid–base disorder. Clinically, four primary acid–base disorders can be recognized: (1) *metabolic acidosis*, (2) *metabolic alkalosis*, (3) *respiratory acidosis*, and (4) *respiratory alkalosis*. Values for an arterial blood gas (ABG) for each primary acid–base disorder are shown in Table 27.1.

Before we analyze each of the above acid–base disorders, it is essential to know the terminology that is used frequently in these acid–base disorders (Table 27.2).

Arterial vs. Venous Blood Sample for ABG

Arterial blood is used most of the time to evaluate an acid–base disorder. However, venous blood samples can be used because there is insignificant difference in ABG values between these two samples (Table 27.3).

Although there is not much difference between the two samples in normal individuals, significant difference can be observed in pathological conditions. For example, large arteriovenous difference can be found in a patient with decreased cardiac output and on mechanical ventilation. In such a patient, the arterial pCO$_2$ remains normal, but central venous pCO$_2$ may be extremely elevated, as more CO$_2$

Table 27.1 Primary acid–base disturbances and their secondary response

Acid–base disorder	pH	Primary change	Secondary change	Mechanism of secondary change
Metabolic acidosis	<7.40	↓ HCO$_3^-$	↓ pCO$_2$	Hyperventilation
Metabolic alkalosis	>7.40	↑ HCO$_3^-$	↑ pCO$_2$	Hypoventilation
Respiratory acidosis	<7.40	↑ pCO$_2$	↑ HCO$_3^-$	↑ HCO$_3^-$ reabsorption
Respiratory alkalosis	>7.40	↓ pCO$_2$	↓ HCO$_3^-$	↓ HCO$_3^-$ reabsorption

© Springer Science+Business Media LLC 2018
A.S. Reddi, *Fluid, Electrolyte and Acid-Base Disorders*,
DOI 10.1007/978-3-319-60167-0_27

Table 27.2 Acid–base terminology

Acidemia: an increase in blood [H⁺]
Alkalemia: a decrease in blood [H⁺]
Acidosis: a pathophysiologic process that tends to acidify body fluids
Alkalosis: a pathophysiologic process that tends to alkalinize body fluids
Arterial blood gas (ABG): includes pH, pCO₂, and calculated serum [HCO₃⁻]
Normocapnia: normal arterial pCO₂ (40 mmHg)
Hypocapnia: a decrease in arterial pCO₂
Hypercapnia: an increase in arterial pCO₂
Normobicarbonatemia: normal serum [HCO₃⁻] (24 mEq/L)
Hypobicarbonatemia: a decrease in serum [HCO₃⁻]
Hyperbicarbonatemia: an increase in serum [HCO₃⁻]
Primary change: an abnormality in either the serum [HCO₃⁻] or arterial pCO₂ resulting from a primary change in body function/metabolism or additions to or losses from body fluids
Secondary change: a compensatory (secondary) response that acts to minimize changes in pH produced by the primary disorder. It is also called compensation
Simple acid–base disorder: presence of one primary disorder with appropriate secondary response
Mixed acid–base disorder: simultaneous occurrence of two or more primary disorders

Table 27.3 Differences between arterial and venous blood samples

ABG value	Arterial blood	Venous blood
[H⁺] (nmol/L)	40	44
pH	7.40	7.36
pCO₂ (mmHg)	40	48
[HCO₃⁻] (mEq/L)	24	26

is added to the perfusing tissue. In low cardiac output states, an arterial ABG is useful in assessing pulmonary gas exchange, and central venous ABG is useful in assessing pH and tissue oxygenation.

Evaluation of an ABG

Three concepts (two of them not defined in Table 27.2) that help you evaluate the acid–base disorders are the *Henderson equation*, the *anion gap*, and the *secondary physiologic response (compensation)*.

Henderson Equation

In clinical practice, the Henderson–Hasselbalch equation is a rather cumbersome way to calculate the pH using logarithms. The same information can be obtained by using the *Henderson equation*, which relates [H⁺] to pH. This equation, which calculates [H⁺], is expressed as:

$$ H^+ \left(nmol/L \right) = 24 \times \frac{pCO_2}{\left[HCO_3^- \right]} $$

As an example of how this equation can be used, consider the following ABG values:

pH = 7.40
pCO_2 = 40 mmHg
HCO_3^- = 24 mEq/L

$$H^+ \left(nmol / L\right) = 24 \times \frac{40}{24} = 40$$

This [H^+] of 40 corresponds to the pH of 7.40. The Henderson equation is thus used clinically to check the validity of pH obtained from the clinical laboratory.

Remember the following approximate [H^+] corresponds to clinically relevant pH values:

pH 7.50 = 30
pH 7.40 = 40
pH 7.30 = 50
pH 7.20 = 60
pH 7.10 = 80
pH 7.00 = 100

The Henderson equation can also be used to calculate the [HCO_3^-]:

$$\left[HCO_3^-\right] \left(mEq / L\right) = 24 \times \frac{pCO_2}{\left[H^+\right]}$$

The HCO_3^- that is reported in the ABG slip is the calculated one from the above equation, and this value is 1–2 mEq/L less than the measured serum HCO_3^-, which is usually called total or TCO_2. TCO_2 includes HCO_3^-, carbonic acid, and dissolved CO_2. For this reason, the measured HCO_3^- is 1–2 mEq higher than the calculated HCO_3^-. In the evaluation of ABG, if there is a large difference between the measured and calculated HCO_3^-, the ABG and electrolytes should be repeated simultaneously or within a few minutes apart.

Anion Gap

In plasma (serum), the number of cations must equal the number of anions to maintain electroneutrality. However, measurement of all of these cations and anions is not done routinely. Among all electrolytes, Na^+, K^+, Cl^-, and HCO_3^- are usually measured. From these measurements, the number of unmeasured anions can be calculated (Table 27.4). Generally, plasma [Na^+] exceeds the sum of plasma [Cl^-] and [HCO_3^-], and the difference is called the *anion gap* (AG). Since the change in serum [K^+] in either health or disease is minimal, this cation is not routinely included in the calculation of AG. Thus, AG is calculated as:

$$AG \left(mEq / L\right) = \left[\left(Na^+\right) - \left(Cl^- + HCO_3^-\right)\right]$$

Table 27.4 Unmeasured anions and cations (particularly anions)

Unmeasured cations (mEq/L)	Unmeasured anions (mEq/L)
K^+: 4.5	Albumin: 12
Ca^{2+}: 5.0	Other proteins: 3
Mg^{2+}: 1.5	
	PO_4^{3-}: 2
	SO_4^{2-}: 1
	Organic acids: 5
Total: 11	Total: 23
AG = 23–11 = 12 ± 4	

Normal AG Values

As shown in Table 27.4, the normal reference range for AG is 12 ± 4. This value was derived from older methods of electrolyte determinations using colorimetry and flame photometry. With the introduction of ion-selective electrode methodology, the normal AG levels are much lower, ranging from 3 to11. These low values are related to high Cl^- determination. Variations in normal values of AG are frequently seen from laboratory to laboratory, and the clinician should follow his or her laboratory values for proper interpretation of AG in clinical medicine. For simplicity, an AG of 10 mEq/L is considered normal.

Hyperglycemia and AG

It is always debated whether or not AG should be calculated using measured serum Na^+ or corrected Na^+ in a patient with severe hyperglycemia. It is suggested that only measured Na^+ should be used for AG and not the corrected Na^+. This suggestion is based on the assumption that Cl^- and HCO_3^- are equally diluted as Na^+ by movement of water from inside to outside of the cell caused by hyperglycemia. When AG is calculated using only corrected Na^+ and not corrected Cl^- and HCO_3^- for hyperglycemia, the AG is overestimated with the implication of underlying high AG metabolic acidosis. Na^+ decreases by 1.6 mEq/dL for each increase in 100 mg/dL glucose above normal glucose levels, but no such number is given for either Cl^- or HCO_3^-. It is, thus, emphasized that only measured Na^+ should be used to calculate the serum AG.

Clinical Use of AG

Traditionally, the AG is useful in classifying metabolic acidosis into high, normal, or low AG metabolic acidosis. High AG is due to accumulation of unmeasured anions, whereas normal AG is usually related to high Cl^- level. Low AG implies a substantial decrease in unmeasured anions, an increase in unmeasured cations, and a spurious decrease in $[Na^+]$ or spurious increases in $[Cl^-]$ or $[HCO_3^-]$.

Mnemonic for High AG Metabolic Acidosis

The mnemonic to remember AG is GOLD MARK (glycols (ethylene and propylene glycols), oxoproline (pyroglutamic acid), L-lactate, D-lactate, methanol, aspirin, renal failure, ketoacidosis). Table 27.5 shows various causes of high AG metabolic acidoses.

Normal AG Metabolic Acidosis

Table 27.6 shows causes for normal (hyperchloremic) AG metabolic acidoses.

Table 27.5 Most common causes of high AG metabolic acidosis

Cause	Unmeasured anions causing high AG
Uremic acidosis (renal failure)	Sulfate, phosphate, urate
Ketoacidosis (diabetes, starvation, alcohol)	Acetoacetate, β-hydroxybutyrate
Lactic acidosis	L-lactate
Small bowl resection	D-lactate
Intoxicants	
Methanol	Formate
Ethylene glycol	Glycolate, oxalate
Aspirin	Salicylate, L-lactate, ketoacids
Acetaminophen (Tylenol)	Pyroglutamate
Paraldehyde	Acetaldehyde or acetic acid
Toluene	Hippurate, benzoate

Table 27.6 Most common causes of normal AG metabolic acidosis

Cause	Mechanism
Diarrhea	Loss of HCO_3^- in stool
Ureterosigmoidostomy, ileal conduit	Loss of HCO_3^- in stool
Carbonic anhydrase inhibitors	Loss of HCO_3^- in urine
Recovery phase of ketoacidosis	Less HCO_3^- synthesis from decreased availability of ketones
Chronic kidney disease (stages 4–5)	Decrease in NH_3 excretion
Proximal renal tubular acidosis (type II)	Loss of HCO_3^- in urine
Distal renal tubular acidosis (type I)	Decreased renal acid secretion
Distal renal tubular acidosis (type IV)	Decreased acid secretion and low NH_3 production
Dilutional acidosis	Increased Cl^- due to normal saline administration
Cholestyramine	Release of Cl^- in exchange for HCO_3^-

Low AG Metabolic Acidosis and Correction for Low Serum Albumin

Other than laboratory error, the most common cause of low AG acidosis in hospitalized patients is hypoalbuminemia. As shown in Table 27.4, albumin is the major contributor for unmeasured anions and thus AG. A decrease in albumin from 4.0 to 2.0 g/dL reduces AG by 5.0 mEq/dL (for each gram decrease in albumin from normal value, the AG decreases by 2.5). Thus, a patient with chronic kidney disease (CKD) stages 4–5 and low albumin may seem to have a normal AG metabolic acidosis, but when corrected for normal albumin, the acid–base disorder is a high AG metabolic acidosis. For example, the above patient with CKD stages 4–5 has a calculated AG of 12, albumin of 2.0 g/dL, and the laboratory reference AG of 10. This shows that the patient has only two excess anions (12−10 = 2). However, when AG is adjusted for hypoalbuminemia, the AG is 17, and Δ AG is 7 (17−10 = 7). Therefore, albumin levels should be obtained whenever an ABG is ordered, particularly in critically ill patients.

In addition to a decrease in unmeasured anions, an increase in unmeasured cations causes low AG. For example, a patient with IgG myeloma will have low AG because IgG molecules carry a positive charge at a pH of 7.4. Also, ingestion of bromide- or iodine-containing medications or intoxication of these halides can raise the concentration of unmeasured anions and lower AG due to measurements of these halides as Cl^-. Salicylate overdose usually gives a negative AG, as high salicylate levels are measured as high as Cl^- levels by certain chloride-sensitive ion-selective electrodes.

Occasionally, patients with severe hypertriglyceridemia may present with low AG due to a different laboratory measurement. Severe hypercalcemia, hypermagnesemia, or lithium toxicity may cause low AG. Some case reports demonstrated low AG in hypotonic hyponatremic patients. Thus, low AG is caused by many conditions.

Use of $\Delta AG/\Delta HCO_3^-$

Not only is AG useful in the classification of metabolic acidosis, but it is also indirectly helpful in analyzing mixed acid–base disorders such as high AG metabolic acidosis and metabolic alkalosis or high AG and normal AG metabolic acidosis. In a simple or uncomplicated high AG metabolic acidosis, the increase in AG above normal (called ΔAG) is equal to the decrease in HCO_3^- from normal value (called ΔHCO_3). In other words, for every 1 mEq/L rise in the AG, there is a concomitant fall of 1 mEq/L in HCO_3^-. This is defined as $\Delta AG/\Delta HCO_3^-$. In a simple high AG metabolic acidosis, the $\Delta AG/\Delta HCO_3^-$ ratio is 1. Any significant deviation from 1 is indicative of a mixed acid–base disorder. For example, a patient with diarrhea typically develops a hyperchloremic or normal AG metabolic acidosis. In this condition, the decrease in HCO_3^- results in a reciprocal increase in Cl^- so that the AG does not change. As a result, the $\Delta AG/\Delta HCO_3^-$ ratio is 0. If this patient develops hypotension and subsequent lactic acidosis, the HCO_3^- decreases even further. In other words, the ΔHCO_3^- is greater than ΔAG, and the $\Delta AG/\Delta HCO_3^-$ ratio is < 1 (above 0 but below 1), indicating a mixed high and normal AG metabolic acidosis.

In pure lactic acidosis, the $\Delta AG/\Delta HCO_3^-$ ratio is usually 1.6 because the lactate anions remain in the extracellular compartment because of low urinary excretion. This raises the AG. However, the HCO_3^- concentration does not decrease as non-HCO_3^- buffers participate in buffering lactate anions. In my opinion, the $\Delta AG/\Delta HCO_3^-$ ratio is usually not helpful in pure lactic acidosis, as lactate levels are available, and the $\Delta AG/\Delta HCO_3^-$ ratio varies from 0.8 to 1.8.

In a mixed high AG metabolic acidosis and metabolic alkalosis, the HCO_3^- level is inappropriately high relative to the increase in AG. As a result, the $\Delta AG/\Delta HCO_3^-$ ratio is >2.

Although the $\Delta AG/\Delta HCO_3^-$ ratio is a useful tool, it should not be used alone in identifying mixed acid–base disorders. Other pieces of evidence such as clinical information about the patient, normal AG range, AG corrected for albumin, and uncovering of hidden acid–base disorder during treatment should be taken into account whenever a mixed acid–base disorder is analyzed. Also, evaluation of volume status is important, as total HCO_3^- content in the ECF compartment may change. An example is diabetic ketoacidosis (DKA). Prior to the development of DKA, the ECF water content in a 70 kg patient is 14 L, and the total HCO_3^- content is 336 mEq (14 L×24 mEq/L = 336 mEq). DKA obligates water loss, and the patient develops volume depletion. As a result, water content decreases presumably to 10 L. At the same time, the HCO_3^- content decreases due to buffering of ketoacids presumably to 15 mEq/L. Now the new total HCO_3^- content is 150 mEq (10 L×15 mEq = 150), a deficit of 186 mEq (336 mEq–150 mEq = 186 mEq). Note that the AG continues to increase because of the addition of ketoacids but the concentration of HCO_3^- decreases. As a result, the $\Delta AG/\Delta HCO_3^-$ ratio will be >2, suggesting the presence of spurious metabolic alkalosis. Thus, one must be cautious in interpreting the $\Delta AG/\Delta HCO_3^-$ ratio.

Secondary Physiologic Response (or Compensatory Response)

It is a physiologic process that minimizes changes in $[H^+]$ brought about by a primary change. In clinical practice, the term compensation rather than secondary physiologic response is usually used. Two types of compensatory responses (secondary physiologic responses) are involved: respiratory and renal. In a metabolic acid–base disorder, the compensatory response is respiratory. For example, in metabolic acidosis, the primary change is a decrease in plasma $[HCO_3^-]$ and an increase in $[H^+]$. The compensatory response is a decrease in pCO_2 due to hyperventilation. This decrease in pCO_2 limits the rise in $[H^+]$, and thus the pH is returned to normal. The observed hyperventilation represents the normal physiologic response to an increase in $[H^+]$. Conversely, hypoventilation is an appropriate physiologic response to metabolic alkalosis (see Table 27.7). In a respiratory acid–base disorder, the compensatory response is renal. In respiratory acidosis, the primary change is an increase in pCO_2 and a decrease in pH or an increase in $[H^+]$. The renal compensation increases the plasma $[HCO_3^-]$ with a resultant increase in pH toward normal. It should be pointed out that these compensatory mechanisms do not increase the pH to normal but rather return the pH toward near normal.

Acid–base disorder	Compensatory response
Table 27.7 Normal compensatory responses to primary acid–base disorders	
Metabolic acidosis	$pCO_2 = HCO_3^- \times 1.5 + 8 \pm 2$, or for each mEq/L decrease in HCO_3^-, pCO_2 decreases by 1.2 mmHg
Metabolic alkalosis	For each mEq/L increase in HCO_3^-, pCO_2 increases by 0.7 mmHg
Respiratory acidosis	
Acute	For each mmHg increase in pCO_2, HCO_3^- increases by 0.1 mEq/L
Chronic	For each mmHg increase in pCO_2, HCO_3^- increases by 0.4 mEq/L
Respiratory alkalosis	
Acute	For each mmHg decrease in pCO_2, HCO_3^- decreases by 0.2 mEq/L
Chronic	For each mmHg decrease in pCO_2, HCO_3^- decreases by 0.4 mEq/L

Pathogenesis of Acid-Base Disorders

It is important to understand the development of acid–base disorders for proper interpretation of the primary acid–base disorder. The following pathophysiology underlies each of the four primary acid–base disorders.

Metabolic acidosis develops because of the following conditions (Chaps. 28, 29, and 30):

1. Loss of HCO_3^- either from the GI tract or kidney
2. Retention of H^+ due to impaired renal function
3. Addition of exogenous or endogenous of strong acids

Metabolic alkalosis develops due to retention of HCO_3^- and/or loss of H^+ (Chap. 31)

Respiratory acidosis results from retention of pCO_2 (Chap. 32).
Respiratory alkalosis develops from hyperventilation (Chap. 33).

With the above background, any acid–base disturbance can be approached with the following steps:

1. Measure electrolytes and ABG simultaneously or within few minutes apart.
2. Check the validity of blood pH—use Henderson equation.
3. Identify the primary disorder—use Table 27.1.
4. Calculate the AG* (correct for low albumin, if indicated).
5. Identify the causes of the primary disorder.
6. Calculate the expected compensation (also called secondary response)—use Table 27.7.
7. Identify the mixed acid–base disorder, if any.

8. Use $\Delta AG/\Delta HCO_3^-$ ratio appropriately.
9. Determine the appropriate treatment.

*Urine AG, urine pH, and plasma osmolal gap will be discussed in other chapters.

How to Evaluate an Acid–Base Disorder

Example A 30-year-old man with a long history of intravenous drug abuse is admitted for weakness and abdominal pain. His respiratory rate is 24/min (normal = 12–14/min). Initial electrolyte and ABG values:

Na^+ = 136 mEq/L	pH = 7.28
K^+ = 5.1 mEq/L	pCO_2 = 30 mmHg
Cl^- = 100 mEq/L	pO_2 = 100 mmHg
HCO_3^- = 14 mEq/L	HCO_3^- = 13 mEq/L
BUN = 120 mg/dL	
Creatinine = 10 mg/dL	
Glucose = 90 mg/dL	

Step 1 Electrolytes and ABG were done simultaneously.
Step 2 Check the validity of blood pH.
Using the Henderson equation, we obtain:

$$\left[H^+\right](nmol/L) = 24 \times \frac{30}{14} = 51.4$$

From the section on Henderson equation, it is evident that the corresponding pH for the [H$^+$] of 51.4 is approximately 7.28. Therefore, the reported pH for the patient is correct.

Step 3 Identify the primary disorder.
From Table 27.1, the primary disorder is metabolic acidosis because both pH and HCO_3^- are less than normal.

Step 4 Calculate the AG.

$$\left[\left(Na^+\right) - \left(Cl^- + HCO_3^-\right)\right]$$

$$136 - (100 + 14) = 22\,(serum\,albumin\,not\,available)$$

Step 5 Identify the cause of the primary disorder.
As the AG is 22, this disorder is a high AG metabolic acidosis. From the causes listed in Table 27.5 and the laboratory values of the patient, it is evident that the cause is renal failure.

Step 6 Calculate the expected compensation.
Since hyperventilation is an appropriate compensatory (secondary physiologic response) response, the pCO_2 should be lower than the normal value of 40 mmHg.

This patient's pCO_2 is 30. The following formula is used to determine whether this value is the expected (or predicted) pCO_2 (Table 27.7):

$$pCO_2 = HCO_3^- \times 1.5 + 8 \pm 2$$
$$= 14 \times 1.5 + 8 \pm 2 = 29$$

If the patient has an appropriate respiratory response for acidemia of 51.4 $[H^+]$, the expected pCO_2 should be between 27 and 31 mmHg. Since the patient's pCO_2 is 30, his respiratory response is appropriate. Therefore, the acid–base disturbance in this patient is a simple high AG metabolic acidosis with appropriate compensatory response.

If the patient's pCO_2 is different from the expected pCO_2, then a coexisting respiratory acid–base disorder is present. For example, if the patient's pCO_2 is lower than the expected pCO_2, a respiratory alkalosis is present in addition to metabolic acidosis. If, on the other hand, the patient's pCO_2 is higher than the expected pCO_2, a coexisting respiratory acidosis is present.

Step 7 Identify the mixed acid–base disorder, if any.

No mixed acid–base disorder is present (this step is not necessary in this patient, as step 6 revealed only one primary acid–base disorder).

Step 8 Use $\Delta AG/\Delta HCO_3^-$ ratio appropriately.

This step is not necessary in this patient.

Step 9 Determine the appropriate treatment.

Generally, the treatment for metabolic acidosis with pH <7.20 is $NaHCO_3$. In this patient, the pH >7.20, and thus no treatment is necessary. The patient is symptomatic from his renal failure and needs dialysis to relieve his symptoms. Dialysis will also improve his plasma $[HCO_3^-]$ and blood pH.

How to Evaluate a Mixed Acid–Base Disorder

It is not uncommon for two or three simple or primary acid–base disturbances to coexist in hospitalized patients. Mixed acid–base disorders should be suspected whenever (see Chap. 34 for details):

1. There is no compensatory response or overcompensation for a primary simple acid–base disorder.
2. The pH and $[HCO_3^-]$ are normal, but the AG is high (mixed metabolic acidosis and metabolic alkalosis).
3. The pH is near normal, but $[HCO_3^-]$ is high (mixed metabolic alkalosis and respiratory acidosis).
4. The pH is near normal, but $[HCO_3^-]$ is low (mixed metabolic acidosis and respiratory alkalosis).
5. The pH is low (<7.4), but $[HCO_3^-]$ is normal (mixed metabolic acidosis and respiratory acidosis).

6. The pH is high (>7.4), but [HCO_3^-] is normal (mixed respiratory alkalosis and metabolic alkalosis).

Example A 31-year-old woman with AIDS is admitted for weakness and poor appetite. Her respiratory rate is 26/min. Lung examination reveals crackles bilaterally, and chest X-ray confirms pulmonary edema. Her electrolyte and ABG values are:

Na^+ = 129 mEq/L	pH = 7.36
K^+ = 3.4 mEq/L	pCO_2 = 22 mmHg
Cl^- = 90 mEq/L	pO_2 = 90 mmHg
HCO_3^- = 12 mEq/L	HCO_3^- = 11 mEq/L
BUN = 82 mg/dL	
Creatinine = 8.2 mg/dL	
Glucose = 100 mg/dL	

To analyze this acid–base disorder, follow the steps 1–9 discussed before.

Step 1 Labs and ABG are available.

Step 2 Check the validity of blood pH.

Using the Henderson equation, the [H^+] is 44, which corresponds to the pH of 7.36.

Step 3 Identify the primary disorder.

The dominant acid–base disturbance is metabolic acidosis because the pH is <7.40 and the HCO_3^- is <24 mEq/L.

Step 4 Calculate the AG.

The AG is 27, which is elevated.

Step 5 Identify the causes of the primary disorder.

From the laboratory values, the cause for the patient's metabolic acidosis is renal failure.

Step 6 Calculate the expected compensation.

For a simple metabolic acidosis, the expected pCO_2 is between 24 and 28 mmHg. However, the patient's pCO_2 is below 24, suggesting the coexistence of respiratory alkalosis. Thus, this patient has a mixed high AG metabolic acidosis and respiratory alkalosis.

Step 7 Identify the mixed acid–base disorder, if any.

This step is not necessary, as step 6 revealed the nature of the acid–base disorder.

Step 8 Use $\Delta AG/\Delta HCO_3^-$ ratio appropriately.

Assuming normal AG is 10, ΔAG is 17, and ΔHCO_3^- is 12; therefore, the $\Delta AG/\Delta HCO_3^-$ ratio is 1.41. Thus, there is no hidden metabolic alkalosis in this patient.

Step 9 Determine the appropriate treatment.

Administration of $NaHCO_3$ to raise serum [HCO_3^-] is not appropriate because of pulmonary edema. The appropriate treatment is renal replacement therapy such as hemodialysis, which not only removes fluid from the lungs but also increases serum [HCO_3^-] and blood pH.

Hydration and Acid–Base Disorder-Induced Changes in Serum [Na⁺] and [Cl⁻]

The normal serum [Na⁺] is 140 mEq/L, and serum [Cl⁻] is 100 mEq/L; therefore the ratio is 1.4:1. This ratio is maintained in states of hydration but altered in acid–base disorders.

Examples In hydration-induced conditions, serum [Na⁺] and serum [Cl⁻] should decrease or increase proportionately to maintain the normal ratio of 1.4:1, as follows:

Overhydration (proportionate decrease in both)

$$\text{Na}^+ \text{ change} : 140 \rightarrow 126 \text{ mEq/L} = 14 \text{ mEq fall or } 10\% \text{ decrease}$$

$$\text{Cl}^- \text{ change} : 100 \rightarrow 90 \text{ mEq/L} = 10 \text{ mEq fall or } 10\% \text{ decrease}$$

Dehydration (proportionate increase in both)

$$\text{Na}^+ \text{ change} : 140 \rightarrow 154 \text{ mEq/L} = 14 \text{ mEq rise or } 10\% \text{ increase}$$

$$\text{Cl}^- \text{ change} : 100 \rightarrow 110 \text{ mEq/L rise or } 10\% \text{ increase}$$

On the other hand, a change in [Cl⁻] without a change in [Na⁺] always represents a disturbance in acid–base alone. Therefore, the ratio of 1.4:1 is disturbed, as follows:

Metabolic alkalosis or respiratory acidosis (disproportionate decrease in Cl⁻ compared to Na⁺)

$$\text{Na}^+ \text{ change} : 140 \rightarrow 140 \text{ mEq/L} = 0 \text{ mEq change or } 0\% \text{ change}$$

$$\text{Cl}^- \text{ change} : 100 \rightarrow 90 \text{ mEq/L} = 10 \text{ mEq/L fall or } 10\% \text{ decrease}$$

Respiratory alkalosis or hyperchloremic acidosis (disproportionate increase in Cl⁻ compared to Na⁺)

$$\text{Na}^+ \text{ change} : 140 \rightarrow 140 \text{ mEq/L} = 0 \text{ mEq change or } 0\% \text{ change}$$

$$\text{Cl}^- \text{ change} : 100 \rightarrow 110 \text{ mEq/L} = 10 \text{ mEq/L rise or } 10\% \text{ increase}$$

Based on the above examples, one can follow the changes in serum [Na⁺] and [Cl⁻] in combined conditions of disturbed hydration and acid–base disorders.

Overhydration and metabolic alkalosis (disproportionate decrease in both; fall in Cl⁻ is additive)

$$\text{Na}^+ \text{ change} : 140 \rightarrow 126 \text{ mEq/L} = 14 \text{ mEq fall or } 10\% \text{ decrease}$$

$$\text{Cl}^- \text{ change} : 100 \rightarrow 80 \text{ mEq/L} = 20 \text{ mEq/L fall or } 20\% \text{ decrease}$$

Dehydration and metabolic alkalosis (disproportionate increase in both; rise in Na⁺>Cl⁻).

$$Na^+ \text{ change}: 140 \rightarrow 168 \text{ mEq}/L = 28 \text{ mEq rise or } 20\% \text{ increase}$$

$$Cl^- \text{ change}: 100 \rightarrow 90 \text{ mEq}/L = 10 \text{ mEq}/L \text{ fall or } 10\% \text{ decrease}$$

Study Questions

Case 1 A 50-year-old man is admitted to the intensive care unit with anterior wall myocardial infarction. Six hours later, he develops shortness of breath. Physical examination and chest X-ray are consistent with pulmonary edema. Electrolytes and ABG values:

Na^+ = 140 mEq/L	pH = 7.36
K^+ = 5.2 mEq/L	pCO_2 = 34 mmHg
Cl^- = 94 mEq/L	pO_2 = 80 mmHg
HCO_3^- = 16 mEq/L	HCO_3^- = 22 mEq/L
BUN = 30 mg/dL	
Creatinine = 1.4 mg/dL	
Glucose = 200 mg/dL	

Question 1 Which one of the following BEST characterizes the acid–base disturbance?

(A) Metabolic acidosis and respiratory alkalosis
(B) Metabolic alkalosis and metabolic acidosis
(C) Respiratory acidosis and metabolic acidosis
(D) Respiratory alkalosis and metabolic alkalosis
(E) None of the above

The answer is E The acid–base disorder should be analyzed systematically. Once the labs are available, the next step is to check whether the pH is correct or not. One must use the Henderson equation to obtain the [H⁺] and then the pH. The Henderson equation is:

$$\left[H^+ \right] = 24 \times \frac{pCO_2}{HCO_3^-}$$

Substituting the values, we obtain:

$$\left[H^+ \right] = 24 \times \frac{34}{16} = 51$$

The [H⁺] of 51 corresponds to a pH of 7.30. Therefore, the pH reported from the lab is incorrect. Also, there is a large difference between the measured and calculated HCO_3^-. In view of this, it is difficult to interpret the ABG. Both electrolytes and ABG should be repeated within few minutes apart. This case emphasizes the need for checking the accuracy or internal consistency of the pH.

Case 2 A 42-year-old man is admitted because of dizziness and weakness. His blood pressure is 120/80 mmHg with a pulse rate of 90 beats/min (sitting) and 100/64 mmHG with a pulse rate of 110 beats/min (standing). He is not on any medications but admits to vomiting. Admitting electrolyte and ABG values:

Na^+ = 129 mEq/L	pH = 7.53
K^+ = 2.5 mEq/L	pCO_2 = 63 mmHg
Cl^- = 58 mEq/L	pO_2 = 62 mmHg
HCO_3^- = 58 mEq/L	HCO_3^- = 58 mEq/L
Creatinine = 1.9 mg/dL	
BUN = 32 mg/dL	
Glucose = 94 mg/dL	

Question 1 Analyze the acid–base disturbance (use steps that are necessary).

Answer To analyze this acid–base disorder, follow the appropriate steps that are necessary.
  Step 1 Check the validity of pH.
  According to the Henderson equation, the [H⁺] is 26, which corresponds to a pH of 7.53. Therefore, the reported pH is correct.
  Step 2 Identify the primary disorder.
  From Table 27.1, the primary acid–base disturbance is metabolic alkalosis.
  Step 3 Calculate the AG.
  The AG is 13, which is normal (calculate AG in all primary acid–base disorders so that the hidden metabolic acidosis is not missed).
  Step 4 Identify the cause of the primary disorder.
  The cause for metabolic alkalosis is vomiting.
  Step 5 Calculate the expected compensation.
  The respiratory compensation is appropriate (Table 27.7), suggesting that this acid–base disturbance is a simple metabolic alkalosis.

Question 2 How would you treat this acid–base disturbance?

Answer The treatment is normal saline with KCl supplementation.

Case 3 A 72-year-old woman with a history of type 2 diabetes mellitus, congestive heart failure (CHF), and renal failure is admitted for nausea, vomiting, and shortness of breath. Her medications include insulin and furosemide. Her weight is 60 kg. Admission electrolyte and ABG values:

Na^+ = 140 mEq/L	pH = 7.40
K^+ = 4.1 mEq/L	pCO_2 = 40 mmHg
Cl^- = 95 mEq/L	pO_2 = 90 mmHg
HCO_3^- = 24 mEq/L	HCO_3^- = 24 mEq/L
Creatinine = 4.1 mg/dL	
BUN = 52 mg/dL	
Glucose = 145 mg/dL	

Question 1 Characterize the acid–base disturbance in this patient.

Answer The electrolytes and ABG values reveal no abnormalities. However, a step-by-step approach reveals that a mixed acid–base disturbance is present.
   Step 1 Check the validity of pH.
   From the Henderson equation, the [H^+] is 40 nmol/L, which is equal to a pH of 7.40.
   Step 2 Identify the primary disorder.
   From ABG values, no apparent acid–base disturbance is present.
   Step 3 Calculate the AG.
   The AG is 21, which suggests the presence of a high AG metabolic acidosis (this case signifies the importance of calculating AG).
   Step 4 Identify the cause of the primary disorder.
   The cause for this metabolic acidosis is renal failure.
   Step 5 Calculate the expected compensation.
   If this were a pure metabolic acidosis, the pH, serum [HCO_3^-], and pCO_2 levels would be lower than normal. Since the patient has vomiting and she is also taking furosemide for her CHF, she developed metabolic alkalosis. The coexistence of metabolic acidosis and metabolic alkalosis normalizes ABG values and gives the impression of no underlying disturbance. The clue for the diagnosis of this mixed metabolic acidosis and metabolic alkalosis is the presence of a high AG. Thus, this case emphasizes the importance of calculating AG in the analysis of any acid–base disturbance.

Question 2 How would you manage her?

Answer Since she has shortness of breath due to CHF, IV furosemide can be tried. If the patient fails to respond, nesiritide can be started alone or in combination with dobutamine. If still unresponsive, two to three treatments of hemodialysis can improve her CHF (the patient's symptoms were relieved by two treatments of hemodialysis with low blood flow).

Case 4 A 65-year-old man with a history of chronic obstructive pulmonary disease (COPD) is admitted for management of shortness of breath. On admission, his electrolyte and ABG values are:

Na^+ = 134 mEq/L	pH = 7.35
K^+ = 3.6 mEq/L	pCO_2 = 64 mmHg
Cl^- = 90 mEq/L	pO_2 = 70 mmHg
HCO_3^- = 34 mEq/L	HCO_3^- = 33 mEq/L
Creatinine = 1.1 mg/dL	
BUN = 12 mg/dL	
Glucose = 100 mg/dL	

Question 1 Characterize the acid–base disorder.

Answer As earlier, follow the step-by-step method to analyze this acid–base disorder.

Step 1 Check the validity of pH.

According to the Henderson equation, the $[H^+]$ is 45 nmol/L, which corresponds to a pH of 7.35.

Step 2 Identify the primary disorder.

From Table 27.1, the primary acid–base disturbance is respiratory acidosis.

Step 3 Calculate the AG.

The AG is 10, which is normal.

Step 4 Identify the cause of the primary disorder.

The cause for this patient's respiratory acidosis is COPD.

Step 5 Calculate the expected compensation.

The compensation for respiratory acidosis is renal reabsorption of HCO_3^-. From Table 27.7, the patient has a primary chronic rather than acute respiratory acidosis.

Step 9 Determine the appropriate treatment.

The immediate treatment is administration of oxygen by nasal cannula and subsequent correction of the precipitating factor.

Case 5 A 51-year-old man is admitted for painless mass in right temporal area for a 3-week period. The only complaint he had was poor appetite with 4 lb weight loss. He has no history of any other chronic disease and was not on any medications. He has not seen a physician in 10 years. Admitting electrolyte and ABG values:

Na^+ = 124 mEq/L	pH = 7.39
K^+ = 3.9 mEq/L	pCO_2 = 39 mmHg
Cl^- = 100 mEq/L	pO_2 = 94 mmHg
HCO_3^- = 23 mEq/L	HCO_3^- = 22 mEq/L
Creatinine = 1.0 mg/dL	
BUN = 16 mg/dL	
Glucose = 102 mg/dL	
Serum osmolality = 284 mOsm/kg H_2O	

Question 1 What is the most clinically evident abnormality in the assessment of acid–base disturbance in this patient?

Answer Calculation of AG is extremely important in this patient. From the electrolytes, it is obvious that the AG is only 1. This is abnormal that warrants further evaluation. Hyponatremia does not lower AG to this extent.

Question 2 What other test is helpful in the analysis of low AG?

Answer Serum albumin is the most common cause of low AG in hospitalized and also in ambulatory patients. Serum albumin level came back as 4.5 g/dL. Therefore, hypoalbuminemia is not the cause for his low AG.

Question 3 What other lab test is pertinent in view of hyponatremia and normal serum osmolality?

Answer Ordering serum total protein is very important at this time. His total protein is 14.2 g/dL, which is elevated.

Serum and urine protein immunoelectrophoresis showed very high IgG levels, suggesting IgG multiple myeloma.

Question 4 How does IgG myeloma cause low AG?

Answer IgG molecules carry a positive charge at pH of 7.4 and thus an increase in unmeasured cations. From Table 27.4, it is evident that an increase in unmeasured cations causes low AG.

Suggested Reading

1. Abelow B. Understanding acid-base. Baltimore: Williams & Wilkins; 1997.
2. Adrogué HJ, Gennari JF, Galla JH, et al. Assessing acid–base disorders. Kidney Int. 2009;76:1239–47.
3. DuBose TD. Disorders of acid-base balance. In: Skorecki K, et al., editors. Brenner & Rector's the kidney. 10th ed. Philadelphia: Elsevier; 2016. p. 511–58.
4. Emmett M. Approach to the patient with a negative anion gap. Am J Kidney Dis. 2016;67:143–50.
5. Gennari JF, Adrogué HJ, Galla JH, Madias NE, editors. Acid-base disorders and their treatment. Boca Raton: Taylor & Francis; 2005.
6. Kamel KS, Halperin ML. Fluid, electrolyte, and acid-base physiology. A problem-based approach. 5th ed. Philadelphia: Elsevier; 2017.
7. Kraut JA, Madias NE. Serum anion gap: its uses and limitations in clinical medicine. Clin J Am Soc Med. 2007;2:162–74.
8. Kurtz I. Acid-base case studies. 2nd ed. Victoria: Trafford Publishing; 2006.

High Anion Gap Metabolic Acidosis

28

In the previous chapter, we presented various causes of high anion gap (AG) metabolic acidosis. For discussion purpose, these causes can be conveniently divided into the following categories:

1. *Acidosis due to kidney injury*
   Acute kidney injury
   Chronic kidney disease (CKD) stages 4–5
2. *Acidosis due to accumulation of organic acids*
   L-Lactic acidosis
   D-Lactic acidosis
   Diabetic ketoacidosis
   Alcoholic ketoacidosis
   Starvation ketoacidosis
3. *Acidosis due to toxins*
   Methanol
   Ethylene glycol
   Propylene glycol
   Isopropyl alcohol
   Salicylates
   5-Oxoproline (pyroglutamic acid)
   Paraldehyde

All of the above acidoses except for acidosis due to CKD stages 4 and 5 are acute in nature, whereas acidosis of CKD is chronic in nature. Acute metabolic acidosis develops in hours to days, moderate to severe in nature, and improves with appropriate therapy. Except for acute hemodynamic instability (see "Clinical Manifestations"), survivors do not experience any long-term complications. On the other hand, patients with chronic metabolic acidosis experience bone disease, muscle weakness, progression of kidney disease, and electrolyte abnormalities. Alkali therapy improves many of these complications.

© Springer Science+Business Media LLC 2018
A.S. Reddi, *Fluid, Electrolyte and Acid-Base Disorders*,
DOI 10.1007/978-3-319-60167-0_28

Clinical Manifestations of Metabolic Acidosis

Metabolic acidosis affects almost all organ systems; however, following are the most important clinical manifestations:

Cardiovascular
  Increased heart rate and contractility at pH <7.2
  Decreased contractility at pH <7.1
  Decreased cardiac responsiveness to catecholamines
  Decreased renal and hepatic blood flow
  Decreased fibrillation threshold
  Increased peripheral vasodilation and hypotension
Neurologic
  Increased sympathetic stimulation
  Altered mental status
  Increased cerebral blood flow
  Decreased cerebral metabolism
Respiratory
  Increased minute ventilation
  Dyspnea
  Decreased diaphragmatic contractility
Other
  Inhibition of anaerobic metabolism
  Increased protein catabolism
  Increased metabolic rate
  Impaired phagocytosis
  Decreased ATP production
  Impaired skeletal growth
  Bone pain

Let us briefly review each of these high AG metabolic acidoses.

Acidosis Due to Kidney Injury

Acute Kidney Injury (AKI)

- AKI other than prerenal azotemia usually causes high AG metabolic acidosis.
- Positive H^+ balance due to decreased excretion of H^+ and accumulation of sulfate and phosphate account for high AG metabolic acidosis.

Treatment If serum $[HCO_3^-]$ is <10 mEq/L, administration of $NaHCO_3$ improves blood pH. Patients not in congestive heart failure (CHF) will tolerate $NaHCO_3$ well. Otherwise renal replacement therapy improves acidosis.

Chronic Kidney Disease Stages 4–5

- High AG metabolic acidosis develops only if GFR is < 15 mL/min.
- Serum $[HCO_3^-]$ does not fall <16 mEq/L in patients with GFR < 10 mL/min because of bone buffering.
- Possible causes of high AG acidosis include:
  1. Decreased NH_4^+ excretion and production by the failing kidney (GFR < 10 mL/min) with positive H^+ balance.
  2. Decreased synthesis of NH_4^+ by hyperkalemia.
  3. Decreased conservation of HCO_3^- by the failing kidney.
  4. Titratable acid (phosphate) excretion may be normal or slightly decreased.
  5. Increased production of anions (sulfate, phosphate).
  6. Increased catabolism in some malnourished patients generating sulfate and phosphate.
  7. Relative hypoaldosteronisms due to diabetes, hypertension, interstitial disease, or drugs, such as ACE-Is, angiotensin receptor blockers, K^+-sparing diuretics, and NSAIDs, may aggravate high AG acidosis by lowering GFR even further.

Treatment Includes protein restriction, $NaHCO_3$, sodium citrate, calcium carbonate, or renal replacement therapy, if indicated.

- In CKD patients, serum $[HCO_3^-]$ should be maintained ≥ 22 mEq/L.

Acidosis Due to Accumulation of Organic Acids

ʟ-Lactic Acidosis

Production
- Lactic acidosis occurs whenever production of lactate exceeds its utilization.
- Lactic acid is formed from pyruvate in the process of glycolysis. The reaction is catalyzed by lactate dehydrogenase (LDH) in the presence of NADH. NADH/NAD^+ ratio determines the conversions between pyruvate and lactate. The normal lactate-to-pyruvate ratio is 10:1.

$$\text{Pyruvate} + \text{NADH} + H^+ \underset{\text{LDH}}{\overset{}{\rightleftharpoons}} \text{Lactate} + NAD^+$$

From the above reaction, excess lactate production can be expected by the following pathophysiologic processes:

1. Increased pyruvate production caused by intravenous (IV) glucose or epinephrine infusion and metabolic or respiratory alkalosis

2. An increase in NADH/NAD⁺ ratio due to hypoxic conditions
3. Combination of above two processes

Causes

- Excess lactic acid production occurs in certain situations, as shown in Tables 28.1 and 28.2.
- Lactic acidosis is divided into two types: type A and type B acidosis.
- Type A acidosis results from generalized or regional tissue hypoxia.
- Type B acidosis results from biochemical abnormalities due to systemic diseases or toxins.
- Note that both type A and type B conditions can be superimposed on one another rather commonly in any patient (metformin use in CHF patient).

Lactic Acidosis Due to Hereditary or Acquired Enzymatic Defects

- Lactic acidosis can occur due to a variety of inherited defects in enzymes involved in glycogen storage diseases, gluconeogenesis, citric acid cycle (pyruvate oxidation), and electron transport (complex I deficiency; complex I, III, and IV deficiency; and complex I and IV deficiency). These are inborn errors associated with "primary" lactic acidosis.
- Disorders associated with "secondary" lactic acidosis include organic acidurias (propionic acidemia, methylmalonic acidemia, etc.), defects in fatty acid oxidation, and urea cycle enzymes.

Table 28.1 Causes of type A lactic acidosis

Cause	Mechanism(s)
Shock	
Septic shock	Hypotension
Hypovolemic shock	$\downarrow O_2$ delivery, $\uparrow$ glycolysis, $\downarrow$ ATP, $\uparrow$ pyruvate production $\rightarrow \uparrow$ lactic acid production
Cardiogenic shock	$\downarrow O_2$ delivery, $\uparrow$ glycolysis, $\downarrow$ ATP, $\uparrow$ pyruvate production $\rightarrow \uparrow$ lactic acid production
Hemorrhagic	$\downarrow O_2$ delivery, $\uparrow$ glycolysis, $\downarrow$ ATP, $\uparrow$ pyruvate production $\rightarrow \uparrow$ lactic acid production
Severe tissue hypoxia	$\downarrow O_2$ delivery, $\uparrow$ glycolysis, $\downarrow$ ATP, $\uparrow$ pyruvate production $\rightarrow \uparrow$ lactic acid production
Severe regional hypoperfusion due to hypotension	$\downarrow O_2$ delivery, $\uparrow$ glycolysis, $\downarrow$ ATP, $\uparrow$ pyruvate production $\rightarrow \uparrow$ lactic acid production
Severe anemia (<4.0 g/dL)	Tissue hypoxia
Severe asthma	Respiratory alkalosis stimulation of glycolysis and lactate production, tissue hypoxia, β-adrenergic stimulation, and lactate production
Carbon monoxide poisoning	Carbon monoxide binds more avidly to Hb than O_2, leading to less delivery to tissues and hypoxia, inhibition of electron transport system, $\downarrow$ ATP, $\uparrow$ anaerobic glycolysis

Table 28.2 Causes of type B lactic acidosis

Causes	Mechanism(s)
Liver disease	↓ Lactate metabolism, ↓ pyruvate dehydrogenase complex (PDC)[a] activity, respiratory alkalosis, and hypoglycemia may precipitate lactate production
Diabetes mellitus	Presence of microvascular disease and atherosclerosis compromising circulation, drug use such as metformin, ↓ PDC activity
Renal failure and renal replacement therapies	Stimulation of lactate production by alkalinization due to HCO_3^-, dialysate baths containing lactate
Malignancy	Lymphomas, leukemias, and carcinomas (breast, lung, colon, pancreas), production of lactate by tumor cells via ↑ anaerobic glycolysis, ↑ cytokine production, hypoxia-inducible factor
ATP depletion	↑ Anaerobic glycolysis
Thiamine deficiency	Inhibits PDC activity, thereby limiting glucose metabolism to glycolysis only
Seizures	Increased muscle activity, compromised blood flow, and tissue hypoxia
Hypoglycemia	Inhibits lactate uptake by the liver, ↑ epinephrine release causing increased production of pyruvate
Drugs/toxins	
Metformin	Promotes lactate production from glucose in the small intestine, ↑ NADH/NAD⁺ ratio, inhibits gluconeogenesis from lactate, inhibition of mitochondrial respiration, patients with renal, hepatic, and cardiac failure are at risk
Ethanol	Impairs gluconeogenesis from lactate to glucose, depletes NAD⁺ favoring lactate accumulation
Methanol	Toxic products of methanol (formaldehyde, formic acid) inhibits oxidative phosphorylation and ATP synthesis
Ethylene glycol	↑ NADH/NAD⁺ ratio during metabolism of ethylene glycol via alcohol dehydrogenase
Propylene glycol	Used as solvent (during infusion of lorazepam, nitroglycerine, or topical application of silver sulfadiazine), produces lactate during its metabolism via alcohol dehydrogenase. This reaction produces high NADH/NAD⁺ ratio
Salicylates	Respiratory alkalosis-stimulated lactate production, inhibition of oxidative phosphorylation
Cyanide poisoning	Inhibition of oxidative phosphorylation, ↓ ATP production, ↑ glycolysis, ↑ NADH/NAD⁺ ratio, leading to pyruvate conversion to lactate production
Catecholamines	Epinephrine increases glycolysis and inhibits pyruvate formation from lactate. Increased vasoconstriction of the skin, skeletal muscle, and splanchnic circulation with high concentrations of epinephrine and norepinephrine. Lactic acidosis may be the initial finding in pheochromocytoma
Cocaine	Increased vasoconstriction
Antiretrovirals (didanosine, zidovudine, stavudine, zalcitabine, tenofovir)	Inhibition of mitochondrial DNA synthesis, ↓ ATP production, ↑ glycolysis

(continued)

Table 28.2 (continued)

Causes	Mechanism(s)
Linezolid	Mitochondrial toxicity
Propofol	Sedative, increased production of lactate on high doses due to uncoupling of oxidative phosphorylation

[a]Pyruvate dehydrogenase complex is an enzymatic system that converts pyruvate to acetyl CoA in the mitochondria and hence to CO_2 and H_2O via citric acid cycle

- Acquired enzyme defects are related to thiamine deficiency (↓ pyruvate dehydrogenase complex activity) and biotin deficiency (↓ pyruvate decarboxylase activity).
- Infants and children are affected the most from inherited defects of enzymes.
- Clinical assessment of skeletal muscle, heart, and hepatic and neurologic functions helps in assessing the enzyme defect.
- Lactate measurement in plasma and CSF and enzyme determinations in cultured fibroblasts, lymphocytes, and muscle biopsies will help in making the final diagnosis.
- Treatment is generally unsatisfactory. Therapies that enhance lactate metabolism are of some help.

Diagnosis
- No unique clinical symptoms and signs can be attributable to lactic acidosis.
- Instead, conditions such as shock and other tissue hypoxic conditions with high AG (>25–30) metabolic acidosis should suggest the presence of lactic acidosis.
- Lactate levels 5–10 mmol/L may not give a high AG acidosis at onset of hypoxic condition, but follow-up lactate levels are indicated.
- $\Delta AG/\Delta HCO_3^-$ of 1.6 is suggestive of lactic acidosis, because lactate anions are buffered by non-HCO_3^- buffers (mostly bone and proteins) sparing HCO_3^-/CO_2 buffer system. Note that this ratio does not always suggest the coexistence of metabolic alkalosis.
- The following laboratory results are unique to lactic acidosis:
  1. Hyperuricemia: lactate competes with urate secretion in the proximal tubule.
  2. Hyperphosphatemia: cellular phosphate efflux due to hypoxia and unreplenished ATP hydrolysis.
  3. Leukocytosis: demargination of white blood cells due to epinephrine release.
  4. Normokalemia: lack of electrical gradient establishment due to lactate permeation into the cell. Therefore, K^+ exit from ICF to ECF does not occur.

Treatment
- Removing or treating the underlying cause improves lactic acidosis. However, it is not that simple to eliminate the cause, particularly in critically ill patients.
- Circulatory support is essential.
- Broad-spectrum antibiotic administration for sepsis is extremely important for SIRS/sepsis syndrome with circulatory support.
- Alkali treatment of metabolic acidosis is important; however, there are several disadvantages with this treatment (Table 28.3).

Table 28.3 Intravenous alkali treatment for metabolic (lactic) acidosis

Alkali	Advantages	Disadvantages
NaHCO$_3$	Rapid effect, inexpensive, easy to administer	Hypertonicity, hypernatremia, ↑ CO$_2$ production, ↑ intracellular acidosis, volume overload, no survival benefit
THAM	No increase in CO$_2$, penetrates cells to buffer intracellular pH, useful in the treatment of mixed metabolic and respiratory acidosis	Respiratory depression, hypoglycemia, hyperkalemia, liver necrosis in children. Avoid in renal failure
Carbicarb	A mixture of 0.33 M Na$_2$CO$_3$ and 0.33 M NaHCO$_3$, less CO$_2$ production	The same as NaHCO$_3$, no clinical benefit and nonavailability

NaHCO$_3$ Requirements
- Decide how much serum [HCO$_3^-$] you need to raise, i.e., ΔHCO$_3^-$.
- Estimate HCO$_3^-$ space as 50% of body weight (kg) in metabolic acidosis. Some authors calculate as 40% (note that HCO$_3^-$ space or deficit increases with an increase in [H$^+$] or a decrease in pH).
- Calculate the amount of NaHCO$_3$ that is needed to raise serum [HCO$_3^-$] to the desired level.

Example

$$\text{Serum}\left[\text{HCO}_3^-\right] = 10\,\text{mEq/L}$$

$$\text{Desired serum}\left[\text{HCO}_3^-\right] = 15\,\text{mEq/L}$$

$$\Delta\text{HCO}_3^- = 5\,\text{mEq/L}$$

$$\text{HCO}_3^-\text{ space in a 70 kg patient} = 70 \times 0.5 = 35\,\text{L}$$

$$\text{Amount of NaHCO}_3\text{ required} = 35 \times 5 = 175\,\text{mEq}$$

- These calculations should be based on an ongoing pathologic process that is causing metabolic acidosis.
- Administer slowly as an isotonic solution at a rate of ~0.1 mEq/kg/min.
- Consider administration of calcium gluconate separately to prevent fall in ionized Ca^{2+} after alkali administration to improve cardiac function.
- Disadvantages of NaHCO$_3$ administration are shown in Table 28.3. However, one important advantage of NaHCO$_3$ administration is that it replaces buffering of lactate by proteins, particularly in the heart and brain. This buffering by NaHCO$_3$ administration restores the functions of proteins in these organs.
- It was also shown that CO$_2$ produced by NaHCO$_3$ administration does not cause intracellular acidosis in those patients with normal lung function compared to those with abnormal lung function.

THAM (Tris-Hydroxymethyl Aminomethane) Requirements
- THAM is an amino alcohol.
- It buffers H$^+$ by virtue of its NH$_3$ moiety in the urine. Therefore, its use is limited only to those with GFR >30 mL/min.
- It does not increase CO$_2$.

- It improves cardiac contractility.
- THAM is given as a 0.3 M solution (300 mEq/L), and its requirements for initial dose are calculated for the above example as:

$$\text{mL of } 0.3\,\text{M solution required}$$
$$=\text{Body weight} \times \text{Base deficit}\left(\Delta HCO_{3^-}\right)70 \times 5 = 350\,\text{mL}$$

- Continue THAM until blood pH >7.20.

Tribonat
- A buffering agent available in Europe.
- It is a mixture of THAM, $NaHCO_3$, acetate, and phosphate.
- It seems to generate less CO_2 and without much effect on intracellular pH.
- Not used in the USA.

Renal Replacement Therapies
- Intermittent hemodialysis is another mode of alkali administration.
- It has been used to avoid $NaHCO_3$-induced hyperosmolality and volume overload.
- Continuous renal replacement therapies [continuous venovenous hemofiltration (CVVH), continuous venovenous hemodialysis (CVVHD), continuous venovenous hemodiafiltration (CVVHDF)] with $NaHCO_3$ replacement fluid was found to be efficacious in improving lactic acidosis (type A) in hemodynamically unstable patients and in type B acidosis due to metformin and other agents.

Thiamine and Riboflavin
- Thiamine is a cofactor for PDC, and activation of PDC may improve lactate levels.
- Riboflavin may provide FAD (flavin adenine dinucleotide), which is required in electron transport system.
- Both of these do not cause any adverse effects, and their use is optional.

Insulin
- Insulin increases the activity of PDC, and its use is beneficial in some patients with mild to moderate hyperglycemia.

Dichloroacetate
- Stimulates PDC and enhances pyruvate oxidation.
- Reduces lactate levels, improves pH, and raises serum $[HCO_3^-]$.
- Despite its beneficial effects on lactic acidemia, there was no survival benefit; therefore, it is not used routinely.
- However, it is effective in some patients with lactic acidosis due to inherited enzyme defects.

Inhibitors of Na/H Exchanger
- In hypoxic conditions with lactic acidosis, there is activation of myocardial Na/H exchanger. As a result, there is accumulation of excess intracellular Na^+ and Ca^{2+},

causing cardiac dysfunction. Inhibitors of Na/H exchanger (sabiporide, caripo-ride) alone or in combination with $NaHCO_3$ improved cardiac function and mortality in animals and one human study. Routine use of these inhibitors awaits further studies.

D-Lactic Acidosis

- D-Lactate is the D-stereoisomer of lactate and not a product of human metabolism.
- Produced by bacteria and ruminants (cows, sheep, goats, etc.).
- In humans, D-lactate is produced by subjects with intestinal bypass surgery for obesity or intestinal resection or patients with chronic pancreatic insufficiency.
- Some patients on prolonged antibiotics may also develop D-lactic acidosis due to overgrowth of gram-positive anaerobes such as D-lactate-producing bacteria (lactobacilli).
- D-Lactate is not detected by the standard method of L-lactate determination.
- Characterized by episodes of neurologic manifestations (confusion, slurred speech, ataxia, memory loss, irritability, or abusiveness), including encephalopathy, and high AG metabolic acidosis with normal L-lactate levels. The neurologic manifestations can last from hours to days.
- High carbohydrate ingestion in subjects with intestinal surgery can precipitate D-lactic acidosis because of large delivery to the colon.
- D-Lactate can be determined by a special technique using D-lactate dehydrogenase.

Treatment Low carbohydrate or starch diet, oral vancomycin, neomycin, or metronidazole.

Diabetic Ketoacidosis (DKA)

- DKA is caused by insulin deficiency and relative glucagon excess.
- DKA presents with a triad of hyperglycemia (glucose >300 mg/dL), ketones in blood and urine, and high AG metabolic acidosis.
- The accumulated ketoacids are acetoacetate and β-hydroxybutyrate (BHB).
- Insulin deficiency promotes lipolysis and fatty acid release, whereas glucagon stimulates the hepatic production of ketoacids from fatty acids.

Diagnosis Diagnosis of DKA is made by high AG metabolic acidosis with documentation of ketones in blood and urine. Volume depletion and many electrolyte abnormalities are commonly associated with DKA.

- The dipstick that is used to detect ketones contains nitroprusside, which reacts strongly (2–4+) with acetoacetate and poorly with BHB (1+). If initial dipstick reaction is 1+ and then 4+ during treatment of DKA, it suggests that severe acidosis initially is due to BHB, and patient's acidosis is improving.
- Use $NaHCO_3$, as previously discussed.
- Follow changes in AG, and adjust the requirement for $NaHCO_3$ administration.

- Changes in AG also indicate the potential HCO_3^- regeneration from ketoacids.
- As AG improves, the HCO_3^- space or deficit decreases.

Treatment Insulin administration and correction of fluids and electrolytes improve high AG acidosis.

- Note that hyperchloremic metabolic acidosis does develop during treatment of DKA in some patients because the regeneration of HCO_3^- from ketones is decreased due to loss of excess ketones in the urine prior to hospitalization.

Alcoholic Ketoacidosis
- Develops following alcohol abstinence as a result of nausea, vomiting, abdominal pain, and possibly starvation.
- Most common in women and diabetics following binge.
- Alcohol withdrawal also precipitates ketoacidosis due to catecholamine release.
- Pathogenesis includes ethanol itself, starvation, insulin deficiency, excess glucagon and catecholamines, and vomiting.
- Ethanol inhibits gluconeogenesis and stimulates lipolysis. It is metabolized to acetaldehyde (catalyzed by alcohol dehydrogenase) and then to acetic acid (catalyzed by aldehyde dehydrogenase). These reactions involve conversion of NAD^+ to NADH, which enhances the production of lactate from pyruvate and BHB from acetoacetate.
- Starvation depletes hepatic glycogen store. Excess glucagon stimulates lipolysis and production of ketoacids from fatty acids.
- Ketoacids are also formed from acetic acid.
- Hypoglycemia is present in some patients.

Treatment Includes fluid replacement with D5W and normal saline, thiamine, and correction of electrolytes.

- Note that hyperchloremic metabolic acidosis develops during the recovery phase of alcoholic ketoacidosis.

Starvation Ketoacidosis
- Starvation ketoacidosis is mild and self-limited.
- Relative decrease in insulin secretion and an increase in glucagon secretion cause ketoacid formation.
- Unlike DKA, the presence of insulin prevents progression of full-blown ketoacidosis.
- Also, insulin secretion is stimulated by ketones and fatty acids during prolonged fasting, thereby minimizing even further the formation of ketoacids.
- Intense ketonuria with a weak serum reaction to nitroprusside test is usually observed in starvation ketosis.

Treatment Resumption of food intake corrects ketoacidosis.

Acidosis Due to Toxins

General Considerations

- Ingestion of alcohols, such as ethanol, methanol, and ethylene glycol, or administration of propylene glycol generates not only hyperosmolality but also metabolic acidosis with high AG. Whenever ingestion of these alcohols is suspected, it is important to measure and calculate serum osmolality to identify osmolal gap.
- *Osmolal gap* is defined as the difference between the measured and calculated serum osmolality. Generally, the measured osmolality is 10 mOsm higher than the calculated osmolality. Values >10 mOsm represent the presence of an osmolal gap.
- Note that in one study, the osmolal gap in healthy volunteers varied from −14 to 10 mOsm, suggesting that >10 is found to be abnormal.
- Elevated osmolal gap suggests the presence of osmotically active substances that are measured, but not included in the calculation of osmolality.
- Lactate and ketoacids also cause high osmolal gap.
- Traditionally, the presence of an osmolal gap and an elevated anion gap is considered to represent the ingestion of toxic alcohols such as methanol, ethylene glycol, and others (Table 28.4) This table shows the number of mOsm contributed by 100 mg/dL of each substance present in the serum.
- Metabolism: the first step in the metabolism of all toxic alcohols is catalyzed by the enzyme alcohol dehydrogenase (ADH), which is the most critical step in metabolism.
- Administration of an antidote to inhibit the enzyme ADH prevents the toxic metabolites of the parent alcohol. Table 28.5 shows metabolic end products that cause toxicity.

Let us discuss each one of these alcohols and others in detail.

Methanol

- Common names: methyl alcohol, wood alcohol, wood spirit, and carbinol.
- Sources: antifreeze, additive to gasoline and diesel oil, windshield wiper fluid (most common abuse in the USA), dyes, varnishes, and cheap alcohols.

Table 28.4 Contribution of some toxic substances to serum osmolality

Serum level (100 mg/dL)	Molecular weight	mOsm/L
Ethanol	46	22
Methanol	32	31
Ethylene glycol	62	16
Propylene glycol	76	13
Isopropanol	60	17
Salicylate	180	6
Acetone	58	17
Paraldehyde	132	8

Table 28.5   Toxic metabolites of alcohols and acetylsalicylate (aspirin)

Substance	Toxic metabolite(s)	Comment
Ethanol	Acetoacetic acid, β-hydroxybutyric acid	Commonly seen in alcoholic intoxication, low mortality
Methanol	Formic acid	Blindness and mortality high, if not recognized and treated early
Ethylene glycol	Glycolic acid, oxalic acid	Acute kidney injury, ↓ cardiac contractility, mortality high, if not treated early
Propylene glycol	Lactic acid	Hospital-acquired lactic acidosis, minimal clinical manifestations
Isopropyl alcohol	Acetone	No acidosis, acetone breath, low mortality
Acetylsalicylic acid (aspirin)	Salicylic acid	Respiratory alkalosis and metabolic acidosis in adults, metabolic acidosis in children

- Lethal dose is 30 mL of absolute methanol.
- Easily absorbed from the gastrointestinal (GI) tract. Other less routes of exposure are inhalation and skin absorption.
- Methanol is not itself toxic, but its metabolites, formaldehyde, and formic acid are extremely toxic.
- Half-life of methanol in low dose is 14–24 h, and in higher doses, the half-life is prolonged to 24–30 h.

Clinical Manifestations Mostly due to formic acid (formate)

- Signs and symptoms of methanol intoxication are related to central nervous and GI systems:
  - Lethargy, headache, confusion, and vertigo are common.
  - Eye pain, blurred vision, photophobia, and blindness are common at presentation in 50% of patients.
  - Dilated pupils, constriction of the visual fields, and papilledema are the ophthalmoscopic findings.
  - Nausea, vomiting, pancreatitis, and abdominal pain are common GI complaints.
- Coingestion of ethanol delays the manifestations of methanol intoxication.

Diagnosis
- Serum electrolytes, BUN, creatinine, glucose, serum osmolality, serum Ca^{2+}, Mg^{2+}, ethanol, ethylene glycol, and ketone levels, urine microscopy, and ABG.
- Visual impairment, high osmolal gap, and high AG metabolic acidosis should alert the physician of methanol intoxication and warrants immediate treatment to prevent blindness. High AG is contributed by formic acid, lactic acid, and ketoacids.

Treatment The criteria for the initiation of therapy in patients with known or suspected methanol poisoning are:

Plasma methanol level of ≥ 20 mg/dL

or

Documented recent history of toxic amounts of methanol ingestion and an osmolal gap >10 mOsm/L

or

Suspected methanol ingestion and at least two of the following criteria:

Arterial pH <7.30

Serum [HCO_3^-] <20 mEq/L

Serum osmolal gap > 10 mOsm/L

- Immediate supportive care includes:
  1. Hydration with normal saline, and glucose for hypoglycemia.
  2. Intravenous $NaHCO_3$ to maintain blood pH >7.2.
  3. Intravenous folinic acid (1 mg/kg) one dose and then folate supplementation to accelerate formate metabolism to CO_2 and water by tetrahydrofolate synthetase. This may benefit some alcoholics with folate deficiency
  4. The American Academy of Clinical Toxicology recommendations are:

Fomepizole (4-methylpyrazole), the drug of choice in the USA.

Ethanol, if fomepizole not available.

Fomepizole is a competitive inhibitor of ADH, and the recommended dosages are as follows:

- *Without dialysis*
- Loading dose: 15 mg/kg
- Maintenance dose: 10 mg/kg Q12 h for four doses
- After 48 h or four doses, 15 mg/kg Q12 h until methanol levels are <20 mg/dL
- *With dialysis*
- The same doses as above except that the drug is given 6 h after the first dose and then Q4 h thereafter

Ethanol is a substrate for ADH, and its administration decreases the metabolism of methanol. It has 10–20 times greater affinity for ADH than other alcohols. Ethanol at a serum concentration of 100 mg/dL inhibits completely the enzyme ADH. The recommended dosage is as follows:

Dose	Absolute alcohol	10% IV solution
Loading	600 mg/kg	7.6 mL/kg
Maintenance (nondrinker)	66 mg/kg/h	0.83 mL/kg/h
Maintenance (drinker)	154 mg/kg/h	1.96 mL/kg/h
Maintenance during dialysis (nondrinker)	169 mg/kg/h	2.13 mL/kg/h
Maintenance during dialysis (drinkers)	257 mg/kg/h	3.26 mL/kg/h

Hemodialysis: With the introduction of fomepizole, routine use of hemodialysis has diminished, and it has become an adjunctive therapy. However, hemodialysis is indicated in the following situations:

1. Ethanol-treated patient with methanol level >50 mg/dL
2. Renal dysfunction

Table 28.6 Advantages and disadvantages of antidotes and dialysis

Treatment modality	Advantages	Disadvantages
Fomepizole	High affinity for alcohol dehydrogenase (ADH). Plasma concentration of 0.8 μg/mL inhibits ADH activity	Not immediately available in all clinical facilities
	Effective at low serum concentrations	Expensive ($4,000–5,000)
	Few adverse effects other than slight increases in AST/ALT	Approved only for methanol and ethylene glycol poisoning
	Admission to intensive care units is not always necessary	No oral form available
	No effect on serum osmolal gap	
Ethanol	Easily available	Lower affinity for ADH than fomepizole
	Inexpensive	ICU monitoring required
	Can be given IV or orally	Maintenance of 100 mg/dL necessary to inhibit ADH
		Ethanol intoxication in some patients
		↑ Serum osmolal gap
Dialysis	Highly efficient to remove both primary alcohol and its metabolites	Invasive
	Improves renal function	Expensive
	Improves acidemia with HCO_3^- dialysis bath	Unavailability in many countries
	Decreases hospital stay	
	Rapid improvement in signs and symptoms of methanol poisoning	

3. Visual impairment
4. Severe acidemia

- It is important to understand the advantages and disadvantages of each of these treatment modalities for judicious use in the management of methanol poisoning (Table 28.6).
- Severe acidemia has a prognostic significance. Serum $[HCO_3^-]$ <20 mEq/L carries 10% mortality, whereas $[HCO_3^-]$ <10 mEq/L has the mortality of 50%. Therefore, maintenance of arterial pH >7.2 is important.

Ethylene Glycol (EG)
- Colorless, odorless, and sweet-tasting alcohol.
- Sources: antifreeze, de-icers, and many industrial products.
- EG intoxication is more common than methanol intoxication.
- Oral ingestion of EG is the most common route of EG intoxication.
- EG is metabolized to glycolic and oxalic acids.
- Glycolic acid is the major cause of high AG acidosis.

- Oxalic acid is the major cause of AKI and myocardial, neurologic, and pulmonary dysfunction due to deposition of calcium oxalate in these organ systems.
- Lethal dose of EG is 1.4 mL/kg.

Clinical Manifestations (Classified into Three Stages)
Stage 1 (0.5–12 h after ingestion): Transient inebriation and euphoria with progression to cerebral edema and coma.

Stage 2 (12–24 h after ingestion): Tachycardia and hypertension, severe metabolic acidosis. ARDS may develop. Most deaths occur during this stage.

Stage 3 (24–72 h after ingestion): Oliguria, anuria, and severe renal dysfunction, requiring hemodialysis.

Note that neurologic, cardiopulmonary, and renal abnormalities can present at the time of admission in some patients.

Coingestion of ethanol delays the manifestations of methanol intoxication.

Diagnosis
- Serum electrolytes, BUN, creatinine, glucose, serum osmolality, serum Ca^{2+}, Mg^{2+}, ethanol, EG, ketones, lactate, urine microscopy, and ABG.
- Severe high AG metabolic acidosis, increased osmolal gap, and, at times, the presence of oxalate crystals in the urine are suggestive of EG intoxication.
- Note that osmolal gap is not always present because of small contribution of osmoles by EG compared to other alcohols and also the absence of glycolic acid due to rapid conversion to oxalic acid.
- Hypocalcemia may be present.
- High AG and high osmolal gap are associated with high mortality.

Treatment The criteria for the initiation of therapy in patients with known or suspected EG poisoning are:

Plasma EG level of ≥20 mg/dL
or
Documented recent history of toxic amounts of EG ingestion and an osmolal gap >10 mOsm/L
or
Suspected EG ingestion and at least two of the following criteria:
Arterial pH <7.30
Serum $[HCO_3^-]$ <20 mEq/L
Serum osmolal gap > 10 mOsm/L
Presence of oxalate crystals in urine

The treatment guidelines for EG ingestion are shown in Table 28.7 [1].

Propylene Glycol (PG)
- PG is used as a diluent in IV and oral drugs, including phenytoin, diazepam, lorazepam, phenobarbital, nitroglycerine, hydralazine, and trimethoprim–sulfamethoxazole.

Table 28.7 Treatment guidelines for EG ingestion

Treatment	Indications
Supportive care	Volume depletion and hypoglycemia: correct volume deficit with normal saline and D5W to improve glucose levels
	NaHCO$_3$, if pH <7.20
	Pyridoxine and thiamine, particularly in alcoholics, to expedite glyoxylate metabolism
	Follow serum EG levels, Ca^{2+}, creatinine, lactate, and ABG
	Ingestion of multiple substances with depressed level of consciousness
Fomepizole	Altered mental status
	Inadequate ICU staffing or laboratory support to monitor ethanol administration
	Relative contraindication to ethanol (liver disease)
	Critically ill patient with high AG metabolic acidosis of unknown etiology and potential exposure to EG
Ethanol	Unavailability of fomepizole
Hemodialysis	Severe metabolic acidosis refractory to fomepizole and ethanol or NaHCO$_3$
	Anuria
	Renal failure

- Most of the cases of PG intoxications are from IV administration of drugs.
- Toxicity of PG occurs at blood concentrations >100 mg/dL.
- Patients with liver and kidney dysfunction are at risk for PG toxicity.

Clinical Manifestations Include disorientation, depression, nystagmus, ataxia, hypotension, and cardiac arrhythmias.

Diagnosis
- Metabolic acidosis with high AG due to lactic acid (both L- and D-forms). Renal failure occurs in some patients.

Treatment Includes discontinuation of the offending agent. Hemodialysis helps in correcting renal failure and lowering PG levels.

Isopropyl Alcohol
- Usually called rubbing alcohol
- Sources: rubbing alcohol, cleaning agents, de-icer, and industrial solvents
- Route of exposure: skin and GI tract absorption as well as inhalation by lungs
- Metabolized to acetone by ADH

Clinical Manifestations Depend on serum levels of isopropanol: levels >150 mg/dL are associated with hypotension and coma, and levels >400 mg/dL carry poor prognosis.

Diagnosis
- High serum osmolality with large osmolal gap and normal acid–base disorder are common findings in subjects with isopropyl alcohol intoxication.

- Acetone breath and positive serum and urine nitroprusside reaction usually mislead to the diagnosis of diabetic ketoacidosis. Only serum glucose levels differentiate between these two conditions.
- If high AG metabolic acidosis is present, suspect lactic acidosis due to hypotension.

Treatment Supportive care, as the intoxication is self-limited. Hemodialysis is indicated in subjects with serum levels >200 mg/dL and hypotension.

Salicylate Intoxication

- Aspirin (acetylsalicylic acid or ASA) is the most commonly used salicylate.
- Exposure is topical and oral forms. ASA is readily absorbed in the GI tract, and salicylate is responsible for systemic toxic effects.
- Intake of ASA is usually accidental in children and suicidal or intentional in adults.
- Serum half-life of salicylate is 2–4 h at low doses, approximately 12 h with therapeutic doses, and can be prolonged to 15–30 h or more with toxic doses.
- Two to 30% of salicylate is excreted unchanged in the urine, with less renal excretion occurring in acidic urine or in patients with renal failure.
- Metabolic effects are:
  1. Uncoupling of oxidative phosphorylation and decreased ATP production.
  2. Inhibition of conversion of α-ketoglutarate to succinate and succinate to fumarate, resulting in lipolysis, ketone formation, and stimulation of glycolysis.
  3. Acid–base disorder in adults: Initially respiratory alkalosis due to stimulation of medullary respiratory center by salicylate and hyperventilation. Subsequently, metabolic acidosis develops due to lactic acid and ketoacid production. Respiratory alkalosis seems to be the main reason for lactic acid production.
  4. In children, metabolic acidosis predominates initially.
  5. Urate excretion is low with low doses of salicylate and high with high doses of salicylate.

Clinical Manifestations Depend on acute or chronic ingestion of ASA.

Acute Manifestations Nausea, vomiting, abdominal pain, hematemesis, tachypnea, tinnitus, deafness, lethargy, confusion, coma, and seizures.

Chronic Manifestations Occur mostly in elderly patients with chronic use of ASA. Most of the manifestations are similar to those of acute intoxication except for GI symptoms. Patients appear ill, and neurologic symptoms are more prominent, including agitation, confusion, slurred speech, coma, and seizures.

Diagnosis

- History is extremely important, if it can be obtained. Type of salicylate, amount ingested, time of ingestion, long-term use, use of other medications, and history of renal, hepatic, cardiac, and psychiatric diseases should help therapeutic decision.
- Fever is common in children.

- Serum electrolytes, BUN, creatinine, glucose, Ca^{2+}, lactate, and ketones should be obtained.
- ABG: Respiratory alkalosis with AG metabolic acidosis with hyperventilation and tinnitus should suggest the diagnosis of salicylate poisoning.
- Urine pH is important, as acid pH increases salicylate toxicity.
- Serial serum salicylate levels are extremely important for therapeutic consideration.
- Obtain chest X-ray for edema and EKG for arrhythmias.

Treatment Four goals for symptomatic acute or chronic toxicity, as there are no antidotes:

1. Supportive care
2. Reduce GI absorption of salicylate
3. Promote renal excretion of salicylate
4. Lowering plasma levels of salicylate by hemodialysis

- *Supportive care*: Should start in the emergency department for the following:
  - Endotracheal intubation for protection of airways, hypoxia, and continuation of hyperventilation to prevent further drop in pH
  - Correction of volume deficit and electrolyte abnormalities to maintain hemodynamic stability
- *Reduce GI absorption of salicylate*: Use oral activated charcoal at 1 g/kg to a maximum of 50 g in children and 100 g in adults. The minimum dose is 30 g. Repeat the dose of charcoal. The use of sorbitol with charcoal is advocated in adults by some physicians. The use of ipecac is controversial.
- *Promote renal excretion of salicylate*: Adequate fluid administration and alkalinization of urine promote the excretion of salicylic acid. Acidosis promotes tissue transfer of salicylate, particularly into the brain, and alkalinization prevents tissue penetration. One way to alkalinize the body fluids and urine is to give 1.5 L of 150 mEq/L of $NaHCO_3$ solution over 4 h. Blood pH should be followed with serum K^+ and Ca^{2+}. Continue urinary alkalinization until serum salicylate levels drop to therapeutic range (30 mg/dL).
- *Lowering plasma levels of salicylate by hemodialysis*: Hemodialysis is indicated for serum salicylate levels >120 mg/dL, refractory acidosis, fluid overload, renal failure, noncardiogenic pulmonary edema, coma, and seizures. Hemoperfusion is efficient in removing salicylate, but may not be that effective in correcting renal failure or fluid overload or severe acidosis. Peritoneal dialysis is not effective. Hemodialysis is also effective in symptomatic patient with chronic overdose and salicylate levels exceed 60–80 mg/dL.

5-Oxoproline (Pyroglutamic Acid)

- Pyroglutamic acid is a degradative product of reduced glutathione (GSH), and its accumulation in blood causes high AG metabolic acidosis (Fig. 28.1).
- The synthesis and degradation of glutathione occurs by reactions of the γ-glutamyl cycle.

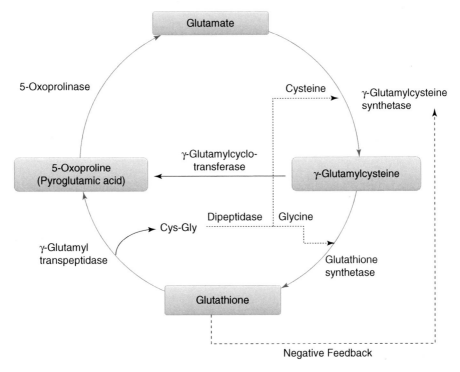

Fig. 28.1 Simplified γ-glutamyl cycle

- Glutathione is a tripeptide, consisting of glutamate, cysteine, and glycine (usually written as L-γ-glutamyl-L-cysteinylglycine). The synthesis and degradation of glutathione involves six enzymes: two enzymes for synthesis (γ-glutamylcysteine synthetase and glutathione synthetase) and four enzymes for degradation (γ-glutamyl transpeptidase, γ-glutamylcyclotransferase, 5-oxoprolinase, and dipeptidase), as shown in Fig. 28.1.
- GSH is found in most cells in high (millimolar) concentrations. It has several functions, including amino acid transport and maintenance of thiol/disulfide balance.
- Under normal circumstances, glutathione inhibits γ-glutamylcysteine synthetase so that excess production of γ-glutamylcysteine is prevented. When glutathione levels decrease, the feedback inhibition is relieved, resulting in accumulation of γ-glutamylcysteine and conversion to pyroglutamic acid by the enzyme γ-glutamylcyclotransferase (Fig. 28.1).
- Elevated levels of pyroglutamic acid in blood cause high AG metabolic acidosis. Initially, pyroglutamic acidemia was described in infants with inherited deficiencies of glutathione synthetase and 5-oxoprolinase.
- These inherited enzyme deficiencies are rather rare, but acquired pyroglutamic acidemia and aciduria have been reported in adults in several clinical settings.
- Clinical conditions associated with pyroglutamic acidosis are sepsis, malnutrition, pregnancy, vegetarian, and modified diets.

- Drugs that cause pyroglutamic acidosis include acetaminophen (paracetamol), vigabatrin, an antiepileptic drug, monosodium glutamate, and antibiotics such as flucloxacillin or netilmicin.
- The common underlying mechanism for pyroglutamic acidemia and aciduria is depletion of tissue glutathione. However, vigabatrin and flucloxacillin seem to inhibit the enzyme 5-oxoprolinase.

Diagnosis
- History of drugs and antibiotics is very important. Chronic clinical conditions, such as rheumatoid arthritis, disc diseases, trauma, neuropathies, and surgeries, can give a clue of pain medication and antibiotic use.
- Unexplained AG metabolic acidosis, like D-lactic acidosis, may be a clue to the diagnosis of pyroglutamic acidosis. Osmolal gap is normal.

Treatment Includes discontinuation of the offending agent. Hemodialysis is needed to improve refractory acidosis and renal failure. N-acetylcysteine (NAC) can provide cysteine to replenish glutathione levels. It is, therefore, suggested that NAC may improve pyroglutamic acidemia.

Toluene
- Other names: methylbenzene or phenylmethane.
- Sources: acrylic paints, varnishes, paint thinners, glues, adhesives, shoe polish, gasoline, transmission fluid, and industrial solvents.
- Poisoning occurs by inhalation to induce euphoria.
- Children and adolescents are common users with male predominance.
- Levels of 200 PPM (parts per million) are dangerous.
- Metabolized to benzyl alcohol, then to benzoic acid, and finally to hippuric acid (hippurate).
- Hippurate is rapidly excreted by the kidneys, if renal function is normal.
- Because of this rapid excretion, hippurate levels are normal at the time of evaluation.

Clinical Manifestations
- Primarily CNS effects, such as euphoria, confusion, dizziness, stupor, and coma. Bronchospasm is common.
- Chronic abuse leads to neuropsychosis, ataxia, optic and peripheral neuropathies, blindness, and decreased cognitive ability.

Diagnosis
- High AG metabolic acidosis is common when serum hippurate levels are high; otherwise, hyperchloremic metabolic acidosis with severe hypokalemia is the common presentation, and serum hippurate levels are normal.
- Hyperchloremic metabolic acidosis and hypokalemia are thought to be due to distal renal tubular acidosis. Some patients also develop Fanconi syndrome.
- Acute kidney injury is also common, which is due to hypotension and/or rhabdomyolysis.

Treatment Includes supportive care and volume expansion with KCl supplementation. There is no antidote. Hemodialysis is recommended for severe renal failure.

Paraldehyde

- Used as a sedative and also for treatment of delirium tremens.
- It is replaced by many other drugs for delirium tremens, so cases of paraldehyde intoxication are rare.
- Metabolized to probably acetaldehyde and acetic acid, causing a high AG metabolic acidosis.
- No osmolal gap is seen.

Treatment Removal of the drug and supportive care.

Study Questions

Case 1 A 54-year-old woman was admitted through the emergency department (ED) for shortness of breath, "unwell" feeling, and weakness of few days duration. Her blood pressure was 114/51 mmHg with a pulse rate of 69 beats per minute. She was afebrile. Her medical history is significant for cervical and lumbosacral disc disease, hypertension, depression, anxiety, ataxia, and chronic pulmonary obstructive disease. She had carpal tunnel and cervical disc surgery, cholecystectomy, and hysterectomy. Her medications included combivent (ipratropium bromide 18 µg and albuterol 90 µg) one puff every 8 h, metoprolol 12.5 mg twice daily, klonopin (clonazepam) 0.5 mg every 8 h, as needed, and vicodin ES (hydrocodone bitartrate 7.5 mg and acetaminophen 750 mg) every 8 h, as needed. The patient was previously admitted with similar complaints and found to have a high AG metabolic acidosis and acute kidney injury, requiring short-term hemodialysis.

Laboratory results are shown in the following table. Hemoglobin was 13.4 g % and a platelet count of 430,000. Serum glucose was 80 mg/dL. ABG: pH of 7.20, pCO_2 15 mmHg, pO_2 91 mmHg, and calculated HCO_3^- of 6 mEq/L. The AG was 16. Other pertinent laboratory results are normal. Serum osmolality was 293 mOsm/L. Serum ketones and lactate were negative, and urinalysis was normal.

Hospital day	Na$^+$ (mEq/L)	K$^+$ (mEq/L)	Cl$^-$ (mEq/L)	HCO$_3^-$ (mEq/L)	Creatinine (mg/dL)	BUN (mg/dL)	AG (mEq/L)	Albumin (g/dL)	pH
Admission	138	4.6	114	8	0.87	10	16	4.4	7.20
Day 2	143	4.8	119	11	0.59	11	13	3.9	7.31
Day 3	141	3.6	109	18	0.55	9	14	3.4	
Day 4	142	3.2	107	25	0.48	8	10	3.3	
Day 5	140	4.1	100	33	0.55	8	7	3.6	

Question 1 Characterize the acid–base disorder in ED.

Answer Based on pH and pCO_2 and serum [HCO_3^-], the acid–base disorder is high AG metabolic acidosis and respiratory alkalosis.

Question 2 Is calculation of osmolal gap important?

Answer Yes. In this patient, the osmolal gap is 6 mOsm/L. Therefore, methanol, ethylene glycol, ketoacidosis, and lactic acidosis (lactate levels are normal) can be excluded.

Question 3 Is aspirin overdose possible in this patient?

Answer Yes. However, the initial acid–base disorder in aspirin overdose is respiratory alkalosis followed by the development of high AG metabolic acidosis. In this patient, serum salicylate levels were normal, excluding the diagnosis of aspirin overdose.

Question 4 How does this acid–base disorder differ from that of toluene inhalation?

Answer Toluene inhalation causes a transient high AG metabolic acidosis and then hyperchloremic (non-AG) metabolic acidosis. In this patient, a slight increase in AG existed until the third day of admission, excluding the possibility of toluene inhalation. Also, the patient did not have any clinical manifestations of toluene inhalation or ingestion.

Question 5 What other laboratory test you order at this time based on her medications?

Answer She is on high doses of acetaminophen (750 mg Q8 h); ordering urinary pyroglutamic acid is appropriate.

Question 6 What is the diagnosis of her high AG metabolic acidosis with normal osmolal gap?

Answer Her urinary pyroglutamic acid level was >11,500 mmol/mol creatinine (reference range 0–100 mmol/mol creatinine). Also, acetaminophen and its metabolites were present. Therefore, the diagnosis was pyroglutamic acidosis due to daily high doses of acetaminophen (Tylenol) use. Tylenol depletes GSH, which promotes pyroglutamic acid production. She was started on fentanyl patch, and her serum [HCO_3^-] has been normal.

Case 2 A 40-year-old woman with history of short-bowel surgery is seen for slurred speech, confusion, weakness, impaired motor coordination, and irritability. She likes ice cream and develops mild neurologic problems following large quantities of ice cream. She is not on any medications or special diets. ABG: pH 7.27, pCO_2 24 mmHg, and calculated HCO_3^- 16 mEq/L. Urine ketones are negative. Serum lactate levels are 1.5 mmol/L. Serum creatinine is normal. The anion gap is 20, but osmolal gap is normal.

Which one of the following is the MOST likely cause of acid–base disturbance in this patient?

(A) L-Lactic acid
(B) Pyroglutamic acid
(C) D-Lactic acid
(D) Methanol
(E) Topiramate

The answer is C Except for topiramate, all other causes generate high AG metabolic acidosis. Topiramate causes non-AG metabolic acidosis due to inhibition of carbonic anhydrase. Serum lactate is normal; therefore, lactic acidosis is excluded. Also, methanol intoxication is excluded based on normal osmolal gap. There is no history of medication (Tylenol or Tylenol-containing narcotics) or antibiotic use. Therefore, pyroglutamic acidosis is ruled out. Based on the surgical history, high carbohydrate intake, and neurologic manifestations, the most likely diagnosis is D-lactic acidosis. Thus, option C is correct.

Case 3 A 17-year-old female student is admitted for confusion and acute kidney injury. She is able to give some history that she had a fight with her boyfriend 2 days ago, and she drank some liquid that was in their garage. She has no other significant medical or illicit drug history. In the ED, her vital signs are stable. Other than altered mental status and confusion, her physical examination is normal. She weighs 60 kg. Laboratory results are as follows:

Serum	Urine
Na^+ = 141 mEq/L	Osmolality = 320 mOsm/kg H_2O
K^+ = 4.2 mEq/L	pH = 5.2
Cl^- = 110 mEq/L	Protein = trace
HCO_3^- = 7 mEq/L	Blood = negative
BUN = 28 mg/dL	Urine sediment = envelope-like crystals
Creatinine = 1.8 mg/dL	
Glucose = 72 mg/dL	
Serum osmolality = 312 mOsm/kg H_2O	
ABG = pH 7.21, pCO_2 17 mmHg, pO_2 94 mmHg, calculated HCO_3^- 6 mEq/L	

Question 1 Characterize the acid–base disorder.

Answer High AG metabolic acidosis with respiratory alkalosis.

Question 2 What is her osmolal gap?

Answer Osmolal gap is the difference between measured serum osmolality and calculated serum osmolality. Therefore, her osmolal gap is 16 (312–296 = 16 mOsm), which is high.

Question 3 What is your diagnosis of this acid–base disorder?

Answer The presence of calcium oxalate crystals (envelope-like) in the urine sediment is the clue for her acid–base disturbance, which is ethylene glycol ingestion. One of the final products of ethylene glycol is oxalic acid, which is excreted as oxalate.

Question 4 What is your initial management?

Answer Antidote for ethylene glycol is fomepizole. The initial dose is 15 mg/kg followed by 10 mg/kg every 12 h for 4 doses. Continue fomepizole, if ethylene glycol levels are not below 20 mg/dL. At the same time, hydration with D5W and three ampules (150 mEq) of $NaHCO_3$ to run at 120 mL/h to improve volume status should be started.

Question 5 Is dialysis needed in this patient?

Answer Yes, if no improvement in renal function and metabolic acidosis following adequate hydration and administration of fomepizole and $NaHCO_3$ (see Table 28.7 for indications of dialysis).

Case 4 A 55-year-old man with chronic alcoholism presents to the ED with agitation, blurred vision, and eye pain. Blood pressure and pulse rate are normal. He is afebrile. He has a high AG metabolic acidosis with an osmolal gap of 26 mOsm/L.
     Which one of the following toxic alcohol ingestions is the MOST likely cause of his symptoms?

(A) Ethanol
(B) Ethylene glycol
(C) Methanol
(D) Toluene
(E) Isopropyl alcohol

The answer is C Only formic acid formed from methanol is toxic to the optic nerve, causing visual impairment, blurred vision, eye pain, and blindness. Therefore, early institution of fomepizole is recommended to inhibit ADH and conversion of methanol to formaldehyde and formic acid.

Case 5 A 60-year-old man is admitted for a 2-week history of cyclic fever, weight loss of 10 lb, nausea, vomiting, and night sweats. He is not on any medications, and he has not seen a physician in years. Physical examination is normal except for a blood pressure of 100/40 mmHg and a pulse rate of 102 beats per minute. There is no lymphadenopathy. He weighs 74 kg. Pertinent laboratory results are as follows:

Serum	ABG
Na$^+$ = 142 mEq/L	pH = 7.20
K$^+$ = 4.2 mEq/L	pCO$_2$ = 20 mmHg
Cl$^-$ = 104 mEq/L	pO$_2$ = 92 mmHg
HCO$_3^-$ = 8 mEq/L	HCO$_3^-$ = 7 mEq/L
BUN = 32 mg/dL	
Creatinine = 1.8 mg/dL	
Glucose = 64 mg/dL	
Measured serum osmolality = 312 mOsm/kg H$_2$O	
Alanine aminotransferase = 60 U/L (normal <38 U/L)	
Aspartate aminotransferase = 58 U/L (normal <41 U/L)	
Lactate dehydrogenase = 690 U/L (normal 115–221 U/L)	
White cell count = 8.2 × 10^3/mm^3	

Question 1 What is the acid–base disturbance?

Answer Based on the pH, serum [HCO$_3^-$], and AG of 30, the primary acid–base disorder is a high AG metabolic acidosis with appropriate respiratory response.

Question 2 Based on the osmolal gap of 14, do you suspect any alcohol intoxication?

Answer No. There are no clinical manifestations that are attributable to toxic alcohol ingestion with such a high AG. The osmolal gap of 14 can be attributable to causes other than alcohols.

Question 3 What other pertinent laboratory tests you order at this time?

Answer Serum lactate and ketones are the appropriate laboratory tests at this time. Serum lactate levels were 14 mmol/L, and ketones were positive. Thus, there are 20 (ΔAG 20; observed AG − normal AG: 30−10 = 20) excess anions in this patient. Of the 20 excess anions, lactate accounts for 14, and the remaining anions are possibly from ketoacids (due to starvation) and sulfate and phosphate from renal failure.

Question 4 Based on clinical presentation and high lactate level, what other consult you request now?

Answer Hematology/oncology consult is extremely important. The hematologist felt that a bone marrow biopsy is valuable in making the diagnosis in the presence of normal white cell count and lymph nodes. The biopsy revealed extranodal T-cell lymphoma, and the lactic acidosis was attributed to lymphoma.

The patient's condition deteriorates, and his pH drops from 7.20 to 7.00 and HCO_3^- from 8 to 6 mEq/L. You intend to start the patient on $NaHCO_3$ drip to raise his serum $[HCO_3^-]$ from 6 to 10 mEq/L.

Question 5 How much $NaHCO_3$ he needs to reach serum $[HCO_3^-]$ of 10 mEq/L?

Answer The HCO_3^- space has increased; therefore, the pH did not improve. The amount of $NaHCO_3$ needed can be calculated as follows:

$$Patient\text{'s weight} = 74 \text{ kg}$$
$$HCO_3^- \text{ space} = 60\%$$
$$\Delta HCO_3^- = 4(10 - 6)$$
$$Amount \text{ of } NaHCO_3^- \text{ needed} = 74 \times 0.6 \times 4 = 178 \text{ mEq}$$

The patient received 180 mEq of $NaHCO_3$, thiamine, and riboflavin, but serum $[HCO_3^-]$ did not change.

Question 6 What is your next approach to improve lactate?

Answer Continuous venovenous hemofiltration (CVVH) with $NaHCO_3$ replacement can be tried, as CVVH is also useful in metformin-induced lactic acidosis.

Case 6 A 28-year-old woman was brought to the emergency department for agitation and respiratory distress, requiring intubation. She required fentanyl and lorazepam for sedation. Renal function was normal. Two days later she had a low serum $[HCO3^-]$ of 12 mEq/L, a drop of 10 mEq/L from baseline value. An ABG shows a high anion gap metabolic acidosis.

Which one of the following acids may have contributed to her anion gap metabolic acidosis?

(A) Acetoacetate
(B) Methanol
(C) Ethylene glycol
(D) Lactic acid
(E) Hippuric acid

The answer is D The patient received lorazepam probably at high doses for sedation. Propylene glycol (PG) is a diluent found in many intravenous and oral drugs, including lorazepam. PG is metabolized by alcohol and aldehyde dehydrogenases to lactic acid. Each milliliter of lorazepam injection contains 828 mg of PG. Thus, high doses of lorazepam administration results in high circulating levels of lactic acid. PG is water soluble and is removed by hemodialysis and also continuous venovenous hemofiltration. Thus, choice D is correct.

Case 7 Match the drug effects of lactic and pyroglutamic acids shown in column A with the mechanisms of action shown in column B.

Column A	Column B
A. Metformin	1. Inhibition of mitochondrial protein synthesis
B. Tenofovir	2. Uncoupling of oxidative phosphorylation
C. Linezolid	3. Inhibition of pyruvate dehydrogenase complex
D. Propofol	4. Inhibition of alcohol dehydrogenase
E. Fomepizole	5. Inhibition of 5-oxoprolinase
F. Flucloxacillin	6. Increase in NADH/NAD⁺ ratio, inhibition of gluconeogenesis from lactate, inhibition of mitochondrial respiration
G. Thiamine deficiency	

Answers A = 6; B = 1; C = 1; D = 2; E = 4; F = 5; G = 3

Reference

1. Barceloux DG, Krenzelok EP, Olson K, et al. American academy of clinical toxicology practice guidelines on the treatment of ethylene glycol poisoning. J Toxicol Clin Toxicol. 1999;37:537–60.

Suggested Reading

2. Cerdá J, Tolwani AJ, Warnock DG. Critical care nephrology: management of acid-base disorders with CRRT. Kidney Int. 2012;82:9–18.
3. Fall PJ, Szerlip HM. Lactic acidosis: from sour milk to septic shock. J Intensive Care Med. 2005;20:255–71.
4. Fenves AZ, Kirkpatrick HM III, Patel VV, et al. Increased anion gap metabolic acidosis as a result of 5-oxoproline (pyroglutamic acid): a role for acetaminophen. Clin J Am Soc Nephrol. 2006;1:441–7.
5. Kraut JA, Madias NE. Treatment of acute metabolic acidosis: a pathophysiologic approach. Nat Rev Nephrol. 2012;8:589–601.
6. Kraut JA, Madias NE. Lactic acidosis. N Engl J Med. 2014;371:2309–19.
7. Kraut JA, Xing SX. Approach to the evaluation of a patient with an increased serum osmolal gap and high-anion gap metabolic acidosis. Am J Kidney Dis. 2011;58:480–4.
8. Kraut JA, Madias NE. Metabolic acidosis: pathophysiology, diagnosis and management. Nat Rev Nephrol. 2010;6:274–85.
9. Hood VL. Lactic acidosis. In: Jennari FJ, Adrogué HJ, Galla JH, Madias NE, editors. Acid-base disorders and their treatment. Boca Raton: Taylor & Francis; 2005. p. 351–82.
10. Laski ME, Wesson DE. Lactic acidosis. In: DuBose TH Jr, Hamm LL, editors. Acid-base and electrolyte disorders. A companion to Brenner & Rector's the Kidney. Philadelphia: Saunders; 2002. p. 83–107.
11. Velez JC, Janech MG. A case of lactic acidosis induced by linezolid. Nat Rev Nephrol. 2010;6:236–40.
12. Kang KP, Lee S, Kang SK. D-lactic acidosis in humans: review of update. Electrolyte Blood Press. 2006;4:53–6.
13. Oh MS, Halperin ML. Toxin-induced metabolic acidosis. In: Jennari FJ, Adrogué HJ, Galla JH, Madias NE, editors. Acid-base disorders and their treatment. Boca Raton: Taylor & Francis; 2005. p. 383–415.
14. Wu D, Kraut JA. Role of NHE1 in the cellular dysfunction of acute metabolic acidosis. Am J Nephrol. 2014;40:26–42.

Hyperchloremic Metabolic Acidosis: Renal Tubular Acidosis

29

Renal tubular acidoses (RTAs) are discrete renal tubular disorders that are characterized by the inability to excrete H^+ in the urine. As a result, there is a positive H^+ balance, causing metabolic acidosis. The net acid excretion (NAE) is decreased, and some of the patients are unable to lower their urine pH <5.5. Despite severe acidosis, the anion gap (AG) remains normal because the decrease in serum $[HCO_3^-]$ is compensated for by a proportionate increase in serum $[Cl^-]$.

There are four types of RTAs:

1. Proximal RTA (type II RTA)
2. Distal RTA (classic or type I RTA)
3. Incomplete RTA (type III RTA)
4. Distal RTA with hyperkalemia

Hyperchloremic metabolic acidosis can also develop following large-volume infusion of normal saline (dilutional acidosis) in chronic kidney disease (CKD) patients with glomerular filtration rate (GFR) ~50 mL/min and during the recovery phase of diabetic ketoacidosis.

NAE or urinary acidification is an important physiologic determinant that is useful in the assessment of metabolic acidosis. In a normal individual, NAE is increased in response to an acid load. Determination of NAE in a patient with hyperchloremic metabolic acidosis can help determine the etiology of this disorder. Simple laboratory tests such as urine pH, urine anion gap (U_{AG}), and urine osmolal gap are helpful during the workup of a patient with RTA. Of the three tests, the first two are routinely performed.

Urine pH

- Normal urine pH varies between 4.5 and 6.0, implying appropriate NAE.
- In patients with proximal RTA, urine pH can be acidic or alkaline (see further).
- In patients with distal RTA, urine pH is *always* >6.5.

© Springer Science+Business Media LLC 2018
A.S. Reddi, *Fluid, Electrolyte and Acid-Base Disorders*,
DOI 10.1007/978-3-319-60167-0_29

- In type III RTA, urine pH is >6.5.
- In patients with hyperkalemic RTA (type IV) with aldosterone deficiency, urine pH is usually <5.5.
- In hyperkalemic distal RTA with variable levels of aldosterone, urine pH is *always* >6.5.

Urine Anion Gap (U_{AG})

- $U_{AG}(U_{Na}+U_K-U_{Cl})$, as discussed in Chap. 2, is an indirect measure of NH_4^+ excretion. It is the best measure to distinguish RTA from hyperchloremic metabolic acidosis due to nonrenal causes such as chronic diarrhea.
- When $U_{Cl}>(U_{Na}+U_K)$, the U_{AG} is negative, indicating adequate NH_4^+ excretion. On the other hand, when U_{AG} is positive [$U_{Cl}<(U_{Na}+U_K)$], NH_4^+ excretion is decreased.
- In conditions such as diabetic ketoacidosis, Cl^- is excreted mostly with ketoanions than with Na^+, K^+, or NH_4^+; therefore, the U_{AG} becomes falsely positive. Therefore, a direct measurement of NH_4^+ is needed. Since direct measurement of NH_4^+ is not available in many clinical laboratories, an indirect measurement can be obtained by calculating the urine osmolal gap.

Urine Osmolal Gap (U_{OG})

- Like serum osmolal gap, U_{OG} is the difference between the measured and calculated urine osmolalities. U_{OG} detects unmeasured anions or cations, and it is an indirect test for NH_4^+ excretion. The U_{OG} is expressed as mOsm/kg H_2O and calculated as follows:

$$U_{OG} = 2\left(Na^+ + K^+\right) + Urea + Glucose\left(all\ in\ mmol\ /\ L\right)$$

- Normal U_{OG} values range from 10 to100 mOsm/kg H_2O.
- U_{NH4} excretion is half of U_{OG} due to the accompanying anions.
- When U_{OG} is <100 mOsm in metabolic acidosis, it indicates impaired NH_4^+ excretion.
- U_{OG} is thus useful in the differential diagnosis of hyperchloremic metabolic acidosis.

Proximal RTA

Characteristics

Proximal RTA is characterized by:

1. Hyperchloremic (non-AG) metabolic acidosis.
2. HCO_3^- wasting in early or initial phase when serum [HCO_3^-] is 20 mEq/L and urine pH is usually >6.5.

3. Urine pH <5.5 in chronic (steady) phase (serum [HCO$_3^-$] is < 18–20 mEq/L.
4. Hypokalemia.
5. Positive U$_{AG}$.
6. Intact distal tubule acidification.

Pathophysiology

Recall from Chap. 26 regarding HCO$_3^-$ handling in the kidney. As stated, 4,320 mEq (serum [HCO$_3^-$] 24 × daily GFR 180 L = 4,320) of HCO$_3^-$ is filtered daily in a normal individual. All of this HCO$_3^-$ is reabsorbed, and virtually none appears in the urine. Approximately 80% of filtered HCO$_3^-$ is reabsorbed in the proximal tubule. In proximal RTA, HCO$_3^-$ reabsoption is reduced. This results in more HCO$_3^-$ delivery to the distal tubules and all HCO$_3^-$ not being reabsorbed. This causes loss of HCO$_3^-$ in the urine, and urine pH becomes alkaline (>6.5). This suggests that there is a certain threshold for HCO$_3^-$ reclamation in the proximal tubule in patients with proximal RTA. When the filtered load of HCO$_3^-$ is reduced because of low serum [HCO$_3^-$] of ~18 to 20 mEq/L, patients with proximal RTA with normal renal function can reabsorb all HCO$_3^-$, and urine is free of HCO$_3^-$ with a pH <5.5 (acid). This acidic pH is due to increased NAE, suggesting that distal acidification is intact. Thus, acidification of urine depends on serum [HCO$_3^-$] in patients with proximal RTA. Table 29.1 explains HCO$_3^-$ handling and urine pH in proximal RTA, which occurs in two phases: initial and steady-state phases.

Hypokalemia

Hypokalemia is extremely common because of excess urinary loss of K$^+$. This is due to the increased delivery of Na$^+$ and HCO$_3^-$ to the distal nephron, where Na$^+$ and K$^+$ exchange occurs. Also, volume depletion-induced aldosterone may contribute to K$^+$ wastage.

Table 29.1 Handling of HCO$_3^-$ in normal subjects and patients with proximal RTA

Subjects	Amount (mEq) of filtered HCO$_3^-$	Amount (mEq) reabsorbed in the proximal tubule	Amount (mEq) delivered to distal segments	Amount (mEq) of HCO$_3^-$ excreted	Urine pH
Normal	4,320	3,456 (80%)	864 (20%)	<3	<5.5
Proximal RTA					
Initial phase	4,320	2,808 (65%)	1,512 (25%)[a]	1,134	>6.5
Steady state	3,600[b]	2,880 (76%)	864 (24%)	<3	<5.5

[a]Maximum reabsorption
[b]Calculated at serum [HCO$_3^-$] of 20 mEq/L

Table 29.2 Causes of proximal RTA

Genetic causes	Acquired causes
Isolated proximal RTA not associated with Fanconi syndrome	*Dysproteinemic states*
Genetic	Multiple myeloma
Autosomal recessive	Light-chain deposition disease
Autosomal dominant	Amyloidosis
Sporadic	*Tubulointerstitial diseases*
Carbonic anhydrase (CA) II deficiency	Sjögren's syndrome
CA IV deficiency	Posttransplantation rejection
Proximal RTA associated with Fanconi syndrome	Medullary cystic disease
Inherited disorders	*Secondary hyperparathyroidism with chronic hypocalcemia*
Cystinosis	Vitamin D deficiency or resistance
Wilson's disease	Vitamin D dependency
Tyrosinemia	*Others*
Hereditary fructose intolerance	Nephrotic syndrome
Lowe syndrome	Paroxysmal nocturnal hemoglobinuria
Galactosemia	*Drugs*
Dent disease	CA inhibitors (acetazolamide, topiramate)
	Anticancer drugs (ifosfamide, cisplatin, carboplatin, streptozotocin, azacitidine, suramin, mercaptopurine)
	Antibacterial drugs (outdated tetracyclines, aminoglycosides)
	Anticonvulsants (valproic acid, topiramate)
	Antiviral agents (DDI, adefovir, cidofovir, tenofovir)
	Others (fumarate, ranitidine, salicylates, alcohol, cadmium)

Causes

Proximal RTA can occur as an isolated defect in HCO_3^- transport (called isolated proximal RTA) or in association with multiple tubular transport defects (called Fanconi syndrome). Table 29.2 shows the causes of proximal RTA.

Clinical Manifestations

- Skeletal abnormalities and osteomalacia are common due to chronic metabolic acidosis and vitamin D deficiency. Hypophosphatemia may also contribute to skeletal abnormalities.
- Vitamin D deficiency is due to decreased formation of $1,25(OH)_2D_3$ from $25(OH)D_3$, as proximal tubular production of 1α-hydroxylase is reduced.
- Osteopenia and pseudofractures occur in adults.
- Nephrocalcinosis and nephrolithiasis are rather uncommon, except in patients treated for epilepsy with topiramate. This drug inhibits carbonic

anhydrase and causes hypercalciuria, hypocitrituria, and alkaline urine pH with resultant formation of calcium phosphate stones.

Specific Causes of Isolated Proximal RTA

Autosomal Recessive Proximal RTA

- Caused by mutations in Na/HCO_3 cotransporter isoform 1 located in the basolateral membrane of the proximal tubule and eyes. Described initially in 2- and 16-year-old females.
- Clinical manifestations include short stature, mental retardation, cataracts, bilateral glaucoma, and band keratopathy. Low HCO_3^-, non-AG acidosis, and acid urine were observed. However, both parents were normal.
- Treatment includes lifelong alkali therapy.

Autosomal Dominant Proximal RTA

- Described only in two brothers belonging to a single Costa Rican family.
- Gene mutation is unknown.
- Clinical manifestations include growth retardation and reduced bone density. Both brothers had low serum $[HCO_3^-]$ with acid urine.
- Treatment is lifelong alkali therapy.

Sporadic Form

- A transient form of inherited proximal RTA, requiring alkali therapy initially, and then discontinuation after several years

Carbonic Anhydrase (CA) Deficiency

- Two isoforms of CA have been described.
- CA II is cytoplasmic and found in the proximal and distal tubule.
- CA IV is located in the apical membrane of the proximal tubule.
- CA II deficiency is caused by mutations in CA II gene and inherited as an autosomal recessive disease.
- CA II deficiency patients are usually Arabic in origin.
- Early manifestations include growth and mental retardation, osteopetrosis, cerebral calcification, hypokalemia, proximal muscle weakness, and other features of both proximal and distal (type III) RTAs.
- CA IV deficiency impairs HCO_3^- reabsorption in the proximal tubule, but a genetic mutation has not been described.

Fanconi Syndrome

Definition

It is defined as a proximal tubular dysfunction, leading to excessive urinary excretion of HCO_3^-, glucose, phosphate, uric acid, amino acids, and to a lesser extent Na^+, K^+, and Ca^{2+}.

Laboratory and Clinical Manifestations

The urinary losses of solutes lead to acidosis, electrolyte abnormalities (hypokalemia, hypophosphatemia, hypouricemia), dehydration with resultant increase in renin–AII–aldosterone production, rickets, osteomalacia, growth, and mental retardation.

Causes

Table 29.2 shows both genetic and acquired causes of proximal RTA associated with Fanconi syndrome. The most common genetic cause of Fanconi syndrome is cystinosis in children and adolescents, whereas multiple myeloma and drugs are important causes in adults.

Diagnosis

- Suspect proximal RTA in an adult with chronic hyperchloremic metabolic acidosis, hypokalemia, and urine pH <5.5 with serum $[HCO_3^-]$ <20 mEq/L.
- Confirmatory tests include:
  1. Positive U_{AG}.
  2. Fractional excretion of HCO_3^- >15% (even >5% may be sufficient in some patients).
  3. HCO_3^- titration test (definitive test): a marked increase in urinary excretion of HCO_3^- and pH occurs, as serum $[HCO_3^-]$ is raised to normal levels (i.e., above renal threshold) by IV administration of $NaHCO_3$.
- Glucosuria in the presence of normal serum glucose levels, phosphaturia, or other solute excretions establish the diagnosis of Fanconi syndrome.
- Growth retardation and rickets in children and osteopenia as well as pseudofractures in adults should alert the physician to consider proximal RTA as one of the diagnoses.

Treatment

The physician should address the cause of proximal RTA and take appropriate steps to improve acidosis and skeletal abnormalities.

Table 29.3 Alkali preparations

Preparation	Amount of HCO_3^- or its equivalent
$NaHCO_3$	4 mEq/325 mg tablet or 8 mEq/650 mg tablet
Baking soda ($NaHCO_3$)	60 mEq/teaspoon (4.5 g) of powder
K-Lyte (K^+ HCO_3/K^+ citrate)	25–50 mEq/tablet
Urocit-K (K^+ citrate)	5–10 mEq/tablet
Kaon (K^+ gluconate)	5 mEq/mL or 1.33 mEq/mL
Shohl's solution, Bicitra (Na^+ citrate/citric acid)	1 mEq/mL
Polycitra (Na^+ citrate/K^+ citrate/citric acid)	2 mEq/mL
Polycitra-K (K^+ citrate/citric acid)	2 mEq/mL

- Alkali therapy is indicated in all the patients (Table 29.3).
- In *children*, the aim is to prevent growth abnormalities. Administration of $NaHCO_3$ or its metabolic equivalent (citrate) to maintain serum [HCO_3^-] to near-normal levels (22–24 mEq/L) is desirable to reestablish normal growth.
- Maintenance of normal serum [HCO_3^-] exacerbates kaliuresis; therefore, high doses of K^+ supplements are necessary.
- Alkali therapy restores growth and volume with suppression of renin–AII–aldosterone system.
- In *adults*, it is not necessary to maintain normal serum [HCO_3^-].
- Adults require between 50 and 100 mEq of alkali daily.
- $NaHCO_3$ and baking soda are inexpensive. Both of them may cause osmotic diarrhea; therefore, small and dividing doses may lower this adverse effect.
- Diuretics such as amiloride may be helpful in some patients by preventing K^+ loss.
- Thiazide and loop diuretics also help in lowering HCO_3^- requirements by volume depletion and increasing HCO_3^- reabsoption in the proximal tubule, but hypokalemia may be aggravated.
- Polycitra-K provides both K and HCO_3 and is recommended by many physicians.
- Active vitamin D_3 and phosphate supplementation help skeletal growth and acidification in patients with low serum phosphate levels.
- Note that citrate increases aluminum absorption.

Hypokalemic Distal (Classic) or Type I RTA

Characteristics

Distal RTA is characterized by:

1. Hyperchloremic (non-AG) metabolic acidosis
2. Inability to acidify urine despite severe acidosis (urine pH >6.5)
3. Hypokalemia
4. Positive U_{AG}

5. Skeletal abnormalities
6. Nephrolithiasis and nephrocalcinosis
7. Intact proximal tubule function

Pathophysiology

The pathophysiology of type I RTA is fairly understood. Two mechanisms seem important in causing hypokalemic distal RTA:

1. Defective H^+ secretion
2. Backleak of H^+

Defective H^+ Secretion Both of the above defects are due to dysfunction of the type A intercalated cell. Recall that acidification of urine occurs by secretion of H^+ via H-ATPase and K/H exchanger. A functional defect in these transport mechanisms results in positive H^+ balance and acidemia. This leads to a decrease in NAE, particularly NH_4^+ excretion, and HCO_3^- wastage with alkaline pH despite severe acidosis.

Patients with distal RTA have low NH_3 secretion, because of the failure to trap NH_3 in the tubular lumen of the collecting duct which has an alkaline pH. Also, secretion of NH_3 is impaired from the medulla due to interstitial disease caused by nephrocalcinosis or hypokalemia. Thus, impaired secretion of NH_3 into the tubular lumen results in decreased NAE and alkaline urine.

Also, a defect in the exit of HCO_3^- via Cl/HCO_3 exchanger (anion exchanger 1 or AE1) results in intracellular alkalinization, which inhibits apical H^+ secretion.

Genetic studies have shown that mutations in B_1 and A_4 subunit of H-ATPase and AE1 cause distal RTA. These genetic defects cause hereditary forms of type I distal RTA (see further).

Backleak of H^+ It is believed that type I RTA is due to altered apical membrane permeability of the type A intercalated cell. An experimental study with amphotericin B has proven this belief. There is no defect in H^+ secretion via H-ATPase transporter. However, the secreted H^+ diffuses back into the cells through the permeable apical membrane. As a result, the luminal pH remains alkaline, and excretion of NAE is substantially decreased.

Causes

Distal RTA can be either hereditary (primary) or acquired. Table 29.4 shows some important causes of distal RTA.

The hereditary forms are rather rare but deserve some discussion. Table 29.5 summarizes genetic abnormalities and clinical manifestations.

Table 29.4 Causes of distal (type I) RTA

Hereditary	Associated with nephrocalcinosis
Autosomal dominant	Hyperparathyroidism
Autosomal recessive with deafness	Primary nephrocalcinosis
Autosomal recessive without deafness	Idiopathic hypercalciuria
Acquired	Vitamin D intoxication
Associated with systemic disease	Medullary sponge kidney
Multiple myeloma	Drugs
Amyloidosis	Amphotericin B
Systemic lupus erythematosus	Toluene
Sjögren's syndrome	Vanadate (?)
Chronic active hepatitis	Lithium
Primary biliary cirrhosis	Analgesics
Cryoglobulinemia	Cyclamate
Thyroiditis	
Posttransplantation rejection	
Balkan nephropathy	

Table 29.5 Clinical characteristics of hereditary distal RTAs

Form	Genetic defect	Age at onset	Clinical features
Autosomal dominant	Mutations in anion exchanger (AE1 or Cl/HCO$_3$ exchanger	Adults	Mild metabolic acidosis
			Mild to moderate hypokalemia
			Mild to moderate bone disease
			Nephrocalcinosis/lithiasis, hypocitrituria, hypercalciuria
			Occasional rickets and osteomalacia
Autosomal recessive with deafness	B1 subunit of H-ATPase	Infancy/childhood	Severe metabolic acidosis
			Vomiting
			Dehydration
			Growth retardation
			Nephrocalcinosis
			Rickets
			Bilateral sensorineural hearing loss
Autosomal recessive without deafness	A4 subunit of H-ATPase	Infancy/childhood	Same as above but without deafness (although late-onset hearing loss in some)

Diagnosis

- Suspect distal RTA in subjects with moderate to severe non-AG metabolic acidosis, hypokalemia, and urine pH >6.5
- Confirmatory urinary acidification tests include:
  1. Positive U_{AG}.
  2. NH$_4$Cl test: in this test, NH$_4$Cl (100 mg/kg) is dissolved in water and given orally. Following ingestion, sequential urine samples are collected for pH over a period of 6 h. At the same time, serum [HCO$_3^-$] before and 3 h after

NH_4Cl ingestion is determined to document systemic acidosis. The normal response is a decrease in urine pH <5.5. In patients with distal RTA, the urine pH is always >6.5. All patients must be screened for urinary tract infection, as urine pH with urease-producing organisms is alkaline. This test is contra-indicated in patients with liver cirrhosis.

3. An alternative test is determination of urine to blood (U–B) pCO_2 difference or gradient. In this test, $NaHCO_3$ (500 mEq/L at 3 mL/min) is infused until bicarbonaturia, and urine pH >7.5 ensues. In a normal individual, urine pCO_2 increases above blood pCO_2 by 20–30 mmHg (U–B pCO_2 gradient 20–30 mmHg). This indicates adequate distal H^+ secretion. However, in a subject with distal RTA, this U–B pCO_2 gradient cannot be achieved, indicat-ing defective distal H^+ secretion. One exception is amphotericin B-induced distal RTA. In this condition, normal U–B pCO_2 can be achieved

Complications

Hypokalemia

Hypokalemia is very common because of increased Na/K cotransporter activity in the distal nephron. Also, dysfunction of H/K-ATPase may contribute to hypokale-mia, as inhibition of this transporter by vanadate causes hypokalemic distal RTA. Loss of Na^+ and HCO_3^- in the urine causes volume depletion, which stimu-lates the renin–AII–aldosterone system and hypokalemia.

Nephrocalcinosis and Nephrolithiasis

One of the major complications of distal RTA is the development of nephrocalcino-sis and nephrolithiasis. The mechanisms are as follows:

1. Chronic metabolic acidosis causes bone buffering and dissolution of bone miner-als, resulting in high Ca^{2+} excretion.
2. In addition, luminal alkalinization inhibits Ca^{2+} reabsorption, promoting an even more excretion of Ca^{2+}.
3. Because of high urine pH, solubility of calcium phosphate stones is decreased, thereby causing their formation.
4. Citrate excretion is reduced in metabolic acidosis, resulting in reduced chelation of free Ca^{2+}.

Treatment

- Treatment in adults is aimed at the correction of primary disease or eliminating the drug that causes distal RTA. Correction of acidosis and hypokalemia should promptly be addressed. Alkali therapy is indicated in all patients.

- NaHCO$_3$ or citrate at 1–1.5 mEq/kg is needed daily. Correction of acidosis reduces K$^+$ wasting and, therefore, does not require K$^+$ supplementation. However, some patients may lose K$^+$. For such patients, K-citrate corrects hypokalemia.
- Patients with severe acidosis and muscle paralysis due to hypokalemia require IV administration.
- Correction of acidosis and hypokalemia improves growth and prevents osteomalacia in adults and rickets in children, hypercalciuria, and nephrocalcinosis as well as nephrolithiasis by improving citrate excretion.

Toluene Ingestion and Distal RTA

- Toluene ingestion causes a high AG metabolic acidosis, if their metabolites (hippuric acid and benzoic acid) are not excreted rapidly due to volume depletion and renal failure.
- When volume is adequate and renal function is normal, these acids are rapidly excreted, and a hyperchloremic metabolic acidosis with hypokalemia develops.
- Possible mechanism includes inhibition of H$^+$ secretion in the distal tubule.
- Treatment is supportive with volume expansion and NaHCO$_3$ therapy. Dialysis is indicated when severe acidosis and renal failure are present.

Incomplete (Type III) RTA

Type III RTA is characterized by both proximal and distal RTAs. Patients with this form of RTA have HCO3$^-$ wastage and inability to acidify their urine <5.5. Generally, the acidification defect is confirmed by one of the urinary acidification tests described earlier.

Clinical characteristics include only mild hyperchloremic metabolic acidosis with near-normal NH$_4^+$ excretion. They may have low citrate excretion because of increased proximal tubule reabsorption and subsequent development of calcium phosphate stones. Conditions that are associated with type III RTA are chronic tubulointerstitial disease, lithium therapy, and medullary sponge kidney. Genetic deficiency of CA II also causes type III RTA.

Distal RTA with Hyperkalemia

Based on the urinary acidification, distal RTA with hyperkalemia can be divided into two subtypes:

1. Hyperkalemic distal RTA (type IV) with urine pH <5.5
2. Hyperkalemic distal RTA with urine pH >5.5 (also called voltage-dependent RTA)

Both subtypes share the following characteristics:

1. More common in adults than in children
2. Hyperkalemic hyperchloremic metabolic acidosis
3. Inhibition of NH_3 synthesis by hyperkalemia in the proximal tubule
4. Decreased urinary NH_4^+ excretion
5. Mild to moderate renal impairment
6. Absence of nephrocalcinosis and nephrolithiasis

Hyperkalemic Distal RTA (Type IV) with Urine pH <5.5

- Patients with type IV RTA have hyperchloremic metabolic acidosis with urine pH <5.5, suggesting decreased NH_4^+ excretion rather than defective H^+ secretion.
- Patients have selective aldosterone deficiency alone.
- Hyporeninemic hypoaldosteronism is also present in some patients.
- NH_3 synthesis is suppressed by both hyperkalemia and aldosterone deficiencies.
- Typically seen in patients with diabetes, who have low renin and aldosterone (hyporeninemic hypoaldosteronism).
- Several drugs that interfere with renin and aldosterone system also cause type IV RTA (Table 29.6).

Hyperkalemic Distal RTA with Urine pH >5.5 (Voltage-Dependent RTA)

- Patients with this form of RTA have hyperkalemic hyperchloremic metabolic acidosis.
- However, these patients cannot lower their urine pH below 5.5.
- The major mechanism includes the inability to maintain lumen negativity (voltage gradient) in the cortical collecting duct. Normally, Na^+ reabsorption occurs via the epithelial sodium channel (ENaC) to maintain favorable voltage gradient for K^+ and H^+ secretion into the lumen. When a defect occurs in Na^+ reabsorption, both K^+ and H^+ are not secreted, resulting in hyperkalemia and inability to acidify urine pH below 5.5.
- Obstructive nephropathy is an important cause of voltage-dependent RTA.
- Also, voltage-dependent RTA has been demonstrated by amiloride, which inhibits ENaC.
- Aldosterone levels may be normal, low, or high, but in most cases, reduced levels have been observed.

Causes of Both Types of Hyperkalemic Distal RTAs

- Causes of distal RTA with hyperkalemia can be due to systemic diseases, acquired or genetic.

Table 29.6 Some causes of distal RTA with hyperkalemia

Hyperkalemic distal RTA (type IV) with urine pH <5.5	Hyperkalemic distal RTA with urine pH >5.5
Primary mineralocorticoid deficiency	*Diseases with both tubulointerstitial and glomerular diseases*
Combined aldosterone and cortisol deficiency	Obstructive nephropathy
Addison disease	Sickle cell disease
Bilateral adrenal destruction (hemorrhage, surgery, or cancer)	Lupus nephritis
21-hydroxylase deficiency	Kidney transplant rejection
Selective aldosterone deficiency	*Drugs*
Idiopathic hypoaldosteronism	ENaC inhibitors
Heparin use in normal and critically ill patients	Amiloride
Primary mineralocorticoid deficiency with hyporeninemic hypoaldosteronism	Trimethoprim
Diabetes mellitus	Pentamidine
Tubulointerstitial diseases	Triamterene
HIV	Na/K-ATPase inhibitors
Nephrosclerosis	Cyclosporine
Drugs causing low renin and low aldosterone	Tacrolimus
NSAIDs	Aldosterone blockers
β-blockers	Spironolactone
Cyclosporine	Eplerenone
Tacrolimus	*Mineralocorticoid resistance and voltage gradient defect*
Drugs causing high renin and low aldosterone	Pseudohypoaldosteronism type I
ACE inhibitors	Pseudohypoaldosteronism type II
Angiotensin II receptor blockers	
Ketoconazole	
Heparin	

- Mechanisms include selective aldosterone deficiency, hyporeninemic hypoaldo-steronism, aldosterone resistance, and drug-induced hypoaldosteronisms (Table 29.6).

Diagnosis of Hyperkalemic Distal RTAs

- Diagnosis of hyperkalemic distal RTA is made on the following observations:
  1. An adult (40–70 years) with hyperchloremic metabolic acidosis and hyperka-lemia (K^+ = 5.5–6.5 mEq/L).
  2. Hyperkalemia is asymptomatic in many, but some patients may have muscle weakness or cardiac arrhythmia.
  3. Serum [HCO_3^-] between 18 and 21 mEq/L.
  4. Decreased NAE.
  5. Estimation of NH_4^+ excretion using U_{AG}.

6. Mild to moderate renal impairment.
7. Urine pH either < 5.5 or > 5.5 (based on etiology).
8. Positive U_{AG}.
9. Low fractional excretion of K^+.

- If clinical diagnosis could not be made on history and laboratory tests, furosemide or bumetanide test can be performed. Loop diuretics deliver more NaCl to the collecting duct, causing Na^+ reabsorption (via ENaC) and K^+ and H^+ secretion into the lumen. This results in the acidification of urine. Amiloride can obliterate these changes.
- Furosemide test: 40–80 mg of furosemide or 1–2 mg of bumetanide is given orally after collecting a urine sample. Urine samples are collected every hour for 4 h. Normal individuals and selective aldosterone deficiency patients lower their urine pH < 5.5. Patients with a defect in voltage gradient cannot lower urine pH < 5.5.
- Figure 29.1 shows an approach to the patient with hyperkalemic distal RTA.

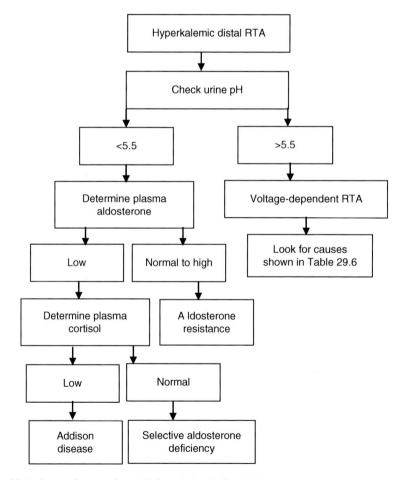

Fig. 29.1 Approach to a patient with hyperkalemic distal RTA

Treatment of Hyperkalemic Distal RTAs

- Inquire about dietary and drug history.
- Review the contributing or precipitating factors, such as hyperglycemia, degree of renal dysfunction, or ingestion of salt substitutes.
- Pharmacologic treatment should be individualized, and decision depends on the severity of hyperkalemia and acidosis after discontinuation of drugs and appropriate management of associated clinical abnormalities.
- Kayexalate (sodium polystyrene sulfate) for hyperkalemia (rule out any GI abnormalities before administration).
- Patiromer can be given, if Kayexalate is contraindicated or unable to tolerate.
- Liberalization of salt intake in patients with euvolemia
- Furosemide or bumetanide to improve hyperkalemia.
- Fludrocortisone alone or in combination with furosemide in patients with low aldosterone levels and normal fluid volume status.
- $NaHCO_3$ or Na citrate to improve acidosis.
- NaCl supplement for patients with pseudohypoparathyroidism type I.
- Hydrochlothiazide for patients with pseudohypoparathyroidism type II.

Distinguishing Features of Various RTAs

So far we have discussed various forms of RTAs. However, it is important to remember the similarities and differences among these RTAs for their easy recognition. Table 29.7 summarizes similarities and differences of these RTAs.

Table 29.7 Comparison of clinical findings among various RTAs

Finding	Proximal RTA	Classic distal RTA	Hyperkalemic RTAs
Serum [K^+]	↓	↓	↑
Urine pH with severe acidosis	<5.5	>5.5	<5.5 (aldosterone deficiency)
Urine acidification	N	↓	↓
NH_4^+ excretion	N	↓	>5.5 (voltage gradient defect)
U_{AG}	+(or −)	+	+
Fanconi syndrome	Yes	No	No
U–B pCO_2	Normal	↓	↓
Hypercalciuria	No	Yes	No
Nephrocalcinosis/lithiasis	No	Yes	No
Citrate excretion	N	↓	N
Bone lesions	Yes	Yes	No
Renal insufficiency	No	No	Yes
Response to alkali therapy	Less	Good	Yes
			Variable

N normal, ↑ increase, ↓ decrease, + positive, - negative

Dilutional Acidosis

- Infusion of large volume of normal (0.9%) saline causes a decrease in serum $[HCO_3^-]$ and $[K^+]$ and an increase in $[Cl^-]$, resulting in hypokalemia and hyperchloremic metabolic acidosis. Serum $[Na^+]$ does not change, as it is being infused. pCO_2 also does not change.
- According to Henderson equation, H^+ increases, resulting in acid pH.
- Dilutional acidosis (preferably called dilutional hyperchloremic acidosis) is transient and improves with discontinuation of saline.
- Carries no morbidity or mortality, but persistent high $[Cl^-]$ may not be desirable.

Acidosis Due to Chronic Kidney Disease

- Loss of kidney function results in metabolic acidosis.
- Hyperchloremic metabolic acidosis typically develops in patients with GFR between 20 and 50 mL/min.
- Serum $[HCO_3^-]$ is reduced to 18–22 mEq/L and maintained around these values because of the bone rather than HCO_3^- buffering of acids.
- The major mechanism of hyperchloremic acidosis is decreased NH_4^+ excretion and its synthesis.
- Because of adaptive increase in K^+ excretion by the collecting duct and colon, normokalemia is maintained until GFR is <15 mL/min.
- Whenever hyperkalemic hyperchloremic acidosis is observed in a patient with GFR between 20 and 50 mL/min, exclude drugs that cause hyperkalemia or severe tubulointerstitial disease.
- Treatment depends on symptoms such as muscle weakness, fatigue, or shortness of breath. Some patients may require $NaHCO_3$ therapy (8 mEq/day) and protein restriction to decrease acid generation.
- High AG metabolic acidosis develops once GFR is < 15 mL/min.

Hyperchloremic Metabolic Acidosis During Treatment of Diabetic Ketoacidosis

- Develops typically during treatment of diabetic ketoacidosis.
- Potential mechanisms include:
  1. Loss of ketoacids in the urine prior or during volume expansion
  2. Lack of ketone absorption by renal tubules
  3. Increase in serum $[Cl^-]$ and no increase in $[HCO_3^-]$ during treatment
- Food intake and maintenance of plasma glucose levels around 100–140 mg/dL improves serum $[HCO_3^-]$.

Study Questions

Case 1 An 18-year-old woman with history of systemic lupus erythematosus (SLE) is admitted to the hospital for worsening weakness and problems with breathing for the last 2 weeks. She loves ice cream since childhood. She states that she had four to six urinary tract infections (UTIs) in recent years, which were treated. She is not on any medications. Admitting laboratory values are:

Serum	Urine
Na^+ = 138 mEq/L	pH = 6.6
K^+ = 1.2 mEq/L	Glucose = negative
Cl^- = 118 mEq/L	Blood = positive (had recent menstruation)
HCO_3^- = 12 mEq/L	Ketones = negative
Creatinine = 0.6 mg/dL	Protein = 3+
BUN = 22 mg/dL	Na^+ = 60 mEq/L
Glucose = 90 mg/dL	K^+ = 100 mEq/L
ANA = positive	Cl^- = 110 mEq/L
Complement = low	
ABG: pH 7.2, pCO_2 26 mmHg, HCO_3^- 11 mEq/L	

Question 1 Which one of the following is the MOST likely cause of her symptoms?

(a) Exacerbation of SLE
(b) Proximal RTA
(c) Distal RTA
(d) Type IV RTA
(e) Hypokalemic periodic paralysis

The answer is C The patient's weakness and respiratory distress are related to hypokalemia rather than exacerbation of SLE. Although glomerular disease is common in SLE, tubular dysfunction is uncommon in the presence of normal renal function. However, hypokalemia-related clinical manifestations have been described prior to the diagnosis of SLE. The serum and urine findings in this patient are suggestive of distal RTA (hyperchloremic metabolic acidosis and alkaline urine pH despite acidosis). A few cases of distal RTA have been reported in the literature. The pathophysiology of distal RTA in lupus patients is unclear; however, destruction of distal nephron by immunoglobulins has been suggested. Proximal RTA in this patient is unlikely as she has no manifestations of Fanconi syndrome. Also, patients with proximal RTA can acidify their urine at a serum $[HCO_3^-]$ of 12 mEq/L. Although type IV RTA has been described in lupus patients, hypokalemia rules out this diagnosis in this patient. Hypokalemic periodic paralysis is also unlikely because of positive ANA, lupus nephritis, and urine [K$^+$] of 100 mEq/L. In hypokalemic periodic paralysis, urine K$^+$ is low because of transcellular distribution.

Question 2 Is urine anion gap (U$_{AG}$) helpful in this patient?

Answer Yes. Calculation of U$_{AG}$ is helpful in the differential diagnosis of hyperchloremic metabolic acidosis. In this patient, the U$_{AG}$ is positive, ruling out diarrhea as a cause of her hyperchloremic metabolic acidosis.

Question 3 Does she require workup for nephrocalcinosis/lithiasis?

Answer Yes. She had several UTIs in the past. Although frequent UTIs are common in young females, she requires minimum workup for nephrocalcinosis/lithiasis as a cause of her UTIs. Patients with distal RTA frequently develop nephrocalcinosis/lithiasis.

Case 2 A 19-year-old thin female student is brought to the emergency department by her friends for altered mental status, euphoria, and dizziness after a rave party. She has no history of drug abuse and is not on any medications. Physical examination is normal except for a blood pressure of 90/60 mmHg with pulse rate of 102 beats/min. Laboratory results on admission and 18 h later are:

On admission	18 h later
Na$^+$ = 142 mEq/L	Na$^+$ = 138 mEq/L
K$^+$ = 3.5 mEq/L	K$^+$ = 2.2 mEq/L
Cl$^-$ = 100 meq/L	Cl$^-$ = 118 mEq/L
HCO$_3^-$ = 12 mEq/L	HCO$_3^-$ = 14 mEq/L
Creatinine = 1.8 mg/dL	Creatinine = 0.9 mg/dL
BUN = 22 mg/dL	BUN = 12 mg/dL
Glucose = 96 mg/dL	Glucose = 100 mg/dL
ABG: pH 7.24, pCO$_2$ 28 mmHg, HCO$_3^-$ 11 mEq/L	ABG: pH 7.31, pCO$_2$ 29 mmHg, HCO$_3^-$ 13 mEq/L
Urine pH = 5.2	Urine pH = 6.5

Question 1 Characterize the acid–base disorder on admission and 18 h later.

Answer On admission, she has a high AG metabolic acidosis with appropriate respiratory compensation, and 18 h later, the acid–base disorder is hypokalemic hyperchloremic metabolic acidosis, and respiratory compensation is appropriate.

Question 2 Which one of the following agents causes these types of acid–base disorders?

(A) Topiramate
(B) Ifosfamide
(C) Toluene
(D) Cisplatin
(E) Tenofovir

The answer is C Toluene is initially metabolized to hippurate, which causes a high AG metabolic acidosis. Subsequently, hippurate is rapidly excreted in the urine with volume expansion, and the AG disappears. The typical acid–base disorder is hyperchloremic metabolic acidosis with severe hypokalemia. Hypokalemia is related to more distal delivery of Na^+ with hippurate, leaving Cl^- behind. Some of the patients are unable to acidify their urine due to impaired H^+ secretion. All other drugs cause proximal RTA with adequate urinary acidification once serum $[HCO_3^-]$ is below 18 mEq/L.

Case 3 A 34-year-old man, brought to the emergency department by his friend, complains of weakness, fatigue, poor appetite, and dizziness for 2 weeks. He has not seen any physician for 5 years. Other than daily cocaine use, he has no significant medical history. He is not on any prescription medications. Physical examination reveals orthostatic blood pressure and pulse changes. Except for anal condyloma acumunata, the remaining examination is unremarkable. Rapid HIV test is positive. Laboratory values on admission are:

Serum	Urine
Na^+ = 126 mEq/L	pH = 5.2
K^+ = 6.5 mEq/L	Glucose = negative
Cl^- = 110 mEq/L	Blood = negative
HCO_3^- = 13 mEq/L	Protein = negative
Creatinine = 2.1 mg/dL	Na^+ = 101 mEq/L
BUN = 42 mg/dL	K^+ = 30 mEq/L
Glucose = 60 mg/dL	Cl^- = 40 mEq/L
ABG: pH 7.29, pCO_2 28 mmHg, HCO_3^- 12 mEq/L	

Question 1 What is the acid–base disorder?

Answer Hyperkalemic hyperchloremic (non-AG) metabolic acidosis with appropriate respiratory compensation

Question 2 Which one of the following is the correct diagnosis?

(A) Proximal RTA (type II)
(B) Distal RTA (type I)
(C) Incomplete RTA (type III)
(D) Type IV RTA with hypoaldosteronism
(E) Hyperkalemic RTA with a defect in voltage gradient

The answer is D Serum and urine chemistry and orthostatic changes suggest Addison disease, which causes type IV RTA. Hypoaldosteronism due to adrenal gland destruction by viruses (HIV, CMV) and bacteria (mycobacterium tuberculosis) or fungal agents has been described. Patients with type IV RTA due to aldosterone deficiency can acidify their urine.

Proximal RTA is unlikely because of hyponatremia and hyperkalemia. Note that the patients with proximal RTA can acidify their urine at this level of serum [HCO_3^-], as all of this HCO_3^- can be reabsorbed and generate an acid urine.

Patients with incomplete RTA cannot acidify their urine even after an acid load. Also, hyperkalemic distal RTA patients with a defect in voltage gradient cannot acidify their urine. Therefore, options A, B, C, and E are incorrect.

Case 4 A 42-year-old man presents to his primary care physician for left flank pain and hematuria. Urinalysis reveals a pH of 6.9 and hematuria only. There is no evidence of UTI. Renal ultrasound shows the presence of kidney stones. He has no deafness. Serum chemistry and ABG show mild hypokalemic hyperchloremic metabolic acidosis. Serum creatinine is normal. He has a family history of kidney stones, and several members have mild hypokalemic hyperchloremic metabolic acidosis.

Question 1 Which one of the following RTAs is the MOST likely diagnosis?

(A) Proximal RTA
(B) Distal RTA
(C) Type IV RTA with aldosterone deficiency
(D) Incomplete RTA
(E) Hyperkalemic RTA with inability to acidy urine

The answer is B This patient has hereditary form of distal RTA with autosomal dominant inheritance. It occurs in adults. Autosomal recessive forms are diagnosed in infancy and childhood with or without deafness. Hyperkalemic RTA with a defect in voltage gradient is seen in patients with mild to moderate renal dysfunction. Type IV RTA patients with aldosterone deficiency have mild renal impairment and can acidify their urine. Patients with incomplete RTA may have a combination of both proximal and distal RTA. They may present with acid urine, but the diagnosis is established only after an acid load. Proximal RTA patients present with severe hypokalemia, but nephrolithiasis is uncommon. Thus, options A, C, D, and E are incorrect.

Question 2 What is the genetic defect in this patient?

(A) Mutations in the gene encoding Cl/HCO3 exchanger (anion exchanger 1, AE1)
(B) Mutations in the gene encoding B1 subunit of H-ATPase
(C) Mutations in the gene encoding a4 subunit of H-ATPase
(D) Mutations in the gene encoding carbonic anhydrase II (CA II) enzyme
(E) Deficiency of Na/H exchanger (NHE3)

The answer is A Autosomal dominant distal RTA is caused by mutations in the gene encoding the basolateral Cl/HCO_3 exchanger. They are unable to acidify their urine. They have mild hypokalemia and mild hyperchloremic acidosis. They have hypercalciuria with hypocitraturia with development of nephrocalcinosis/lithiasis later in life.

Gene mutations stated in options B and D cause autosomal recessive distal RTA with or without deafness, respectively. Deficiency of CA II enzyme causes distal RTA with osteopetrosis and cerebral calcifications. It occurs mostly in Arab populations of the Middle East. At times patients present with clinical manifestations of both proximal and distal RTAs. Deficiency of Na/H exchanger causes possibly autosomal dominant form of proximal RTA, and so far no gene mutations have been reported. Thus, options B, C, D, and E are incorrect.

Case 5 A 32-year-old woman with seizure disorder and migraine is consulted for hyperchloremic metabolic acidosis with serum [HCO_3^-] of 19 mEq/L. Her urine pH is 6.4.

Question 1 Which one of the following medications causes this acid–base disorder?

(A) Phenytoin
(B) Topiramate
(C) Levetiracetam
(D) Carbamazepine
(E) Gabapentin

The answer is B Except for topiramate, all other drugs are not known to cause hyperchloremic metabolic acidosis. Topiramate is a neuromodulator that is approved for use in the treatment of seizure activity and for migraine prophylaxis. Initially, it was observed that topiramate causes type II RTA and hyperchloremic metabolic acidosis in children. Since then, a number of case reports in adults have been described. Discontinuation of the drug improves serum [HCO_3^-] with resolution of RTA.

Question 2 Why is her urine pH alkaline?

Answer Topiramate is an inhibitor of carbonic anhydrase, causing HCO_3^- loss in the urine. This results in alkaline urine pH.

Case 6 A 65-year-old woman with type 2 diabetes is referred to by a primary care physician for evaluation of hyperkalemia. Other than hypertension, she has no significant medical history. Her medications include hydrochlorothiazide 25 mg QD, sitagliptin 50 mg QD, glipizide 5 mg QD, and lisinopril 20 mg

QD. Her blood pressure is 144/84 mmHg with a pulse rate of 82 beats/min. She has a trace pedal edema. The rest of the examination is normal. Recent laboratory results are:

Serum	Urine
Na^+ = 136 mEq/L	pH = 5.4
K^+ = 6.1 mEq/L	Glucose = negative
Cl^- = 110 mEq/L	Blood = negative
HCO_3^- = 19 mEq/L	Protein = 2+
Creatinine = 1.9 mg/dL (eGFR = 49 mL/min)	Protein/creatinine ratio = 1
BUN = 22 mg/dL	Na^+ = 80 mEq/L
Glucose = 120 mg/dL	K^+ = 30 mEq/L
A1c = 7.9%	Cl^- = 60 mEq/L

Question 1 What is the reason for her hyperkalemia with eGFR of 49 mL/min?

Answer Hyperkalemia is disproportionate to her renal dysfunction. From several studies, it is clear that diabetic patients develop hyperkalemia due to hyporeninemic hypoaldosteronism. In this patient, lisinopril, an ACE-I, can raise renin levels, but her aldosterone levels can be low. Table 29.8 shows some clinical features of hyporeninemic hypoaldosteronism.

Question 2 What is your suggestion for the management of her hyperkalemia?

Answer As stated before, type IV RTA can be managed by several ways. In this patient, switching diuretic to furosemide (discontinuation of hydrochlorothiazide) and restricting K^+ in diet may be sufficient to manage hyperkalemia. Also, better control of glucose (A1c 7–7.5%) and blood pressure is necessary.

Table 29.8 Clinical features of hyporeninemic hypoaldosteronism

Feature	Approximate prevalence
Age (year)	>50%
Presence of diabetes	50%
Hyperkalemia	75%
eGFR	>75%
Type IV RTA	>50%
Serum [HCO_3^-]	75%
Serum [HCO_3^-] <13 mEq/L	<1%
Hypertension	75%
Congestive heart failure	50%
Arrhythmias	24%

Case 7 A 44-year-old woman with Sjögren's syndrome with hypergammaglobu-linemia and tubulointerstitial disease is referred to renal clinic for evaluation of documented hypokalemic hyperchloremic metabolic acidosis. She was treated with corticosteroids for tubulointerstitial disease. Her serum $[HCO_3^-]$ is 16 mEq/L and eGFR is 56 mL/min. Serum phosphate, uric acid, and glucose levels are normal.

Question 1 What other pertinent lab test you order at this time?

(A) Arterial blood gas
(B) Renal biopsy to know the extent of interstitial disease
(C) Urine analysis
(D) Serum renin and aldosterone levels
(E) None

The answer is C It is important to know whether the patient is able to acidify or alkalin-ize her urine. Patients with Sjögren's syndrome can develop type I or type II RTA. At times, they can present with both type I and type II RTAs. Urine pH is an important deter-minant in the diagnosis of the type of RTA. All other tests are not important at this time.

Question 2 When urine pH is 6.8, what type of RTA does this patient have?

Answer Classic distal RTA (type I). Proximal or type II RTA patients can acidify their urine at serum $[HCO_3^-]$ of 16 mEq/L because all this HCO_3^- can be reabsorbed and the urine pH will be acidic.

Question 3 What is the mechanism of classic distal RTA in patients with Sjögren's syndrome?

Answer To my knowledge, there are two case reports that showed absence of H-ATPase in the cortical collecting duct on renal biopsies in these patients. This suggests that patients with Sjögren's syndrome are unable to secrete H^+ and acidify their urine.

Case 8 Match the following causes with their RTAs:

Cause	RTA
A. Obstructive uropathy	1. Classic distal RTA
B. Spironolactone	2. Hyperkalemic distal RTA with alkaline urine
C. Valproic acid	3. Hyperkalemic distal (type 4) RTA with acid urine
D. Ifosfamide	4. Proximal RTA
E. Amiloride	
F. Cyclosporine	
G. NSAIDs	
H. Medullary sponge kidney	

Answers A=2; B=3; C=4; D=4; E=2; F=1; G=3; H=1.

Suggested Reading

1. Batlle D, Haque SK. Genetic causes and mechanisms of distal renal tubular acidosis. Nephrol Dial Transplant. 2012;27:3691–704.
2. Golembiewska E, Ciechanowski K. Renal tubular acidosis-underrated problem? Acta Biochim Pol. 2012;59:213–7.
3. Haque SK, Ariceta G, Batlle D. Proximal renal tubular acidosis: a not so rare disorder of multiple etiologies. Nephrol Dial Transplant. 2012;27:4273–87.
4. Izzedine H, Launay-Vacher V, Isnard-Bagnis C, et al. Drug-induced Fanconi syndrome. Am J Kidney Dis. 2003;41:292–309.
5. Karet FE. Mechanisms in hyperkalemic renal tubular acidosis. J Am Soc Nephrol. 2009;20:251–4.
6. Kraut JA, Madias NE. Treatment of acute metabolic acidosis: a pathophysiologic approach. Nat Rev Nephrol. 2012;8:589–601.
7. Moorthi KMLST, Batlle D. Renal tubular acidosis. In: Gennari FJ, Adrogué HJ, Galla JH, Madias NE, editors. Acid-base disorders and their treatment. Boca Raton: Taylor & Francis; 2005. p. 417–67.
8. Reddy P. Clinical approach to renal tubular acidosis in adult patients. Int J Clin Pract. 2011;65:350–60.
9. Rodriguez-Soriano J. Renal tubular acidosis: the clinical entity. J Am Soc Nephrol. 2002;13:2160–70.

Hyperchloremic Metabolic Acidosis: Nonrenal Causes

30

In the previous chapter, we discussed both hypo- and hyperkalemic hyperchloremic metabolic acidoses due to renal causes. In this chapter, we will discuss hypokalemic hyperchloremic metabolic acidosis due to nonrenal causes, mostly gastrointestinal (GI) disorders. Table 30.1 shows nonrenal causes of hyperchloremic metabolic acidosis.

Before we discuss the pathophysiology of diarrhea, it is essential to understand water and electrolyte handling by the GI tract.

Water Handling

Figure 30.1 illustrates approximate daily water handling by the GI tract following a meal, which is summarized as follows:

- Daily intake of water from diet and drinking amounts to 2 L.
- Secretions from saliva, stomach, bile, pancreas, and small intestine amount to 7 L.

Table 30.1 Causes of nonrenal hyperchloremic metabolic acidosis

Intestinal	Diarrhea
	Biliary fistula
	Pancreatic fistula
	Villous adenoma
Gastrointestinal (GI)–ureteral connections	Ureterosigmoidostomy
	Ureterojejunostomy
	Ureteroileostomy
Drugs	Laxatives
	Cholestyramine

© Springer Science+Business Media LLC 2018
A.S. Reddi, *Fluid, Electrolyte and Acid-Base Disorders*,
DOI 10.1007/978-3-319-60167-0_30

Fig. 30.1 Water handling
by the normal
gastrointestinal tract

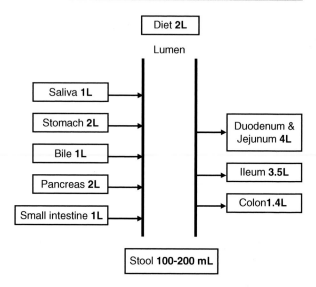

- Thus, the daily total handling of water by the GI tract is 9 L.
- Of these 9 L, 4 L are absorbed by the duodenum and jejunum, 3.5 L by the ileum, and 1.4 L by the colon, leaving 100–200 mL in the stool.

Intestinal Electrolyte Transport

Na⁺ and Cl⁻ Transport (Jejunum)

- The epithelial cells lining the small intestine and colon absorb most of the delivered electrolytes and water in isoosmolar concentrations. Thus, the fluid that is absorbed is always *isosmotic*. The absorption of Na⁺ and Cl⁻ in the small intestine is similar to that of the proximal tubule and involves the following transport mechanisms:

  1. Na⁺ transport coupled with solutes.
  2. Na/Cl cotransporter.
  3. Na⁺ transport alone via water channels.
  4. Na/H-ATPase with generation and absorption of HCO_3^-.
  5. Na⁺ exits via Na/K-ATPase.

Na⁺ and Cl⁻ Transport (Ileum)

- Same transport mechanisms as those in the jejunum and additionally a Cl/HCO₃ exchanger, which facilitates absorption of Cl⁻ and secretion of HCO_3^- into the lumen, are used.
- Thus, HCO_3^- absorption occurs in the jejunum, whereas its secretion occurs in the ileum.

Na⁺ and K⁺ Transport (Colon)

- Like principal cells, the epithelial cells of the colon contain Na^+ and K^+ channels separately.
- Absorption of Na^+ and secretion of K^+ occur via their respective channels.
- Aldosterone regulates both Na^+ and K^+ transports.

Intestinal Secretion of Cl⁻

- The epithelial cells lining the intestinal crypts secrete both electrolytes and water.
- The apical membrane of crypt cells contains Cl^- channels, and the basolateral membrane contains Na/K-ATPase, Na/K/2Cl cotransporter, and a K^+ channel. Na^+, K^+, and Cl^- enter the cells from blood via these transporters. Cl^- is secreted into the lumen via Cl^- channel, whereas Na^+ enters the lumen passively via the paracellular pathway. Subsequently, water moves into the lumen following NaCl secretion.
- Usually, Cl^- channels are closed but remain open following activating substances. These substances bind to their receptor at the basolateral membrane, leading to the stimulation of adenylate cyclase and production of cAMP in crypt cells. cAMP then keeps Cl^- channel open, facilitating its secretion into the lumen.

HCO₃⁻ Handling in the Colon

- Although HCO_3^- is secreted in the colon, all of it is not excreted in the stool. Most of this HCO_3^- is used up by the production of organic acids such as propionic acid, butyric acid, acetic acid, and lactic acid. These acids are the products of unabsorbed carbohydrates that are fermented by bacteria.
- Titration of these acids by $NaHCO_3$ generates sodium propionate, sodium butyrate, and other organic acids, which enter the liver for regeneration of HCO_3^-. Therefore, the stool contains low HCO_3^-.

Volume and Electrolyte Concentrations of GI Fluids

- Table 30.2 shows the normal values of electrolytes in various fluids of the GI tract. The information is useful in assessing the acid–base disturbances due to GI disorders.
- It is evident from Table 30.2 that the GI tract as a whole absorbs all the secreted Na^+ and Cl^-, leaving very few milliequivalents in the stool.
- More specifically, the jejunum absorbs about 100 mEq of Na^+ and 3 L of water, whereas the ileum absorbs 400 mEq each of Na^+ and Cl^- as well as 3.5 L of water.

Table 30.2 Volume and concentrations of electrolytes in fluids of normal GI tract

Source	Volume (L/day)	Na$^+$ (mEq/L)	K$^+$ (mEq/L)	Cl$^-$ (mEq/L)	HCO$_3^-$ (mEq/L)
Saliva (meal stimulated)	1	50–88	20	50	60
Gastric fluid (stimulated)	2	10–20	5–14	130–160	0
Bile	1	135–155	5–10	80–110	20
Pancreatic fluid	2	120–160	5–10	30–76	70–120
Small intestinal fluid	1	75–120	5–10	70–120	30
Stool	0.1–0.2	20–30	55–75	15–25	30

- Finally, the colon is the most efficient segment of the intestine, absorbing >90% of 200 mEq of Na$^+$, 100 mEq of Cl$^-$, and 1.4 L of water delivered to it. Because of this tremendous absorptive capacity of the colon, the stool contains <100–200 mL of water and low quantities of Na$^+$, Cl$^-$, and HCO$_3^-$; however, K$^+$ concentration in stool is more than the other electrolytes because of its secretion in the colon.

Diarrhea

Water and Electrolyte Loss

- Diarrhea is defined when stool weight exceeds 200 g/day or 200 mL/day, when secretions of fluids exceed their absorption.
- Diarrhea is the most common nonrenal cause of hyperchloremic metabolic acidosis.
- Unlike renal acidoses where hyperchloremic metabolic acidosis is due to defects in transport mechanisms, diarrhea or GI disorder-induced hyperchloremic metabolic acidosis is due to loss of HCO$_3^-$ and other electrolytes in the stool.
- The composition of the diarrheal fluid varies depending on the etiology of diarrhea (Table 30.3).

Types of Diarrhea

- Diarrhea is usually classified into the following types:

  1. Osmotic diarrhea (due to laxatives, poorly absorbed carbohydrates such as lactulose) characterizes loss of more water than electrolytes.
  2. Secretory diarrhea (increased secretions of water and electrolytes due to cholera, *Escherichia coli*-induced enterotoxin, or hormones such as vasointestinal polypeptide, or bile acids) causes more electrolyte than water loss
  3. Inflammatory diarrhea (due to loss of intestinal absorptive surface, cytokines).

Table 30.3 Volume and electrolyte composition of diarrheal fluid

Etiology of diarrhea	Volume (L/day)	Na^+ (mEq/L)	K^+ (mEq/L)	Cl^- (mEq/L)	HCO_3^- (mEq/L)
Stool (normal)	0.1–0.2	20–30	55–75	15–25	30
Osmotic	1–5	5–20	20–30	5–10	10
Secretory	1–20	75–140	15–40	75–105	30–75
Inflammatory (due to bowl disease) or infectious	1–3	50–100	15–20	50–100	10

4. Infectious diarrhea (due to loss of intestinal absorptive surface, cytokines).
- Table 30.3 shows the diarrheal fluid volume and electrolyte composition in various types of diarrhea.

It is evident from Table 30.3 that diarrhea causes the following:

1. Na^+ loss and volume depletion: hypernatremia in osmotic diarrhea if no water intake and hyponatremia in secretory diarrhea with water intake.
2. HCO_3^- loss in the stool: colonic HCO_3^- secretion is increased in secretory diarrhea; however, in other types of diarrhea, colonic loss may be offset by regeneration by the kidney. Persistent stool losses as well as inability of the kidney to secrete H^+ in the urine due to severe volume depletion can cause acidosis.
3. K^+ loss in the stool: hypokalemia occurs due to stool and renal loss mediated by aldosterone. Also, less K^+ intake may contribute to hypokalemia.

Diagnosis

- History, physical examination, and medications are important.
- Serum electrolytes, Ca^{2+}, Mg^{2+}, phosphate, albumin, and arterial blood gas (ABG).
- Urine anion gap (U_{AG}) is helpful in distinguishing between renal and nonrenal acidoses. U_{AG} is negative in diarrhea and positive in renal acidoses.
- Urine pH is <5.5 in moderate diarrhea and >6.5 in severe diarrhea because of volume depletion and increased urinary excretion of NH_4^+.
- Stool osmolal gap is not routinely calculated but is helpful in diagnosing the type of diarrhea.

Method of Calculating Stool Osmolal Gap

- Centrifuge at least 1.5 g of fresh stool, and separate supernatant from precipitate.
- Measure osmolality and electrolytes in supernatant.
- Calculate osmolal gap (mOsm/kg) as follows:
- Osmolal gap (mOsm/kg) = measured osmolality $-2 \times (Na^+ + K^+)$, where 2 accounts for the unmeasured anions accompanying the measured cations.

Interpretation

A positive value ≥50 mOsm/kg indicates unmeasured osmoles suggestive of osmotic diarrhea.

A negative value or a smaller positive value indicates secretory diarrhea.

Types of Acid–Base Disorders in Diarrhea

- In mild to moderate diarrhea, only hyperchloremic metabolic acidosis occurs (a decrease in serum [HCO$_3^-$] is accompanied by a proportionate increase in serum [Cl$^-$]), resulting in normal AG.
- However, mixed acid–base disorders are commonly seen in diarrheal states in the following clinical situations:

  1. Uncomplicated diarrhea: hyperchloremic metabolic acidosis (HCMA)
  2. Diarrhea + hypovolemia + hypotension or sepsis: HCMA + lactic acidosis
  3. Diarrhea + vomiting: HCMA + metabolic alkalosis
  4. Diarrhea + hyperventilation (gram-negative enteric pathogen): HCMA + respiratory alkalosis
  5. Diarrhea + sepsis + pneumonia: HCMA + lactic acidosis + respiratory alkalosis

- Figure 30.2 illustrates the pathogenesis of HCMA and other acid–base disorders in diarrhea.

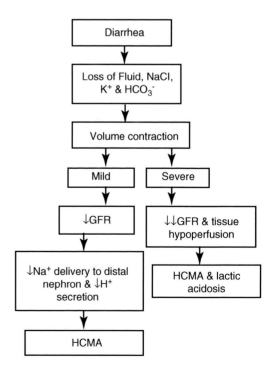

Fig. 30.2 Pathogenesis of hyperchloremic metabolic acidosis (*HCMA*) and combined lactic acidosis and HCMA in diarrhea. *GFR* glomerular filtration rate

Treatment

- Normal saline is required to replace volume loss, if there is mild volume depletion.
- Correction of volume deficit is crucial to improve renal function and facilitate H^+ secretion for regeneration of HCO_3^- by the kidney.
- Provide 0.45% saline with 75 mEq of $NaHCO_3$ to improve serum $[HCO_3^-]$ for severe acidemia. Treat hypokalemia with KCl prior to $NaHCO_3$ infusion, as $NaHCO_3$ lowers serum $[K^+]$ even further. Ringer's lactate can be used in selected patients following volume replacement.
- Treat the underlying cause of diarrhea simultaneously with replacement of fluid and electrolytes.
- In patients with acute or chronic noncholera diarrhea, oral replacement solution may be required. The standard World Health Organization Oral Rehydration Solution (311 mOsm/L) contains Na^+ (90 mEq/L), Cl^- 80 mEq/L), K^+ (20 mEq/L), glucose (111 mmol/L), and citrate (10 mEq/L). Some studies have shown that low osmolality solutions are associated with reduction in stool volume and duration of diarrhea.

Biliary and Pancreatic Fistulas

- Recall that bile and pancreatic secretions amount to 3 L and the $[HCO_3^-]$ is approximately 200–300 mEq.
- Consequently, any enterocutaneous fistulas or catheters draining any of these secretions can generate HCMA by losing HCO_3^- in excess of Cl^-.

Villous Adenoma

- Usually found in the colon with capacity to undergo malignant transformation.
- Interestingly, one tumor produces HCMA, and another tumor produces metabolic alkalosis by losing Cl^-.
- Prevention of severe volume depletion and resection of the tumor improve the acid–base disorder

Urinary Intestinal Diversions

- When the ureter or bladder is damaged, a diversion for urine to pass through a segment of the GI tract is created.
- The urine that enters the GI tract facilitates Cl^- absorption and HCO_3^- secretion via the Cl/HCO_3 exchanger present in the colon. This exchange is accentuated when the urine remains for a long period of time in the bowl.
- Loss of HCO_3^- in the stool and accumulation of Cl^- in blood result in HCMA.

- HCMA is common in ureterosigmoidostomy and less common with ureteroileostomy, because of rapid drainage of urine into ileostomy bag.
- Another way of HCMA development is absorption of NH_4^+ derived from urine and urea by the colon. Absorbed NH_4^+ is converted to NH_3 and H^+, and NH_3 is subsequently converted into urea. When a disturbance of this conversion occurs, acidosis develops.
- Note that patients with ureteral diversions may have other causes such as obstructive uropathy for HCMA.
- Hypokalemia results from active Na^+ absorption with creation of a favorable voltage gradient for K^+ secretion and also from secondary hyperaldosteronism.
- Treatment of HCMA depends on the severity of acidosis and volume status.

Laxative Abuse

- Laxative abuse is rather common mostly in younger women.
- Mild to moderate hypokalemic HCMA develops.
- Some patients may also develop metabolic alkalosis.
- Diagnosis is usually suspected when patients complain of alternating constipation and diarrhea, HCMA, and hypokalemia.
- The above clinical manifestations and hypermagnesemia suggest the use of Mg^{2+}-containing laxatives. Urine pH is >7 in these subjects.
- Phenolphthalein-containing laxatives stain pink with either NaOH or KOH.
- Treatment is correction of volume depletion and stopping laxative abuse by education as well as addressing psychiatric issues, if any.

Cholestyramine

- As an anion-exchange resin, cholestyramine is used to treat hypercholesterolemia. It also binds bile acids.
- As a resin, it adsorbs HCO_3^- and releases Cl^-, which is subsequently reabsorbed, resulting in HCMA.

Study Questions

Case 1 An 18-year-old female student is admitted for weakness, tiredness, and loose stools for 1 week. She denies diarrhea or any type of medications but admits to frequent urination. Physical examination reveals that she is thin with no apparent distress. Blood pressure is 100/60 mmHg with a pulse rate of 94 beats/minute with orthostatic changes. She is afebrile. Lungs and heart are normal. Abdomen is soft with no tenderness. There is no peripheral edema. Laboratory results:

Serum	Urine
Na^+ = 132 mEq/L	pH = 6.4
K^+ = 2.8 mEq/L	Osmolality = 800 mOsm/kg H_2O
Cl^- = 115 mEq/L	Na^+ = 20 mEq/L
HCO_3^- = 15 mEq/L	K^+ = 15 mEq/L
Creatinine = 1.5 mg/dL	Cl^- = 55 mEq/L
BUN = 30 mg/dL	
Glucose = 90 mg/dL	
Albumin = 4.2 g/dL	
ABG: pH = 7.32; PCO_2 = 30 mmHg; PO_2 = 98 mmHg	
HCO_3^- = 14 mEq/L	

BUN blood urea nitrogen, *ABG* arterial blood gas

Question 1 What is the acid–base disturbance in this patient?

Answer HCMA with appropriate respiratory response

Question 2 Which one of the following best describes the observed abnormalities in serum chemistry?

(A) Distal renal tubular acidosis (RTA)
(B) Diuretic abuse
(C) Laxative abuse
(D) Proximal RTA
(E) Surreptitious vomiting

The answer is C On the basis of the urine pH and HCMA, distal RTA can be considered; however, urine electrolytes do not support this diagnosis. Diuretic abuse may cause volume depletion and orthostatic changes, but urine pH, osmolality, and electrolyte pattern do not support diuretic abuse. Also, diuretics such as furosemide and hydrochlorothiazide cause metabolic alkalosis rather than metabolic acidosis. Carbonic anhydrase inhibitors such as acetazolamide cause HCMA with alkaline urine pH and proximal RTA; however, urine lytes do not support acetazolamide abuse. Proximal RTA is also unlikely because the urine pH is usually <5.5 with serum [HCO_3^-] of 15 mEq/L. Urine pH and electrolytes do not suggest late vomiting, as early and late vomiting cause low Cl^- and high K^+ excretion. During early vomiting, the urine pH is alkaline because of HCO_3^- excretion, and during late vomiting, pH is acidic because of H^+ secretion. Thus, options A, B, D, and E are incorrect.

The patient agrees to laxative abuse, which is confirmed by stool testing with NaOH. Laxative abusers will have diarrhea-induced volume depletion and the electrolyte abnormalities as described earlier.

Question 3 Why is her urine pH alkaline rather than acidic as in diarrhea?

Answer Generally, diarrhea causes acidic urine pH. However, when volume depletion is severe owing to diarrhea, NH_4^+ excretion is increased, which raises urine pH.

Question 4 Is there any evidence in this patient that NH_4^+ excretion increased?

Answer Yes. The U_{AG} is negative ($U_{Na} + U_K - U_{Cl}$ or $20 + 15 - 55 = -20$), suggesting high NH_4^+ excretion. This test also rules out both proximal and distal RTAs.

Case 2 A 55-year-old man with HIV is admitted for profuse diarrhea, volume depletion, and weakness. Despite highly active antiretroviral therapy (HAART) medications, diarrhea developed 10 days ago with gradual worsening of his symptoms. Blood pressure, electrolytes, and ABG were similar to case 1, except for pH of 7.20.

Question 1 How would you manage this patient?

Answer There are three major diarrhea-induced complications in this patient: (1) volume depletion, (2) hypokalemia, and (3) severe metabolic acidosis.

Volume Depletion and Hypokalemia Normal saline is the fluid of choice, as he has orthostatic blood pressure and pulse changes. Hypokalemia should be corrected before infusion of normal saline, as volume expansion improves glomerular filtration rate (GFR) and promotes K^+ excretion. Oral KCl is always preferred to IV KCl if the patient can take it by mouth. Otherwise, IV KCl 20 mEq/L/h can be given. Another way (some physicians prefer) is adding 75 mEq of KCl to 0.45% saline to make the fluid isotonic. Infusion of 200–250 mL/h for 4 h will improve volume and blood pressure status. This regimen should be continued with less infusion of fluid until serum $[K^+]$ is >3.5 mEq/L, and then assess the need for KCl supplementation.

Some physicians prefer Ringer's lactate to replenish electrolytes, but volume expansion and correction of Na^+ are less than normal saline. Intravenous K citrate can also be given once renal function is normalized.

Correction of Acidosis Once hypokalemia and volume are partially corrected, serum $[HCO_3^-]$ decreases. Therefore, $NaHCO_3$ should be given to improve $[HCO_3^-]$ and pH. One needs to calculate ΔHCO_3^-, and then $NaHCO_3$ should be given, as shown in the following example:

$$\text{Body weight} = 70\,\text{kg}$$
$$HCO_3^- \text{ space} = 50\%$$
$$\Delta HCO_3^- = 4\,(\text{increase from 15 to 19 mEq})$$
$$\text{Required NaHCO}_3 \text{ to raise serum HCO}_3^- \text{ from 15 to 19 mEq/L:}$$
$$70 \times 0.5 \times 4 = 140\,\text{mEq}$$

Add 140–150 mEq of $NaHCO_3$ to 5% dextrose in water (D5W), and infuse over 6–8 h, provided serum $[K^+]$ is >3.5 mEq/L; otherwise, hypokalemia develops.

The cause of diarrhea should be investigated and treated appropriately. Osmotic diarrhea will improve with fasting but not secretory diarrhea.

Question 2 Match the following electrolyte and ABG values with the case histories:

(A) Patient with simple diarrhea
(B) Patient with diarrhea and vomiting
(C) Patient with diarrhea and lactic acidosis
(D) Patient with diarrhea and respiratory alkalosis due to pneumonia

Option	Na^+ (mEq/L)	K^+ (mEq/L)	Cl^- (mEq/L)	HCO_3^- (mEq/L)	pH	pCO_2 (mmHg)
1	138	2.4	120	9	7.32	18
2	140	3.2	116	5	7.13	14
3	134	2.8	104	23	7.40	38
4	136	3.1	114	12	7.28	26

Answers A = 4; B = 3; C = 2; D = 1. Calculation of serum AG is helpful, because lactic acidosis is associated with elevated AG. The serum AG in option 2 is 19 and therefore associated with case C. All other cases have normal serum AG.

Patient with diarrhea and vomiting should have near-normal serum [HCO_3^-] compared with other cases, because vomiting is associated with low serum [Cl^-]. Serum pH should be normal (diarrhea causes low pH and vomiting raises pH. When both coexist, the pH becomes normal). Thus, option 3 corresponds to case B.

Patient with diarrhea and respiratory alkalosis should have relatively low HCO_3^-, high Cl^-, and near-normal pH. Electrolytes and ABG described in option 1 are consistent with case D.

Uncomplicated diarrhea is associated with moderate acidemia, and electrolyte and ABG pattern is consistent with option 4.

Suggested Reading

1. Atia AN, Buchman AL. Oral rehydration solutions in non-cholera diarrhea: a review. Am J Gastroenterol. 2009;104:2596–604.
2. Batlle DC. Hyperchloremic metabolic acidosis. In: Seldin DW, Giebisch G, editors. The regulation of acid-base balance. New York: Raven Press; 1989. p. 319–51.
3. Charney AN, Danowitz M. Gastrointestinal influences on hydrogen ion balance. In: Gennari FJ, Adrogué HJ, Galla JH, Madias NE, editors. Acid-base disorders and their treatment. Boca Raton: Taylor & Francis; 2005. p. 209–40.
4. Field M. Intestinal ion transport and the pathophysiology of diarrhea. J Clin Invest. 2003;111:931–43.
5. Gennari FJ, Weise WJ. Acid-base disturbances in gastrointestinal disease. Clin J Am Soc Nephrol. 2008;3:1861–8.
6. Kent AJ, Banks MR. Pharmacological management of diarrhea. Gastroenterol Clin N Am. 2010;39:495–507.
7. Kunzelmann K, Mall M. Electrolyte transport in the mammalian colon: mechanisms and implications for disease. Physiol Rev. 2002;82:245–89.
8. Wesson DE, Laski M. Hyperchloremic metabolic acidosis due to intestinal losses and other nonrenal causes. In: Gennari FJ, Adrogué HJ, Galla JH, Madias NE, editors. Acid-base disorders and their treatment. Boca Raton: Taylor & Francis; 2005. p. 487–99.

Metabolic Alkalosis

<big>**31**</big>

Metabolic alkalosis is defined as a primary increase in serum $[HCO_3^-] > 26$ mEq/L with pH >7.45. Hypoventilation with an increase in arterial pCO_2 is an appropriate respiratory response for an increase in serum $[HCO_3^-]$. Thus, metabolic alkalosis is characterized by an elevated pH, an increase in serum $[HCO_3^-]$, and an elevated pCO_2.

Course of Metabolic Alkalosis

The course of metabolic alkalosis is divided into three phases: generation phase, maintenance phase, and recovery phase.

Generation Phase

Generation occurs either by loss of H^+ from the body or addition of alkali by any one of the causes shown in Table 31.1.

© Springer Science+Business Media LLC 2018
A.S. Reddi, *Fluid, Electrolyte and Acid-Base Disorders*,
DOI 10.1007/978-3-319-60167-0_31

Table 31.1 Causes of metabolic alkalosis

Chloride-responsive alkalosis	Chloride-resistant alkalosis
Gastrointestinal (GI) and renal-associated	*Hypertension-associated*
Vomiting	Primary aldosteronism
Nasogastric suction	11β-hydroxysteroid dehydrogenase type 2 deficiency
Congenital chloride diarrhea	Licorice, chewing tobacco, and carbenoxolone
Villous adenoma	Fludrocortisone administration
Posthypercapnia	Cushing syndrome
Contraction alkalosis[a]	Glucocorticoid-remediable aldosteronism
Cystic fibrosis	Hyperreninism and hyperaldosteronism (malignant and renovascular hypertension, renin-secreting tumors)
Severe K^+ deficiency	Liddle syndrome
Milk–alkali syndrome	*Normotension-associated*
Gastrocystoplasty	Bartter syndrome
Zollinger–Ellison syndrome	Gitelman syndrome
Drug-associated	*Others*
Loop diuretics	Hypercalcemia
Thiazide diuretics	Hypoparathyroidism
Poorly reabsorbable anions (carbenicillin, penicillin, phosphate, sulfate)	Post-feeding alkalosis
$NaHCO_3$ (baking soda)	
Sodium citrate, lactate, gluconate, and acetate	
Antacids	
Transfusions	

[a]The term contraction alkalosis should not be used routinely since it implies that serum $[HCO_3^-]$ increases because of loss of water. This increase in serum $[HCO_3^-]$ alone does not generate metabolic alkalosis, but contraction (volume depletion) does maintain alkalosis

Maintenance Phase

Following generation, persistence of metabolic alkalosis is maintained by volume depletion (Cl^- responsive), Cl^- deficiency, K^+ deficiency, low glomerular filtration rate (GFR), or excess mineralocorticoid activity.

Cl^- depletion sustains metabolic alkalosis by the following mechanisms (Fig. 31.1):

1. Cl^- depletion inhibits K^+ reabsorption in the thick ascending limb of Henle's loop (TALH) via Na/K/2Cl cotransporter.
2. Along with K^+, Na^+ reabsorption is also impaired in the TALH. This causes more delivery of Na^+ to the cortical collecting duct (CCD), where it is reabsorbed via the luminal epithelial Na^+ channel (ENaC). Reabsorption of Na creates a negative lumen potential, resulting in K^+ and H^+ secretion.
3. Cl^- depletion causes decreased delivery of Cl^- to the CCD where HCO_3^- secretion is reduced via apical Cl/HCO_3 exchanger located in the intercalated type B

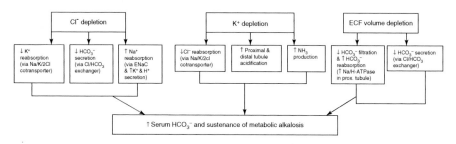

Fig. 31.1 Factors that generate and maintain metabolic alkalosis

cell. Thus, Cl⁻ depletion maintains metabolic alkalosis by causing hypokalemia and hyperbicarbonatemia.

K^+ depletion maintains metabolic alkalosis by the following mechanisms (Fig. 31.1):

1. A decrease in intracellular pH due to movement of H^+ into the cell to replace K^+ loss
2. An increase in HCO_3^- reabsorption by enhanced activities of luminal Na/H⁻ ATPase and basolateral Na/HCO_3 cotransporters in the proximal tubule
3. An increase in distal tubule acidification by activating H-ATPase in response to the increased production of NH_3
4. A decrease in Na/K/2Cl cotransporter activity due to Cl⁻ depletion in the TALH
5. Reduction of GFR by both K^+ and Cl⁻ depletion

Recovery Phase

Correction of Cl⁻, K^+, and treatment of underlying cause improves metabolic alkalosis.

Figure 31.1 summarizes the mechanisms for generation and maintenance of metabolic alkalosis. Cl⁻ loss with Na^+ induces volume contraction. Also, Cl⁻ depletion causes K^+ loss. Therefore, NaCl administration corrects certain cases of metabolic alkalosis. Mineralocorticoid excess stimulates Na^+ reabsorption and, in turn, promotes K^+ and H^+ secretion. Volume status is variable (↑ in primary aldosteronism and ↓ in Gitelman syndrome).

Respiratory Response to Metabolic Alkalosis

An increase in pCO_2 due to hypoventilation is a normal response to metabolic alkalosis, so that extremely dangerous levels of blood pH are avoided. On average, pCO_2 increases by 0.7 mmHg (above normal pCO_2 of 40 mmHg) for each mEq/L increase in serum $[HCO_3^-]$ (above normal $[HCO_3^-]$ of 24 mEq/L). The following example shows the appropriate respiratory response to an increase in pCO_2 in metabolic alkalosis.

$$\underline{pH} \quad \underline{HCO_3^-} \quad \underline{pCO_2}$$

Normal : 7.40   24 mEq / L   40 mmHg

Patient : 7.47   34 mEq / L   ?

Example

$$\Delta HCO_3^- = 34 - 24 = 10$$
$$\text{Expected } pCO_2 = 10 \times 0.7 = 7$$
$$40 + 7 = 47$$

Classification

Clinically, metabolic alkalosis is divided into:

1. Chloride (saline)-responsive alkalosis
2. Chloride (saline)-resistant alkalosis

Causes

The most important causes of metabolic alkalosis are shown in Table 31.1.

Pathophysiology

For simplicity, the pathophysiology of metabolic alkalosis is discussed in selective conditions and under two major mechanisms: renal and gastrointestinal (GI).

Renal Mechanisms

Renal Transport Mechanisms

Since retention of HCO_3^- and secretion of H^+ are responsible for the development of metabolic alkalosis, it is important to recall the normal cellular mechanisms involved in their renal handling (Chap. 26). Disturbances in these transport mechanisms cause metabolic alkalosis by retention of HCO_3^- and secretion of H^+. Table 31.2 summarizes the transport mechanisms and their modifiers for HCO_3^- reabsorption and sustenance of metabolic alkalosis.

Table 31.2 Renal mechanisms for increased HCO_3^- reabsorption

Tubule	Transporter	Mechanism for HCO_3^- reabsorption
PT	Na/H-ATPase	$\downarrow$ K$^+$ (hypokalemia) stimulates H$^+$ secretion
	H-ATPase	$\downarrow$ K$^+$ stimulates H$^+$ secretion
TALH	Na/K/2Cl cotransporter	(1) $\uparrow$ Delivery of NaCl to CCD, resulting in $\uparrow$ Na$^+$ reabsorption with subsequent $\uparrow$ K$^+$ and H$^+$ secretion due to the loop diuretic inhibition of cotransporter
		(2) Bartter syndrome due to mutation in cotransporter
		(3) $\downarrow$ K$^+$ inhibition of cotransporter
		(4) Cl$^-$ depletion by above mechanisms
DCT	Na/Cl cotransporter	(1) $\uparrow$ Delivery of NaCl to CCD, resulting in $\uparrow$ Na$^+$ reabsorption with subsequent $\uparrow$ K$^+$ and H$^+$ secretion due to thiazide diuretic inhibition of cotransporter
		(2) $\downarrow$ K$^+$ inhibition of cotransporter
		(3) Gitelman syndrome due to mutation in cotransporter
CCD		
Principal cell	ENaC	Liddle syndrome due to mutation in ENaC
β-intercalated cell	Pendrin (Cl/HCO$_3$ exchanger)	(1) Hypokalemia downregulates pendrin, resulting in the maintenance of metabolic alkalosis
		(2) Loss-of-function mutation of gene encoding pendrin aggravates metabolic alkalosis
		(3) Thiazide therapy aggravates metabolic alkalosis in Pendred syndrome
α-intercalated cell	H-ATPase	$\uparrow$ H$^+$ secretion in response to $\uparrow$ Na$^+$ delivery to ENaC due to loop diuretics
	H/K-ATPase	Same as above

PT proximal tubule, *TALH* thick ascending limb of Henle's loop, *DCT* distal convoluted tubule, *CCD* cortical collecting duct, $\uparrow$ increase, and $\downarrow$ decrease

Genetic Mechanisms (See Chap. 15 for Details)

- *Bartter syndrome*: caused by genetic defects in the apical or basolateral membrane transport mechanisms of the thick ascending limb of Henle's loop.
- Behaves similarly to a patient on loop diuretics.
- Generation phase is due to increased loss of H$^+$ in the urine.
- Maintenance phase is due to K$^+$ and Cl$^-$ loss, volume depletion, and secondary hyperaldosteronism.
- Characterized by hypokalemia, metabolic alkalosis, and normal blood pressure or at times hypotension.
- Treatment includes chronic supplementation of K$^+$. Spironolactone, amiloride, ACE-inhibitors, and nonsteroidal anti-inflammatory drugs have been tried with variable results.

- *Gitelman syndrome*: caused by mutations in the distal tubule Na/Cl cotransporter.
- Behaves similarly to a patient on thiazide diuretics.
- Generation and maintenance phases are similar to those of Bartter syndrome.
- Characterized by hypokalemia, hypomagnesemia, metabolic alkalosis, and normal blood pressure.
- Treatment includes lifelong liberal salt intake, K^+ and Mg^{2+} supplementation (KCl, $MgCl_2$), as well as K^+-sparing diuretics (spironolactone, amiloride, aldosterone-receptor blocker)
- *Liddle syndrome*: An autosomal dominant disorder, caused by mutations in the subunits of ENaC.
- Generation of metabolic alkalosis is caused by increased K^+ and H^+ loss, and maintenance is due to hypokalemia and hypochloremia.
- Aldosterone levels are low because of Na^+ reabsorption and volume expansion.
- Characterized by hypokalemia, metabolic alkalosis, and hypertension.
- Hypertension does not respond to spironolactone. Amiloride is the drug of choice.
- *Glucocorticoid-remediable hyperaldosteronism (GRA)*: Also called familial hyperaldosteronism type I.
- Caused by fusion of two enzymes: aldosterone synthase and 11β-hydroxylase.
- Patients present with hypokalemia, metabolic alkalosis, and hypertension.
- Administration of glucocorticoid improves hypokalemia, metabolic alkalosis, and hypertension.
- *Apparent mineralocorticoid excess (AME) syndrome*: Cortisol is not converted into inactive cortisone by the mutated enzyme 11β-hydroxysteroid dehydrogenase type 2.
- Patients present with hypokalemia, metabolic alkalosis, and hypertension.
- Treatment with spironolactone or amiloride improves hypokalemia, alkalosis, and hypertension.
- AME can also be acquired. Ingestion of licorice, chewing tobacco, bioflavonoids, or carbenoxolone can cause AME. These agents contain glycyrrhetinic acid, which is a competitive inhibitor of 11β-hydroxysteroid dehydrogenase type 2.
- Clinical manifestations are similar to the genetic type of AME.

Acquired Causes

- *Primary aldosteronism*: caused by autonomous secretion of aldosterone by adrenal adenoma or hyperplasia of the adrenal gland.
- Alkalosis is generated by K^+ and H^+ loss due to the increased delivery of NaCl to the distal nephron.
- Hypokalemia, hypochloremia, and persistent aldosterone activity maintain metabolic alkalosis.
- Characterized by hypokalemia, hypertension, and metabolic alkalosis.

- Removal of adenoma or treatment with K^+-sparing diuretics (spironolactone) corrects metabolic abnormalities and hypertension.
- *Malignant hypertension*: a disorder of high-renin-AII-aldosterone activity.
- Characterized by hypertension, hypokalemia, and metabolic alkalosis.
- *Renal artery stenosis*: clinically similar to malignant hypertension with high-renin-AII-aldosterone activity.
- Patients present with severe hypokalemia, hypertension, and metabolic alkalosis.
- Removal of stenosis by stents or surgery improves hypokalemia, metabolic alkalosis, and hypertension.
- *Drugs other than diuretics*: Exogenous alkali causes metabolic alkalosis only when the subject is hypovolemic with compromised renal function. Dialysis patients develop metabolic alkalosis due to the use of HCO_3^- in the dialysate bath.
- One study showed that daily ingestion of 140 g (1667 mEq) of baking soda ($NaHCO_3$) for up to 3 weeks raises serum $[HCO_3^-]$ and causes metabolic alkalosis.
- Metabolic alkalosis resolves following discontinuation of $NaHCO_3^-$ provided hypokalemia and volume depletion are absent; however, it continues once renal failure develops.
- Delivery of nonreabsorbable anions such as sodium penicillin to the distal tubule promotes K^+ secretion, resulting in hypokalemia and metabolic alkalosis.
- *Diuretics*: Diuretics other than acetazolamide and K^+-sparing diuretics generate metabolic alkalosis
- Mechanisms include:
  1. Relative volume depletion by loss of NaCl
  2. Hypokalemia
  3. Hypochloremia
  4. Increased net acid secretion due to hyperaldosteronism (most important)
- Note that urine Cl^- may be a variable; high when diuretic action is maximum and low after 24 h of diuretic ingestion.
- *Posthypercapnic metabolic alkalosis*: This condition results in patients with chronic respiratory acidosis with high HCO_3^- and pCO_2.
- When such patients require intubation and pCO_2 is acutely lowered, blood pH goes up without a change in serum $[HCO_3^-]$.
- Since the kidneys cannot excrete HCO_3^- immediately, the pH should be corrected by any one or all of the following treatments:
  1. Increase pCO_2.
  2. Lower serum $[HCO_3^-]$ by administration of normal saline and/or acetazolamide.
  3. To lower pH acutely, some physicians use HCl administration, but this option is rarely required.

Table 31.3 summarizes various laboratory tests that are useful in the differential diagnosis of metabolic alkalosis.

Table 31.3 Serum renin, aldosterone (aldo), urine electrolytes, and pH in metabolic alkalosis

Condition	Renin	Aldo	Na$^+$ (mEq/L)	K$^+$ (mEq/L)	Cl$^-$ (mEq/L)	HCO$_3^-$ (mEq/L)	pH	Volume status
Bartter syndrome	↑	↑	↑	↑	↑	↓	↓ (acid)	↓
Gitelman syndrome	↑	↑	↑	↑	↑	↓	↓	↓
Liddle syndrome	↓	↓	N↑	↑	↑	↑	↓	↑
Licorice	↓	↓	↑	↑	↑	↓	↓	↑
AME	↓	↓	↑	↑	↑	↓	↓	↑
GRA	↓	↑	↑	↑	↑	↓	↓	↑
Primary aldosteronism	↓	↑	↑	↑	↑	↓	↓	↑
Malignant and renovascular HTN	↑	↑	↑	↑	↑	↓	↓	↓
Diuretics (loop and thiazide)	↑	↑	↓↑^{a}	↑	↑	↓	↓	↓

AME apparent mineralocorticoid excess syndrome, *GRA* glucocorticoid-remediable hyperaldosteronism, *N* normal, ↑ increase, and ↓ decrease
^{a}Variable

GI Mechanisms

Vomiting and Nasogastric Suction

These are the most common causes of metabolic alkalosis besides diuretic use.

- On average, gastric fluid contains the following electrolytes in mEq/L:

$$H^+ \quad = 100$$
$$Cl^- \quad = 120$$
$$Na^+ \quad = 15$$
$$K^+ \quad = 10$$
$$Volume = 1L$$

- Generation of alkalosis starts with the loss of HCl, resulting in addition of HCO$_3^-$ and loss of Cl$^-$.
- Glomerular filtration of Cl$^-$ is reduced.
- Initially, the kidney gets rid of HCO$_3^-$, which obligates Na$^+$ and K$^+$ excretion.
- Because of bicarbonaturia, the urine pH is alkaline (>6.5).

Table 31.4 Urinary electrolyte (mEq/L) pattern and pH in vomiting

Vomiting	Na⁺	K⁺	Cl⁻	HCO₃⁻	pH
Early (1–2 days)	↑	↑	↓	↑	↑
Late (> 2 days)	↓	↑	↓	↓	↓

- If vomiting or gastric suction continues, loss of Na^+ and water results in volume depletion. Na^+ and HCO_3^- reabsorption increases, and their excretion is decreased.
- Na^+ reabsorption is accompanied by the secretion of H^+ and K^+, resulting in net acid excretion, and urine pH becomes acidic (Table 31.4).
- Metabolic alkalosis is, therefore, maintained by hypokalemia and volume depletion.
- Table 31.4 shows urinary electrolyte pattern in early (1–2 days) and late (>2 days) vomiting.
- Treatment: Both volume repletion with normal saline and correction of hypokalemia with KCl improve metabolic alkalosis.
- Correction of the cause of vomiting should be addressed to prevent metabolic alkalosis.
- Urine $Cl^->40$–50 mEq/L and urine pH >6.5 during treatment are indications of volume expansion as well as improvement in metabolic alkalosis.

Congenital Chloride Diarrhea

This is inherited as an autosomal recessive disease.

- Cl^- absorption in the ileum and colon is decreased due to mutations in the Cl/HCO_3 exchanger, resulting in stool loss of Cl^-.
- Extremely large fecal losses of Na^+, K^+, and water result in hypokalemia, volume depletion, and metabolic alkalosis.
- Secondary hyperaldosteronism increases body volume by Na^+ and water reabsorption while promoting maintenance of alkalosis by secretion of K^+ and H^+.
- Urinary Cl^- and K^+ levels are low because of their loss in the stool.
- Neonatal abdominal distention due to intestinal dilatation and maternal polyhydramnios are the clues to the diagnosis of this disease.

Villous Adenoma

Metabolic acidosis is common; however, some patients develop metabolic alkalosis.

- Fecal loss of NaCl and HCO_3^- and water seem to generate and maintain metabolic alkalosis.

Laxative Abuse

Similar to villous adenoma, laxative abuse causes hyperchloremic metabolic acidosis. However, some case reports documented metabolic alkalosis simulating Bartter syndrome.

- Urine Cl^- and K^+ are low.
- Hydration with NaCl, K^+ supplementation, and discontinuation of laxative improves metabolic alkalosis.

Clinical Manifestations

Severe metabolic alkalosis affects several organ systems, including central nervous system and neuromuscular, cardiovascular, and pulmonary systems. In addition, several metabolic abnormalities have been reported. Table 31.5 summarizes these manifestations.

Table 31.5 Clinical manifestations of metabolic alkalosis

Central nervous system
Reduction in blood flow
Confusion
Obtundation
Reduced seizure threshold
Neuromuscular
Increased excitability
Tetany
Cardiovascular
Reduced cardiac output
Reduced coronary blood flow
Arteriolar vasoconstriction
Increased heart rate
Predisposition to refractory ventricular and supraventricular arrhythmias
Pulmonary
Hypoventilation
Hypercapnia
Hypoxia
Metabolic
Hypokalemia
Decreased ionized Ca^{2+}
Hypophosphatemia
Hypomagnesemia
Stimulation of glycolysis and production of lactate

Diagnosis

Step 1

- History of diuretic use, exogenous intake of antacids, Ca^{2+} supplements, laxatives, licorice, and inquiries into vomiting, bulimia, family, or personal history of hypertension are extremely important.
- Complaint of alternating diarrhea and constipation is suggestive of laxative abuse.

Step 2

- Physical examination includes:
  1. Blood pressure
  2. Volume status
  3. Examination of teeth enamel (usually black due to gastric HCl)
  4. Examination of the dorsum of the hand for scarring and hypertrophy of salivary glands (habitual vomiting)
  5. Peripheral edema in young women unrelated to pregnancy and menstruation (suspect diuretic use for idiopathic edema)

Step 3

- Laboratory tests:
  - Serum electrolytes, including creatinine, BUN, Ca^{2+}, Mg^{2+}, phosphate, and albumin.
  - ABG to exclude chronic respiratory acidosis.
  - Urine electrolytes and pH (see Tables 31.3 and 31.4).
  - Of all urine electrolytes, urine Cl^- is the most important electrolyte that distinguishes Cl^--responsive from Cl^--resistant alkalosis.
- Figure 31.2 illustrates the use of urine Cl^- determination in the evaluation of metabolic alkalosis.

Serum anion gap (AG) is increased in metabolic alkalosis due to (1) an increase in albumin with negative charge on it and (2) an increase in glycolysis due to stimulation of the rate-limiting enzyme, phosphofructokinase, and lactic acid production. Although the AG up to 8 mEq/L has been observed, its clinical importance has never been appreciated in metabolic alkalosis.

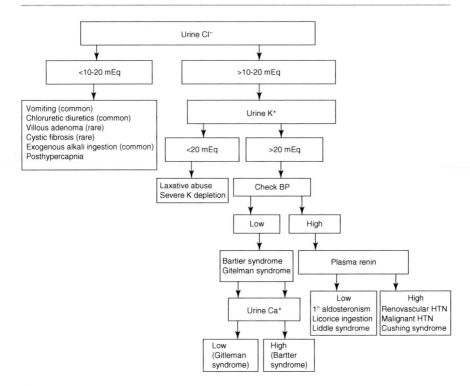

Fig. 31.2 Evaluation of metabolic alkalosis

Treatment

Treatment includes:

1. Address the specific cause, and correct it.
2. Volume depletion: common in many patients with metabolic alkalosis. Administration of normal saline is the appropriate therapy in such patients. It replaces volume and Cl^- loss.
3. Administer KCl orally or IV for severe hypokalemia.
4. Avoid Ringer's lactate, as lactate is converted into HCO_3^- and worsens alkalosis.
5. Intravenous HCl (0.1 or 0.2 M) is indicated when NaCl and KCl administrations are contraindicated, blood pH >7.5, or hypervolemic.
6. HCl should be infused via a large vein to avoid extravasation at <0.2 mEq/kg/h. The amount of HCl needed to lower serum $[HCO_3^-]$ from 40 to 34 mEq/L is calculated as follows:

$$\text{Weight (kg)} = 70$$
$$H^+ \text{ space} = 50\%$$
$$\Delta HCO_3^- = 6 (\text{decrement from 40 to 34 mEq/L})$$
$$70 \times 0.5 \times 6 = 210 \text{ mEq}$$

7. An alternative to HCl is NH_4Cl or arginine HCl. NH_4Cl is contraindicated in hepatic and renal failure.
8. Acetazolamide (250 mg BID or TID) is used to improve metabolic alkalosis in patients with volume overload and normal renal function.
9. When a renal failure patient fails to respond to Cl^- repletion, renal replacement therapy (hemodialysis, peritoneal dialysis, or hemodiafiltration) is indicated.
10. Occasionally, in patients with protracted vomiting or prolonged nasogastric suction, H_2 blockers such as cimetidine or ranitidine or H/K-ATPase inhibitor such as omeprazole can blunt acid production in the stomach and reduce HCl loss.
11. Omeprazole is effective in the treatment of alkalosis in patients with gastrocystoplasty.
12. Octreotide is used to control hypergastrinemia in Zollinger–Ellison syndrome.

Study Questions

Case 1 A 42-year-old man is admitted for dizziness and weakness. His blood pressure is 120/80 mmHg with a pulse rate of 90 beats per minute (sitting) and 100/64 mmHg with a pulse rate of 110 beats per minute (standing). He is not on any medications but admits to vomiting. Admitting laboratory data:

Electrolytes	ABG
Na^+ = 129 mEq/L	pH = 7.53
K^+ = 2.5 mEq/L	pCO_2 = 63 mmHg
Cl^- = 58 mEq/L	HCO_3^- = 57 mEq/L
HCO_3^- = 58 mEq/L	
Creatinine = 1.9 mg/dL	
BUN = 32 mg/dL	
Glucose = 94 mg/dL	

Question 1 Analyze the acid–base disturbance.

Answer To analyze this acid–base disorder, follow the steps 1–5 shown in Chap. 27.

Step 1 According to the Henderson equation, the $[H^+]$ is 26, which corresponds to a pH of 7.53. Therefore, the reported pH is correct.

Step 2 Based on elevated pH and serum $[HCO_3^-]$, the primary acid–base disturbance is metabolic alkalosis.

Step 3 The AG is 13, which is slightly elevated due to alkalemia.

Step 4 The cause for metabolic alkalosis is vomiting.

Step 5 The respiratory compensation is appropriate, suggesting that this acid–base disturbance is an uncomplicated metabolic alkalosis.

Question 2 What other laboratory test should you order?

Answer The laboratory test that is pertinent to this acid–base disorder is the determination of urinary Cl^-, which is 5 mEq/L. The patient, therefore, has Cl^--responsive metabolic alkalosis.

Question 3 Why did the patient develop hypokalemia, if he had only vomiting?

Answer There are two mechanisms for hypokalemia: (1) volume depletion-induced hyperaldosteronism and (2) adequate delivery of Na^+ with HCO_3^- to the cortical collecting duct where Na^+ is reabsorbed and K^+ is secreted.

Question 4 How would you treat this acid–base disturbance?

Answer The patient is volume depleted with orthostatic blood pressure and pulse changes. The appropriate IV fluid is normal (0.9%) saline with K^+ supplementation, which replenishes both volume and Cl^-.

Case 2 The patient is a 65-year-old man who was brought to the Emergency Department (ED) after being found on the floor at home due to a fall. He was awake and alert but oriented to place and time only. He was then noted to have a draining wound of his left foot that was wrapped in plastic. The patient complained of generalized weakness with muscle cramps and poor appetite for a few days. He also admitted to difficulty in walking from his foot ulcer. While in the ED, the patient became agitated, requiring intubation for airway protection. Past medical history included only foot ulcers for 2 years. He was hospitalized 2 weeks prior to this admission at another hospital. He was treated with intravenous antibiotics for 1 week and discharged. He was not on any medications.

On admission, his blood pressure was 131/77 mmHg with a regular pulse rate of 82 per minute. He was afebrile. His body mass index was 18.2. He was well developed but poorly nourished. Except for a well-demarcated left lower foot ulcer with unclean margins extending from distally one-third of the foot to the toes, the rest of the physical examination was unremarkable. The ulcers were foul smelling with serous but not purulent discharge and wrapped with white powder in plastic cover.

Laboratory value	Day 1	Day 2	Day 3	Day 4	Day 5
Na^+ (mEq/L)	148	142	140	137	138
K^+ (mEq/L)	1.8	2.9	2.9	2.5	3.6
Cl^- (mEq/L)	73	92	92	96	100
HCO_3^- (mEq/L)	54	45	40	38	32
Creatinine (mg/dL)	3.4	2.7	2.4	1.6	1.2
Albumin (g/dL)	2.7	–	–	–	–
Lactate (mmol/L)	2.2	–	–	–	–
Urine (U) pH	6.0	6.0	–	8.0	–
U_{Na} (mEq/L)	21	27	43	74	–
U_K (mEq/L)	58	90	59	4	–
U_{Cl} (mEq/L)	<10	<10	26	37	–
Ketones	Negative	–	–	–	–
ABG					
pH	7.69	7.55	7.48	7.48	7.46
pCO_2	45	56	59	51	34
pO_2	48	218	134	101	94
CK (U)	5,604	1,846	1,335	771	–
Tropinin	28.32	5.16	–	–	–

Chest X-ray was unremarkable. The EKG showed normal sinus rhythm with a pulse rate of 80 beats per minute, normal axis, first degree AV block, QT prolongation (536 ms), one VPC, ST depression in V3–V6, and inferior leads. Because of agitation, a CT scan of the head was done, which was negative. Initial and subsequent laboratory data are shown in the table.

Question 1 What is the acid–base disturbance on day 1?

Answer Based on elevated pH and HCO_3^-, the primary acid–base disorder is metabolic alkalosis.

Question 2 What other acid–base disorders are present?

Answer Calculation of respiratory compensation and AG would help to characterize the acid–base disturbance in this patient. From Table 27.7, it is evident that the expected pCO_2 should be 61; however, the reported pCO_2 is 45. This indicates that the patient is hyperventilating and, therefore, respiratory alkalosis is also present.

The AG is 25 (corrected for normal albumin level), which is not due to entirely metabolic alkalosis. Despite volume depletion, his albumin is only 2.7 g/dL, which could not account for elevated AG. Also, ketoacidosis or lactic acidosis is not the cause. We believe that either renal insufficiency or other organic acid may have caused elevated AG.

Thus, the acid–base disorder is a primary metabolic alkalosis with superimposed respiratory alkalosis and a high AG metabolic acidosis.

Question 3 What would have been his pH, if his pCO_2 were 61 mmHg?

Answer If the patient had a pCO_2 of 61, his pH would have been 7.53 instead of 7.69 (calculation based on Henderson equation and assuming serum HCO_3^- of 54 mEq/L).

Question 4 Based on urine electrolytes, what is your differential diagnosis?

Answer Based on low urine Cl^-, the patient has Cl^--responsive metabolic alkalosis. Vomiting, thiazide diuretic use, milk-alkali syndrome (although serum Ca^{2+} was 8.2 mg/dL), or exogenous alkali intake were considered.

Urine Cl^- is always low in both early and late vomiting, but its level is usually high in recent diuretic use and relatively low in remote use. Urine pH is alkaline in early vomiting but acidic in late vomiting and diuretic use. Based on urine electrolytes, we excluded the diagnosis of diuretic use in our patient. However, low urine Na^+, high K^+, low Cl^-, and acidic pH are consistent with late vomiting. Milk-alkali syndrome was ruled out when previous serum creatinine of 0.8 mg/dL was available later that day. Thus, either habitual vomiting or exogenous alkali intake was considered initially in our patient.

Question 5 How would you manage the patient?

Answer First, normal saline with KCl supplementation is needed to improve volume status and serum [K^+]. Volume expansion improves GFR and promotes HCO_3^- excretion. Second, acetazolamide (250 or 500 mg QD or BID) can be tried. Third, HCl administration can be considered, if there is no improvement in pH despite volume and K^+ correction, fourth, cardiology consult and, finally, adequate oxygenation and trial of extubation.

In a 24-h period, the patient received a total of 7 L of 0.9% saline, 2 L of 0.45% saline, 360 mEq of KCl, and 8 mEq of $MgSO_4$. BP improved. The patient received only one dose of acetazolamide 250 mg, after adequate hydration. In a 4-day period, the patient received a total of 7 L of 0.9% saline, 19 L of 0.45% saline, and 960 mEq of KCl. The EKG abnormalities had resolved, and an ECHO showed no wall motion or valvular abnormalities.

Question 6 What is the final diagnosis?

Answer After extubation, the patient admitted to eating baking soda (a palm full with water) and covering the foot ulcer with adequate amount of baking soda for a year and a half. The final diagnosis was severe metabolic alkalosis as a primary acid–base disorder due to the chronic ingestion of baking soda ($NaHCO_3$).

Case 3 A 17-year-old Caucasian medical student is seen in the ED for persistent headache for a 2-week duration. She has no history of hypertension, migraine, or diabetes. She has been healthy and not on any medication. There is no family history of hypertension other than obesity. Physical examination shows a blood pressure of 200/142 mmHg and pulse rate of 94 beats per minute. Her BP was normal 6 months ago. Funduscopic examination reveals hypertensive retinopathy without papilledema. There are no crackles, S_4 or S_3, abdominal bruits, or edema. Neurologic examination is normal. Laboratory data:

Serum	Urine
Na^+ = 136 mEq/L	pH = 6.2
K^+ = 2.8 mEq/L	Osmolality = 1,000 mOsm/kg H_2O
Cl^- = 84 mEq/L	Na^+ = 80 mEq/L
HCO_3^- = 35 mEq/L	K^+ = 55 mEq/L
Creatinine = 1.5 mg/dL	Cl^- = 75 mEq/L
BUN = 32 mg/dL	
Glucose = 92 mg/dL	
Albumin = 4.2 g/dL	
ABG	
pH = 7.48	
pCO_2 = 47 mmHg	
HCO_3^- = 34 mEq/L	

Question 1 What is the acid–base disturbance?

Answer Both blood pH and serum [HCO_3^-] are increased; therefore, the primary acid–base disturbance is metabolic alkalosis with appropriate respiratory response.

Question 2 What is the significance of the urine Cl^-?

Answer Urine Cl^- determination is very important to distinguish Cl^--responsive from Cl^--resistant metabolic alkalosis. This patient has Cl^--resistant metabolic alkalosis.

Question 3 What is the differential diagnosis of her metabolic alkalosis with hypertension?

Answer From Table 31.1, the causes of Cl^--resistant metabolic alkalosis with hypertension are:

1. Primary aldosteronism
2. 11β-hydroxysteroid dehydrogenase type 2 deficiency
3. Licorice, chewing tobacco, and carbenoxolone
4. Fludrocortisone administration
5. Cushing syndrome
6. Glucocorticoid-remediable aldosteronism
7. Hyperreninism and hyperaldosteronism (malignant and renovascular hypertension, renin-secreting tumors)
8. Liddle syndrome

Question 4 What tests would you order to distinguish the above clinical syndromes?

Answer Plasma renin and aldosterone levels are very helpful. Both of them are high.

Question 5 What is the diagnosis in this patient?

Answer Malignant hypertension is unlikely in view of normal blood pressure 6 months ago. Although retinopathy supports the diagnosis of long-standing hypertension, the absence of papilledema does not support the diagnosis of malignant hypertension.

Renin-secreting tumor is a possibility; however, patients with this tumor have resistant hypertension prior to the diagnosis of this tumor. Although the occurrence of this tumor in many case reports is in young patients (18–24 years), they all had prior hypertension. Also, retinopathy has not been described (to my knowledge). After the exclusion of the above conditions, possible renovascular hypertension has been entertained.

Question 6 What diagnostic test would you order to confirm renovascular hypertension?

Answer After volume expansion and controlling BP, an MR angiography is preferred because of its 100% sensitivity and 94% specificity for detecting renovascular stenosis.

This patient was found to have unilateral renal artery stenosis due to fibromuscular dysplasia.

Case 4 A 22-year-old woman visits her primary care physician for weakness, fatigue, and occasional dizziness. She has no history of hypertension, diabetes, or irregular eating habits but practices weight reduction methods. She is not on any medications. Physical examination reveals a thin but well-nourished woman. Blood pressure is 100/68 mmHg with a pulse rate of 88 beats per minute (sitting) and 98/66 mmHg with a pulse rate of 102 beats per minute (standing). Except for trace edema, the rest of the examination is normal. Laboratory data:

Serum	Urine
Na^+ = 134 mEq/L	pH = 7.58
K^+ = 2.9 mEq/L	Na^+ = 40 mEq/L
Cl^- = 86 mEq/L	K^+ = 30 mEq/L
HCO_3^- = 36 mEq/L	Cl^- = 42 mEq/L
Creatinine = 1.1 mg/dL	
BUN = 32 mg/dL	
Glucose = 122 mg/dL	
Albumin = 4.2 g/dL	
ABG	
pH = 7.48	
pCO_2 = 48 mmHg	
HCO_3^- = 35 mEq/L	

Question 1 What is her acid–base disturbance?

Answer Since both pH and serum [HCO_3^-] are elevated, she has metabolic alkalosis as her primary acid–base disorder. The expected pCO_2 from respiratory compensation is 48 mmHg, which is in agreement with the reported pCO_2. Therefore, there is no additional acid–base disorder superimposed on metabolic alkalosis.

Question 2 Are urine electrolytes consistent with Cl^--resistant alkalosis?

Answer Yes. However, she has orthostatic pulse changes, suggestive of mild volume depletion. Therefore, she has Cl^--responsive alkalosis, and a drug use such as a diuretic should be suspected. The recent use of a thiazide or loop diuretic can cause urine electrolyte pattern, as shown in the table of laboratory results. If urine electrolytes are repeated 24 h later, Cl^- level will be low.

Case 5 A 42-year-old man presents to the ED with complaints of headache, weakness, fatigue, and shortness of breath. He has hypertension for 2 years. His medications include hydrochlorothiazide 25 mg QD, lisinopril 20 mg QD, metoprolol 50 mg BID, and KCl 40 mg QD. His blood pressure is 190/110 mmHg with a pulse of 74 beats per minute. There are no orthostatic changes. Pertinent physical examination reveals crackles in both lung fields and trace edema in lower extremities. Laboratory data:

Serum	Urine
Na^+ = 145 mEq/L	pH = 5.9
K^+ = 2.6 mEq/L	Na^+ = 100 mEq/L
Cl^- = 92 mEq/L	K^+ = 56 mEq/L
HCO_3^- = 34 mEq/L	Cl^- = 102 mEq/L
Creatinine = 1.1 mg/dL	
BUN = 10 mg/dL	
Glucose = 102 mg/dL	
Albumin = 4.0 g/dL	
ABG	
pH = 7.52	
pCO_2 = 40 mmHg	
HCO^{3-} = 33 mEq/L	

Question 1 What is his acid–base disturbance?

Answer Both the pH and serum $[HCO_3^-]$ are elevated; therefore, he has metabolic alkalosis as his primary acid–base disorder. The expected pCO_2 from respiratory compensation is 47 mmHg, but the reported pCO_2 is 40 mmHg due to hyperventilation. Therefore, respiratory alkalosis is superimposed on metabolic alkalosis. Hyperventilation is due to shortness of breath.

Question 2 In addition to urine electrolytes, what other tests would you order to make the diagnosis?

Answer Plasma renin and aldosterone levels can help in the differential diagnosis of hypertension-associated metabolic alkalosis.

Twenty-four hours later, the results were available. Renin level was 0.01 (normal: 1–3 ng/mL/h), and aldosterone levels were 44 (range 5–20 ng/dL), suggesting primary aldosteronism as a cause of his metabolic alkalosis. After stabilization of the patient with furosemide and KCl supplementation, the patient was started on spironolactone 100 mg QD initially, and his BP improved. CT of the adrenal gland revealed a unilateral adenoma, which was surgically removed. His BP was subsequently controlled with diet.

Case 6 A 17-year-old man, a garbage collector for the city, is admitted for weakness, fatigue, dizziness, and occasional left knee pain. He craves Chinese food. He has no history of hypertension and does not use illicit drugs or alcohol. Blood pressure is 102/66 mmHg with a pulse rate of 88 beats per minute (sitting) and 88/60 mmHg with a pulse rate of 112 beats per minute (standing). Except for left knee tenderness, the rest of the examination is normal. Laboratory data:

Serum	Urine
Na^+ = 126 mEq/L	pH = 5.9
K^+ = 1.8 mEq/L	Na^+ = 180 mEq/L
Cl^- = 82 mEq/L	K^+ = 86 mEq/L
HCO_3^- = 36 mEq/L	Cl^- = 232 mEq/L
Creatinine = 0.7 mg/dL	Ca^{2+} = 0.008 mg/mg creatinine (normal: 0.06–1.0)
BUN = 20 mg/dL	24-h urine Ca^{2+} = 52 mg (range 150–200 mg)
Glucose = 90 mg/dL	FE_{Mg} = 2.8% (range 1.2–2.4%)
Ca^{2+} = 8.2 mg/dL	
Mg^{2+} = 0.8 mg/dL	
Albumin = 4.4 g/dL	
ABG	
pH = 7.5	
pCO_2 = 46 mmHg	
HCO_3^- = 35 mEq/L	

Which one of the following options is the MOST likely diagnosis in this patient?

(A) Bartter syndrome
(B) Gitelman syndrome
(C) Liddle syndrome
(D) Diuretic abuse
(E) Licorice ingestion

The answer is B The patient's clinical manifestations, serum chemistry, and ABG suggest either Bartter or Gitelman syndrome. However, five findings distinguish Gitelman syndrome from Bartter syndrome:

1. Hypomagnesemia
2. Hypocalciuria
3. Hypermagnesuria
4. Normal prostaglandin E_2 levels
5. Chondrocalcinosis (pseudogout)

In Bartter syndrome, urine Ca^{2+} and Mg^{2+} excretions are normal. Hyperprostaglandinemia E_2 is characteristic of Bartter syndrome. Also, pseudogout is absent in Bartter syndrome. Both syndromes are characterized by very high urine levels of Na^+ and Cl^-.

Liddle syndrome and licorice ingestion are associated with hypertension and volume expansion. Diuretic abuse can present with similar clinical findings, but the urine electrolyte levels do not suggest diuretic abuse. Also, mild hypercalcemia is seen in diuretic users. Elevation of uric acid and gouty attack can be observed with diuretic use; however, normocalcemia rules out the possibility of diuretic use. Thus, option B is correct.

Case 7 A 24-year-old man was referred to the renal clinic for evaluation of recent onset hypertension noted on a routine physical checkup. He has a strong family history of hypertension at an early age. He is not on any medications. Blood pressure is 190/104 mmHg with a pulse rate of 74 beats per minute. There are no orthostatic changes. His laboratory test results are consistent with hypokalemic metabolic alkalosis. He has high urine Cl^- relative to Na^+ and K^+, which are also high. His plasma renin and aldosterone levels are extremely low.

Question 1 Which one of the following is the MOST likely diagnosis in this patient?

(A) Primary aldosteronism
(B) Renal artery stenosis
(C) Liddle syndrome
(D) Gitelman syndrome
(E) Bartter syndrome

The answer is C Primary aldosteronism and renal artery stenosis are associated with hypertension and high aldosterone levels. Patients with Gitelman and Bartter syndromes present with normal to low blood pressure. Renin and aldosterone levels are high rather than low in these syndromes. Therefore, the patient has Liddle syndrome, which is a genetic disorder due to mutations in ENaC. Renin and aldosterone levels are usually low, but normal values have also been reported. These low levels have been attributed to volume expansion and/or sclerosis of renin-producing cells in the juxtaglomerular apparatus.

Question 2 Which one of the following drugs is APPROPRIATE for this patient?

(A) Spironolactone
(B) Eplerenone
(C) Hydrochlorothiazide
(D) Metolazone
(E) Amiloride

The answer is E Patients with Liddle syndrome respond only to amiloride or triamterene and not to the other drugs mentioned above. In contrast, patients with primary aldosteronism respond to both spironolactone and amiloride. Thus, control of hypertension with spironolactone or eplerenone suggests the diagnosis of primary aldosteronism, whereas failure to control blood pressure suggests either Liddle syndrome or essential hypertension. Blood pressure improves with amiloride in Liddle syndrome, whereas it may not improve in essential hypertension. The latter requires probably more than one drug.

Case 8 Match the serum and urinary electrolyte pattern with patient history.

	Serum [Na⁺]ᵃ	Serum [K⁺]	Serum [Cl⁻]	Serum [HCO₃⁻]	Blood pH	Urine [Na⁺]	Urine [K⁺]	Urine [Cl⁻]	Urine [Ca²⁺]ᵇ	Urine pH
A	136	3.0	89	28	7.48	100	40	15	200	7.2
B	135	2.8	86	32	7.50	40	30	15	150	5.8
C	136	3.0	86	32	7.51	80	44	60	250	6.1
D	137	2.9	84	30	7.48	120	80	60	50	6.2

ᵃmEq/L
ᵇmg/24 h

1. An 18-year-old man with a craving for salty food and a mutation in Na/Cl cotransporter
2. A 12-year-old boy with a documented mutation in Na/K/2Cl cotransporter
3. A 27-year-old woman with vomiting for <2 days
4. A 40-year-old man with protracted vomiting for >7 days

Answers A = 3, B = 4, C = 2, and D = 1.

The 18-year-old man carries the diagnosis of Gitelman syndrome, whereas the 12-year-old boy has Bartter syndrome. Clinically, both syndromes behave similarly. The level of urinary excretion of Ca²⁺ is the most important determinant of these syndromes. Hypocalciuria characterizes the Gitelman syndrome, whereas Ca²⁺ excretion is normal in Bartter syndrome (see Case 6). Laboratory data shown in D and C are consistent with Gitelman and Bartter syndromes, respectively.

From the above table, it is evident that early and late vomiting can be diagnosed based only on the urine electrolytes and urine pH. In early vomiting, the kidneys try to get rid of excess Na⁺ and HCO₃⁻ in the urine to maintain near normal serum levels of these electrolytes. The urine pH is alkaline because of the presence of HCO₃⁻. If this vomiting continues, the intravascular volume is depleted, and metabolic alkalosis is sustained. This causes Na⁺ and HCO₃⁻ reabsorption, resulting in low levels of these electrolytes and acidification of urine pH. During the correction phase of metabolic alkalosis, urine pH becomes alkaline because of HCO₃⁻ excretion. Thus, laboratory data shown in A and B correspond to early and late vomiting, respectively.

Case 9 Match the following serum values with the clinical diagnoses:

Case	Na⁺	K⁺	HCO₃⁻	Renin	Aldosterone
A	↑	↓	↑	↓	↑
B	N/↑	↓	↑	↓	↑
C	↓	↓	↑	↑	↑

↑ increase, ↓ decrease, and *N* normal

1. Primary aldosteronism
2. Glucocorticoid-remediable aldosteronism (GRA)
3. Renal artery stenosis

Answers A = 1, B = 2, and C = 3.

Primary aldosteronism is the most common hypertensive disorder that is associated with low renin and high aldosterone levels. High levels of aldosterone are due to increased secretion of this hormone by either adrenal cortical adenoma or bilateral hyperplasia of the gland. Aldosterone promotes Na^+ reabsorption and K^+ secretion in the distal nephron. As a result, plasma volume is increased with an increase in serum $[Na^+]$ and volume-dependent hypertension. Hypernatremia may also be caused by relative suppression of ADH due to volume expansion. Plasma renin level is low because of volume expansion. Primary aldosteronism is commonly seen in young patients with refractory hypertension, hypokalemia, hypernatremia, and saline-resistant metabolic alkalosis. Spironolactone or amiloride is the drug of choice for hypertension management. Laboratory data shown in A are consistent with primary aldosteronism.

Glucocorticoid-remediable hyperaldosteronism (GRA), also called familial hyperaldosteronism type I, is caused by fusion of two enzymes: aldosterone synthase and 11β-hydroxylase. Some patients with GRA may have severe hypertension, hypokalemia, and metabolic alkalosis. Plasma renin is suppressed, but aldosterone levels are increased. Aldosterone secretion is stimulated by ACTH and not by angiotensin II. Therefore, administration of glucocorticoid suppresses excessive aldosterone secretion and improves hypertension. Laboratory data shown in B are consistent with GRA.

Patients with renal artery stenosis present with severe hypertension, hyponatremia, hypokalemia, and saline-resistant metabolic alkalosis. Hyponatremic hypertensive syndrome is characteristic of unilateral renal artery stenosis, but this syndrome has also been described in patients with bilateral renal artery stenosis. The pathophysiologic mechanism is that renal ischemia causes an increase in renin-AII-aldosterone, which in turn raises blood pressure. This increase in blood pressure causes pressure natriuresis through the nonstenotic kidney, resulting in volume depletion and orthostatic hypotension. High levels of AII stimulate thirst and water consumption, finally leading to hyponatremia.

Hyponatremic hypertension can also be seen in patients with malignant hypertension, renin-secreting tumors, and CKD and those on diuretics. In young patients, renal artery stenosis is predominantly due to fibromuscular dysplasia, and in subjects aged >50 years, it is the atherosclerosis of the renal artery that causes hypertension. Laboratory data shown in C are consistent with renal artery stenosis.

Case 10 A 36-year-old woman was admitted for weakness, dizziness, and inability to walk for 2 weeks. She has a childhood history of hypothyroidism and sensorineural deafness. She denied vomiting. Her medications include synthroid for hypothyroidism and hydrochlorothiazide (HCTZ) for endolymph excess in the ear. Except for palpable goiter and low blood pressure, her physical examination is otherwise normal. Two months ago, her labs were normal. Current labs:

Serum	Urine
Na$^+$ = 134 mEq/L	pH = 6.0
K$^+$ = 2.6 mEq/L	Osmolality = 400 mOsm/kg H$_2$O
Cl$^-$ = 84 mEq/L	Na$^+$ = 40 mEq/L
HCO$_3^-$ = 36 mEq/L	K$^+$ = 50 mEq/L
Creatinine = 1.1 mg/dL	Cl$^-$ = 20 mEq/L
BUN = 10 mg/dL	
Glucose = 90 mg/dL	
Albumin = 4.0 g/dL	
ABG	
pH = 7.48	
pCO$_2$ = 47 mmHg	
HCO$_3^-$ = 35 mEq/L	

Which one of the following transport mechanisms is IMPLICATED for her childhood disease and metabolic alkalosis?

(A) Na/H-ATPase
(B) Na/K/2Cl cotransporter
(C) Na/Cl cotransporter
(D) Epithelial Na$^+$ channel (ENaC)
(E) Cl/HCO$_3$ exchanger

The answer is E This patient carries the diagnosis of Pendred syndrome, which is an autosomal recessive disorder. This disorder is characterized by sensorineural deafness and goiter due to defect in iodide organification. Pendred syndrome is caused by biallelic mutations in the solute carrier family 26A4 gene, which encodes pendrin. In the kidney, pendrin functions as a Cl/HCO$_3$ exchanger in the β-intercalated cell where Cl$^-$ is reabsorbed and HCO$_3^-$ is excreted into the lumen (Chap. 26). This suggests that pendrin may protect against the development of either salt loss or metabolic alkalosis under basal conditions because excess generation of HCO$_3^-$ from any source is transported into the lumen and Cl$^-$ is reabsorbed.

Under basal conditions, patients with Pendred syndrome do not develop any electrolyte or acid-base abnormalities. This suggests that there is a compensatory mechanism that prevents these abnormalities. Studies have shown that thiazide-sensitive Na/Cl cotransporter in the distal tubule takes over the function of pendrin as a Cl$^-$ transporter. Conversely, when Na/Cl cotransporter is inhibited by a thiazide, pendrin expression and activity are increased. When both transporters are inhibited, volume depletion and metabolic alkalosis develop due to loss of NaCl in the urine. This happens when a Pendred syndrome patient is treated with a thiazide diuretic for endolymph accumulation in the ear. The mechanism by which this cross talk between Na/Cl cotransporter and Cl/HCO$_3$ exchanger occurs is not completely understood.

Our patient with Pendred syndrome developed hypokalemia, hypochloremia, metabolic alkalosis, and volume depletion (low blood pressure) because of mutation in pendrin and inhibition of Na/Cl cotransporter by HCTZ. Discontinuation of HCTZ and hydration with normal saline and KCl would improve her electrolyte abnormalities and metabolic alkalosis. Thus, choice E is correct. Although pendrin interacts with other transporters, their deficiency or activation does not cause Pendred syndrome. Thus, choices A–D are incorrect.

Suggested Reading

1. Galla JH. Metabolic alkalosis. J Am Soc Nephrol. 2000;11:369–75.
2. Gennari FJ. Metabolic alkalosis. In: Mount DB, Sayegh MH, Singh AJ, editors. Core concepts in the disorders of fluid, electrolytes and acid-base balance. New York: Springer; 2013. p. 275–96.
3. Gennari FJ. Pathophysiology of metabolic alkalosis: a new classification based on the centrality of stimulated collecting duct ion transport. Am J Kidney Dis. 2011;58:626–36.
4. Kandasamy N, Fugazola L, Evans M, et al. Life-threatening metabolic alkalosis in pendred syndrome. Eur J Endocrinol. 2011;165:167–70.
5. Reimann D, Gross P. Chronic, diagnosis-resistant hypokalaemia. Nephrol Dial Transplant. 1999;14:2957–61.
6. Soleimani M. The multiple roles of pendrin in the kidney. Nephrol Dial Transplant. 2015;30:1257–66.
7. Wall SM, Laza-Fernandez Y. The role of pendrin in renal physiology. Annu Rev Physiol. 2015;77:363–78.

Respiratory Acidosis

32

Physiology

As stated in Chap. 26, respiratory acid–base disorders are due to changes in pCO_2. In normal individuals, the arterial partial pressure of carbon dioxide (pCO_2) is maintained at approximately 40 mmHg. This consistency of pCO_2 is maintained by the alveolar ventilation. Lungs are the only organs that eliminate (excrete) CO_2. Several physiologic mechanisms participate in the maintenance of CO_2 balance (see below). Disturbance in any one of these mechanisms leads either to retention (hypercapnia or an increase in pCO_2) or excessive elimination (hypocapnia or a decrease in pCO_2) of CO_2. The respiratory acid–base disorder that is associated with hypercapnia is called respiratory acidosis, whereas that associated with hypocapnia is known as respiratory alkalosis.

In a normal individual, CO_2 balance is maintained by the following mechanisms:

1. CO_2 production
2. CO_2 transport
3. CO_2 excretion
4. Control of ventilation by central nervous system (CNS)

CO$_2$ Production

- CO_2 is produced by metabolism of carbohydrates and fats.
- Approximately 15,000 mmol of CO_2 are produced daily.
- Heavy exercise generates several-fold higher quantity of CO_2 than when the body is in resting state.
- Lungs are the only organs that excrete all the CO_2 that is produced.

© Springer Science+Business Media LLC 2018
A.S. Reddi, *Fluid, Electrolyte and Acid-Base Disorders*,
DOI 10.1007/978-3-319-60167-0_32

CO$_2$ Transport

- The CO$_2$ that is produced during metabolism is transported by the blood (plasma and red blood cells) to the lungs via the pulmonary arteries.
- The pCO$_2$ difference (gradient) between the tissues and alveoli is only 6 mmHg.
- In red blood cells, CO$_2$ is converted to carbonic acid (H$_2$CO$_3$) in the presence of carbonic anhydrase.
- H$_2$CO$_3$ then dissociates into H$^+$ and HCO$_3^-$. It is this HCO$_3^-$ that diffuses into the plasma via Cl/HCO$_3$ exchanger and is carried to the lungs, where it is converted back to CO$_2$.

CO$_2$ Excretion

- Alveolar ventilation is the major determinant of CO$_2$ excretion.
- A decrease in alveolar ventilation causes retention of CO$_2$, resulting in an increase in total body CO$_2$ balance.
- Other determinants include blood flow through the aerated lung, diffusion of CO$_2$ from the capillary to the alveolar space, and physiologic dead space.

CNS Control of Ventilation

In a normal individual, variations in pCO$_2$, partial pressure of oxygen (pO$_2$), and pH are minimized and kept within normal limits by the respiratory control system, which includes the following:

1. Sensors (chemoreceptors)
2. Central controller (medulla and pons)
3. Effectors (respiratory muscles)

Sensors
Two types of chemoreceptors are involved in ventilation:

1. Central chemoreceptors, located in the medulla, are surrounded by the interstitial and cerebrospinal fluid and respond to changes in [H$^+$] or pCO$_2$. For example, an increase in [H$^+$], i.e., a decrease in pH, stimulates respiration and decreases pCO$_2$. These responses, in turn, raise pH. On the other hand, a decrease in [H$^+$] or an increase in pH depresses alveolar ventilation and causes retention of pCO$_2$, so that the pH is returned to near normal. An increase in pCO$_2$ stimulates ventilation, whereas a decrease depresses ventilation.
2. Peripheral chemoreceptors are located in the carotid body and aortic arch. They respond to decreases in pO$_2$ and pH and increases in pCO$_2$. The sensitivity to changes in pO$_2$ begins at around 500 mmHg, but little response occurs until pO$_2$ is <70 mmHg.

Medullary Center

1. Central controller includes neurons located in the medulla and pons, which are referred to as respiratory centers.
2. Medullary respiratory center has two identifiable areas of cells. One group of cells is located in the dorsal region of the medulla. It is called the dorsal respiratory group, which is involved in inspiration. The other group of cells, the ventral respiratory group, controls expiration.

Effectors

1. Once changes are sensed in the medullary respiratory center, they are transmitted through nerves to the muscles of respiration (diaphragm, intercostal muscles, abdominal muscles, and sternocleidomastoid muscles). It is the coordinated effort of these muscles that is responsible for ventilation.
2. Any disturbance in sensing and signaling results in either hypercapnia or hypocapnia, leading to either respiratory acidosis or respiratory alkalosis, respectively. Let us discuss respiratory acidosis.

Respiratory Acidosis

Respiratory acidosis, also called primary hypercapnia, is initiated by an increase in arterial pCO_2. This increase is related to decreased excretion relative to the production of CO_2. Whenever pCO_2 increases, the pH falls. The excess H^+ is immediately (within minutes) buffered by nonbicarbonate buffers, such as hemoglobin, phosphates, and plasma proteins, so that HCO_3^- is not used up. During this buffering, some HCO_3^- is also formed from dissociation of H_2CO_3. The acute nonbicarbonate buffer response is completed within 10–15 min, and a steady-state condition persists for 1 h. If hypercapnia continues for >12 h, the kidneys generate additional HCO_3^- by excretion of H^+, and the maximum level of HCO_3^- generation is completed within 3–5 days. Thus, respiratory acidosis can be classified into acute (<12 h) or chronic (>5 days) types. Both acute and chronic hypercapnias are associated with hypoxemia.

Secondary Physiologic Response to Hypercapnia

As stated earlier, the renal and extrarenal mechanisms respond to an increase in pCO_2 by preventing loss of HCO_3^- so that dangerous decreases in pH are avoided. Although acute respiratory acidosis causes low pH, chronic respiratory acidosis maintains pH at slightly low but near-normal levels because of renal regeneration of HCO_3^-. The secondary responses to both acute and chronic respiratory acidosis are given below:

Acute respiratory acidosis: For each mmHg increase in pCO_2, HCO_3^- increases by 0.1 mEq/L.

Table 32.1 Relationship between hypercapnia, secondary response, and pH

Type	pCO$_2$ (mmHg)	Expected secondary response (compensation)	Expected serum [HCO$_3^-$]	pH (calculated from Henderson equation)
Normal	40	–	24	7.40
Acute	70[a]	For each mmHg increase in pCO$_2$, HCO$_3^-$ increases by 0.1 mEq/L, ΔpCO$_2$ = 30 (70–40 = 30×0.1=3)	27 (24+3=27)	7.10
Chronic	70[a]	For each mmHg increase in pCO$_2$, HCO$_3^-$ increases by 0.4 mEq/L, ΔpCO$_2$ = 30 (70–40=30×0.4=12)	36	7.34

[a]Arbitrary value

Chronic respiratory acidosis: For each mmHg increase in pCO$_2$, HCO$_3^-$ increases by 0.4 mEq/L.

Table 32.1 shows the relationship between rise in pCO$_2$, secondary response (compensation), and arterial pH in acute and chronic respiratory acidoses.

Acute Respiratory Acidosis

Causes
- There are several causes of acute respiratory acidosis, as shown in Table 32.2.

Clinical Manifestations
As stated earlier, acute respiratory acidosis causes hypoxemia, resulting in several organ dysfunctions.

CNS manifestations predominate and include the following:

1. Signs and symptoms: Nausea, vomiting, restlessness, headache, confusion, seizures, and coma.
2. Cerebral blood flow: Increases acutely due to cerebral vasodilation of the capillaries and venules. This cerebral vasodilation is mediated by nitric oxide.
3. Intracranial pressure: Hypercapnia increases intracranial pressure due to increased blood volume and increased vascular pressure caused by vasodilation.

Cardiac manifestations include an increase in blood pressure and heart rate secondary to increased sympathetic tone. Cardiac output increases. Also, coronary blood flow increases due to hypercapnia-induced vasodilation. Both peripheral vasodilation (due to hypercapnia) and vasoconstriction (due to increased sympathetic tone) occur in patients with acute respiratory acidosis. Arrhythmias are also common.

Renal effects include renal vasodilation with mild hypercapnia and vasoconstriction at pCO$_2$ >70 mmHg. Renin–angiotensin II (AII)–aldosterone axis is stimulated by hypercapnia-induced sympathetic tone. Antidiuretic hormone (ADH) secretion is also increased.

Table 32.2 Causes of acute respiratory acidosis

Depression of medullary respiratory center
Drugs: anesthetics, sedatives, opiates
Cerebral trauma or infarct
Central sleep apnea
Cardiac arrest
Failure of motor functions of respiratory muscles and chest wall
Drugs: succinylcholine, curare, aminoglycosides
High cervical cordotomy
Myasthenia crisis
Guillain–Barrè syndrome
Status epilepticus
Tetanus
Acute botulism poisoning
Familial hypokalemic periodic paralysis
Severe hypophosphatemia
Airway obstruction
Aspiration
Laryngospasm
Severe bronchospasm
Obstructive sleep apnea
Ventilatory defects
Flail chest
Pneumothorax
Hydrothorax
Adult respiratory distress syndrome
Acute pulmonary embolism
Acute pulmonary edema
Severe asthma
Severe pneumonia
Mechanical ventilation: increased production of CO_2 due to high carbohydrate feedings and fixed minute ventilation

Other effects include skeletal muscle contraction, particularly diaphragmatic movement is reduced.

Also, acute and chronic hypercapnias increase the production of gastric acid.

Diagnosis

- History of cough, shortness of breath, fever, asthma, congestive heart failure, or trauma to head or back, drug use, and other medical conditions should be obtained.
- Physical examination should include vital signs, breathing pattern, body habitus, teeth (dentures, if any), mouth for any foreign material, chest exam for shape and accessory muscle use, auscultation of the lungs for crackles, wheezing, tactile fremitus, movement of the diaphragm, cardiac examination for an S_3 and an S_4, abdomen for muscle use, lower extremities for edema, upper extremities for clubbing, and a good neurologic examination.

- Laboratory results:
    1. Arterial blood gas (ABG): Low pH (<7.25), slightly elevated serum HCO_3^- (<30 mEq/L), and elevated pCO_2 (>60 mmHg) characterize acute respiratory acidosis; pH, expected $[HCO_3^-]$, and pCO_2 shown in Table 32.1 distinguish acute respiratory acidosis from chronic respiratory acidosis.
    2. Serum chemistry, including Ca^{2+}, Mg^{2+}, phosphate, and hemoglobin.
    3. A slight increase in serum Na^+ (2–4 mEq/L) is observed.
    4. A slight increase in serum K^+ (~0.1 mEq/L for 0.1 unit decrease in pH) is common.
    5. A slight decrease in serum Cl^- is seen because of Cl^- entry into red blood cells in exchange for HCO_3^- (chloride shift).
    6. Hyperphosphatemia is common due to release of phosphate from tissues (not present in chronic respiratory acidosis).
    7. Ca^{2+} and Mg^{2+} are usually normal, but slight increases have been reported.
    8. Normal anion gap.
    9. Acidic urine pH (<5.5).
    10. Chest X-ray and electrocardiogram (EKG).
    11. Calculation of alveolar–arterial (A–a) gradient for gas exchange.

Treatment

Correction of the underlying cause should be attempted whenever possible. Immediate treatment should include the following:

1. Establishing a secure patent airway in both awake and obtunded patients.
2. Hypercapnic encephalopathy may occur in patients with narcotic overdose and in those with chronic hypercapnia and superimposed acute respiratory acidosis.
3. Administration of O_2 to improve hypoxemia. This is more important than lowering pCO_2 and raising pH. Assisted ventilation should be initiated promptly in severely obtunded, comatose patients, or patients with pH <7.10. If a patient is awake and hemodynamically stable, O_2 by nasal cannula or by high-flow Venturi face mask may be sufficient. The aim of O_2 therapy is to achieve pO_2 of 60–70 mmHg or an O_2 saturation >88%.
4. Mechanical ventilation is indicated in apneic, obtunded, and hemodynamically unstable patients with pH <7.10 and pCO_2 >80 mmHg. Lowering pCO_2 may be sufficient to raise pH, but $NaHCO_3$ is needed in some patients.
5. Loop diuretics may be needed in a patient with crackles.
6. Antibiotics, β_2-agonists, and other bronchodilators, as well as corticosteroids, may be necessary in patients with infection and wheezing, to improve ventilation.
7. Carbohydrate feedings in ventilator-dependent patients should be minimized to prevent excess CO_2 generation. Calories from fat emulsions should be encouraged.

Remember that clinical assessment and proper use of pharmacotherapy are extremely important in the management of acute respiratory acidosis.

Chronic Respiratory Acidosis

Steady-state hypercapnia is achieved in 3–5 days following secondary renal adaptive changes that increase serum [HCO_3^-] by 0.4 mEq/L for each mmHg increase in pCO_2 above the normal level. Thus, the acid–base pattern of chronic acidosis is different from that of acute acidosis.

Causes
Table 32.3 shows various causes of chronic respiratory acidosis.

Clinical Manifestations
- Less severe compared to patients with acute respiratory acidosis because of near-normal pH.
- Hypoxemia and associated symptoms are common.
- CNS manifestations include tremors, ataxia, and poor appetite. Cerebral vasodilation and blood flow are increased but not to the extent of acute hypercapnia.
- Cardiovascular effects are pulmonary hypertension (cor pulmonale), peripheral edema, and supraventricular as well as ventricular arrhythmias. Cardiac output is normal or near normal.

Table 32.3 Causes of chronic respiratory acidosis

Depression of medullary respiratory center
Chronic sedative and opiate addiction
Brain tumors
Primary alveolar hypoventilation
Obesity-hypoventilation syndrome
Bulbar poliomyelitis
Failure of motor functions of respiratory muscles and chest wall
Spinal cord injury
Multiple sclerosis
Muscular dystrophy
Amyotrophic lateral sclerosis
Myxedema
Poliomyelitis
Diaphragmatic paralysis
Airway obstruction
Chronic obstructive pulmonary disease (COPD) (most common cause)
Ventilatory defects
Hydrothorax
Fibrothorax
Kyphoscoliosis
Interstitial lung fibrosis
Severe chronic pneumonia
Extreme obesity

- Glomerular filtration rate (GFR) is normal.
- Bone disease is present but less severe compared with metabolic acidosis. Hypercalciuria is less common or absent.

Diagnosis

- As in acute respiratory acidosis, history and physical findings are important in chronic respiratory acidosis. Body habitus, deformed chest, and clubbing are prominent findings.
- Laboratory results:
    1. ABG: pH near normal (>7.30), elevated HCO_3^- (>32 mmHg), and elevated pCO_2 (>60 mmHg) usually characterize chronic respiratory acidosis.
    2. Serum Na^+ is slightly elevated.
    3. K^+ is normal.
    4. Cl^- decreases proportionately with the increase in HCO_3^-.
    5. Ca^{2+} and Mg^{2+} are normal.
    6. When K^+ is low, suspect superimposed metabolic alkalosis or excessive β_2-agonist therapy.
    7. AG is normal; when high, suspect superimposed metabolic acidosis such as lactic acidosis.
    8. Urine pH is <5.5.
    9. Secondary polycythemia is common.
    10. Chest X-ray if infection is suspected and for evaluation of chronic pneumonia.

Treatment

- Treatment of chronic respiratory acidosis is different from that of acute respiratory acidosis.
- Address the cause of chronic respiratory acidosis and treat appropriately.
- The primary goal of treatment is to maintain adequate oxygenation as well as alveolar ventilation and amelioration of hypoxemia.
- In contrast to acute respiratory acidosis, excessive oxygenation should be avoided in order to prevent CNS depression.
- Avoid long-term sedatives and sleeping pills because they depress CNS drive.
- Do not treat the acidic pH; however, patients with cor pulmonale and lower extremity edema receive diuretics, and their pH may be slightly elevated.
- Antibiotics for infections are indicated.
- Bronchodilator therapy should be continued.
- Weight reduction methods should be suggested for obese individuals.
- Dietary modification is needed to reduce CO_2 production.
- If severe hypoxemia (arterial pO_2 <50 mmHg) persists, continuous low-flow O_2 therapy may improve pulmonary circulation and gas exchange through reduction in pulmonary vasoconstriction.
- The goal of O_2 therapy is to maintain pO_2 between 60 and 70 mmHg and O_2 saturation of 88–93%.

- Mechanical ventilation is not necessary for a patient who is alert and able to cough and follow medical therapy.
- Obtunded patients and patients with superimposed acute respiratory acidosis may require mechanical ventilation. Minute ventilation should be raised to achieve baseline pH and pCO_2. Sudden drop in pCO_2 may induce posthypercapnic metabolic alkalosis.

Study Questions

Case 1 A 65-year-old man with a history of chronic obstructive pulmonary disease (COPD) is admitted for evaluation of shortness of breath. On admission, his laboratory values are as follows:

Serum	ABG
Na^+ = 134 mEq/L	pH = 7.35
K^+ = 3.6 mEq/L	pCO_2 = 64 mmHg
Cl^- = 90 mEq/L	pO_2 = 70 mmHg
HCO_3^- = 34 mEq/L	HCO_3^- = 33 mEq/L
Creatinine = 1.1 mg/dL	
BUN = 12 mg/dL	
Glucose = 100 mg/dL	

Question 1 Characterize the acid–base disorder.

Answer Follow step-by-step approach given in Chap. 27 to analyze this acid–base disorder.

Step 1 According to the Henderson equation, the [H⁺] is 45 nmol/L and corresponds to a pH of 7.35.

Step 2 On the basis of low pH and elevated pCO_2 and HCO_3^-, the primary acid–base disturbance is respiratory acidosis.

Step 3 The AG is 10, which is normal.

Step 4 The cause for this patient's respiratory acidosis is COPD.

Step 5 The compensation for respiratory acidosis is renal reabsorption of HCO_3^-. Gathering from Table 32.1, the patient has a primary chronic rather than an acute respiratory acidosis.

Step 6 The immediate treatment is administration of low-flow O_2 by nasal cannula and subsequent correction of the precipitating factor.

Case 2 A college-going, healthy student is brought to the Emergency Department (ED) in obtunded condition by his friends, 24 h after a birthday party. He has a low respiratory rate, requiring elective intubation. His blood pressure is 120/78 mmHg with a pulse rate of 86 beats per minute. Chemistry 7 is normal except for HCO_3^- of 27 mEq/L. AG is normal. ABG prior to intubation: pH 7.09, pCO_2 70 mmHg, pO_2 88 mmHg, HCO_3^- 26 mEq/L.

Question 1 Characterize the acid–base disorder.

Answer On the basis of low pH and high pCO_2 and HCO_3^-, the acid–base disturbance is an uncomplicated respiratory acidosis.

Question 2 Is it acute or chronic respiratory acidosis?

Answer It is acute respiratory acidosis, as the expected HCO_3^- is 27 mEq/L. In acute respiratory acidosis, HCO_3^- increases by 0.1 mEq/L for each mmHg increase in pCO_2.
 Thus, the excess pCO_2 is 30 mmHg (70–40 = 30), which elevates serum HCO_3^- to 27 mEq/L.

Question 3 Why is his respiratory rate decreased?

Answer On the basis of his history of attending a birthday party, one can assume that he may have taken a drug that depressed the respiratory center. Urine toxicology showed the presence of opiates.

Case 3 A 42-year-old man with a history of kyphoscoliosis and right heart failure is admitted for progressive shortness of breath and worsening peripheral edema. He is on furosemide for heart failure. Blood pressure is 140/82 mmHg and a pulse rate is 88 beats per minute. Respiratory rate is 18 per minute. Pertinent findings are distant breath sounds bilaterally and 1+ pitting edema in lower extremities. Laboratory results:

Serum	ABG
Na^+ = 137 mEq/L	pH = 7.34
K^+ = 4.2 mEq/L	pCO_2 = 68 mmHg
Cl^- = 91 mEq/L	pO_2 = 52 mmHg
HCO_3^- = 35 mEq/L	HCO_3^- = 34 mEq/L
Creatinine = 0.9 mg/dL	
BUN = 14 mg/dL	
Glucose = 90 mg/dL	
Albumin = 4.5 g/dL	

Question 1 What is the acid–base disturbance?

Answer The increases in both HCO_3^- and pCO_2 with relatively low pH indicate that the acid–base disorder is respiratory acidosis.

Question 2 Is it a mixed acid–base disorder?

Answer No. On the basis of the renal response to hypercapnia, the expected HCO_3^- should be 35 ($68 - 40 = 28 \times 0.4 = 11.2$), which coincides with the reported HCO_3^- of 35 mEq/L. Therefore, the acid–base disorder is chronic respiratory acidosis. Also, low Cl^- is consistent with chronic respiratory acidosis. The AG is 11, suggesting that no other metabolic acid–base disorder is present.

One month later, the patient comes back with cough and yellowish sputum production. Chest X-ray shows bilateral infiltrates. He is confused and lethargic. Laboratory results:

Serum	ABG
Na$^+$ = 140 mEq/L	pH = 7.28
K$^+$ = 3.5 mEq/L	pCO$_2$ = 88 mmHg
Cl$^-$ = 100 mEq/L	pO$_2$ = 48 mmHg
HCO$_3^-$ = 34 mEq/L	HCO$_3^-$ = 32 mEq/L
Creatinine = 0.9 mg/dL	
BUN = 12 mg/dL	
Glucose = 84 mg/dL	
Albumin = 4.5 g/dL	

Question 3 Characterize the acid–base disorder.

Answer Compared with previous laboratory results, the current laboratory results show an increase in pCO$_2$, a decrease in pH, and worsening hypoxemia. This patient has acute respiratory acidosis superimposed on chronic respiratory acidosis.

Question 4 Does this patient need NaHCO$_3$ administration to improve pH?

Answer No. The patient requires intubation and an increase in minute ventilation. Lowering of pCO$_2$ to 66 mmHg raises his pH from 7.28 to 7.34, assuming no change in serum [HCO$_3^-$]. Actually, administration of NaHCO$_3$ increases pCO$_2$ and worsens pH.

Case 4 A 64-year-old woman with COPD develops diarrhea of 1 week duration. She says that she took enough fluids "to keep up with diarrhea," but abdominal cramps and slight dizziness brought her to the ED. She is alert and oriented. Her blood pressure is 120/60 mmHg with a heart rate of 96 per minute. Respiratory rate is 19 per minute. She has orthostatic blood pressure and pulse changes. Laboratory results:

Serum	ABG
Na$^+$ = 136 mEq/L	pH = 7.27
K$^+$ = 3.2 mEq/L	pCO$_2$ = 62 mmHg
Cl$^-$ = 100 mEq/L	pO$_2$ = 88 mmHg
HCO$_3^-$ = 28 mEq/L	HCO$_3^-$ = 27 mEq/L
Creatinine = 1.0 mg/dL	
BUN = 24 mg/dL	
Glucose = 92 mg/dL	

Question 1 What is the acid–base disturbance?

Answer Low pH and high pCO$_2$ and HCO$_3^-$ indicate that the primary acid–base disorder is chronic respiratory acidosis. If she had acute respiratory acidosis, her serum HCO$_3^-$ would have been 26 (24 + 2) rather than 28 mEq/L.
    The pH and serum [HCO$_3^-$] are low for chronic respiratory acidosis. Since she has diarrhea, she developed non-AG metabolic acidosis, which lowered HCO$_3^-$ and

pH. Note that pCO_2 may have been slightly lowered because of mild increase in respiratory rate. Thus, the patient has chronic respiratory acidosis and non-AG metabolic acidosis.

Case 5 A 56-year-old man with a history of COPD and essential hypertension is admitted for recently exacerbated shortness of breath and easy fatiguability. He is on bronchodilators and hydrochlorothiazide (HCTZ). Laboratory results:

Serum	ABG
Na^+ = 134 mEq/L	pH = 7.42
K^+ = 3.6 mEq/L	pCO_2 = 59 mmHg
Cl^- = 91 mEq/L	pO_2 = 62 mmHg
HCO_3^- = 37 mEq/L	HCO_3^- = 36 mEq/L
Creatinine = 0.9 mg/dL	
BUN = 14 mg/dL	
Glucose = 90 mg/dL	
Albumin = 4.5 g/dL	

Question 1 What is the acid–base disturbance?

Answer The increase in HCO_3^- and pCO_2 with slightly elevated pH indicates that the acid–base disorder is metabolic alkalosis.

Question 2 Is it a mixed acid–base disorder?

Answer Yes. On the basis of the respiratory response for metabolic alkalosis, the expected pCO_2 should be (ΔHCO_3^- = 13 (37–24)×0.7 = 13) 53 (40 + 13) mmHg. However, the reported pCO_2 is 59 mmHg. Therefore, the acid–base is metabolic alkalosis superimposed on chronic respiratory acidosis. The coexistence of metabolic alkalosis is due to HCTZ.

Suggesting Reading

1. Adrogué HJ. Diagnosis and management of severe respiratory acidosis: a 65-year-old man with a double lung transplant and shortness of breath. Am J Kidney Dis. 2010;56:994–1000.
2. Adrogué HJ, Madias NE. Management of life-threatening acid-base disorders [1 of 2 parts]. N Engl J Med. 1998;338:26–34.
3. Adrogué HJ, Madias NE. Respiratory acidosis. In: Gennari FJ, Adrogué HJ, Galla JH, Madias NE, editors. Acid-base disorders and their treatment. Boca Raton: Taylor & Francis; 2005. p. 597–639.
4. Bruno CM, Valenti M. Acid-base disorders in patients with chronic obstructive pulmonary disease: a pathophysiological review. J Biomed Biotechnol. 2012;2012:915150. (Article ID 915150, 2012)
5. Elliott CG, Morris AH. Clinical syndromes of respiratory acidosis and alkalosis. In: Seldin DW, Giebisch G, editors. The regulation of acid-base balance. New York: Raven Press; 1989. p. 483–521.

Respiratory Alkalosis

33

The physiology section of Chap. 32 applies to this chapter as well. Respiratory alkalosis, also called primary hypocapnia, is characterized by low pCO_2 and high pH (>7.40). Primary hypocapnia reflects pulmonary hyperventilation. The resultant alkalinization of body fluids is ameliorated by a decrease in serum $[HCO_3^-]$. Secondary hypocapnia should be distinguished from primary hypocapnia, as the former occurs in response to metabolic acidosis. As soon as respiratory alkalosis develops, a decrease in serum $[HCO_3^-]$ occurs within minutes. This is due to nonbicarbonate buffering as well as H^+ release from tissues. Lactate is also produced by alkalemia. This buffering from various sources persists for several hours, and the resultant acid–base disturbance is called acute respiratory alkalosis. During acute hypocapnia, the H^+ secretion in both proximal tubule and cortical collecting duct is suppressed. When alkalemia persists, renal compensation starts with a decrease in both H^+ secretion and basolateral exit of HCO_3^- in the proximal tubule. This lowers serum $[HCO_3^-]$ even further, due to which the pH is maintained close to normal. The full renal compensation takes 2–3 days for completion, and a new steady state is established, which is called chronic respiratory alkalosis.

As stated in Chap. 32, both central and peripheral receptors, medullary respiratory center, and respiratory muscles sense changes in pCO_2, O_2, and pH and respond appropriately.

Secondary Physiologic Response to Respiratory Alkalosis (Hypocapnia)

As stated earlier, the renal and nonrenal mechanisms respond to a decrease in pCO_2 by lowering $[HCO_3^-]$, so that dangerous increases in pH are avoided. Although acute respiratory alkalosis causes high pH, chronic respiratory alkalosis maintains pH at slightly high but near normal levels by further lowering serum

© Springer Science+Business Media LLC 2018
A.S. Reddi, *Fluid, Electrolyte and Acid-Base Disorders*,
DOI 10.1007/978-3-319-60167-0_33

Table 33.1 Relationship between hypocapnia, renal response, and pH

Type	pCO$_2$ (mmHg)	Expected renal response (compensation)	Expected serum [HCO$_3^-$]	pH (calculated from Henderson equation)
Normal	40	–	24	7.40
Acute	20[a]	For each mmHg decrease in pCO$_2$, HCO$_3^-$ decreases by 0.2 mEq/L, ΔpCO$_2$ = 20 (40–20 = 20 × 0.2 = 4)	20 (24–4 = 20)	7.56
Chronic	20[a]	For each mmHg decrease in pCO$_2$, HCO$_3^-$ decreases by 0.4 mEq/L, ΔpCO$_2$ = 20 (40–20 = 20 × 0.4 = 8)	16 (24–8 = 16)	7.50

[a]Arbitrary value

[HCO$_3^-$]. The secondary responses to both acute and chronic respiratory alkalosis are shown below:

Acute respiratory alkalosis: For each mmHg decrease in pCO$_2$, HCO$_3^-$ decreases by 0.2 mEq/L
Chronic respiratory alkalosis: For each mmHg decrease in pCO$_2$, HCO$_3^-$ decreases by 0.4 mEq/L

Table 33.1 shows the relationship between pCO$_2$, expected secondary response (compensation), and arterial pH in acute and chronic respiratory alkalosis.

Causes of Acute and Chronic Respiratory Alkalosis

With few exceptions, all causes are associated with both acute and chronic respiratory alkaloses. Acute respiratory alkalosis is generally caused by anxiety-hyperventilation syndrome, pain, and acute illnesses such as pneumonia, acute asthmatic attack, septicemia, pulmonary embolism, pulmonary edema, salicylate ingestion, or increased minute ventilation in mechanically ventilated patients. Therefore, acute respiratory alkalosis is rather common in general wards and intensive care units. Table 33.2 shows the most important causes of respiratory alkalosis.

Clinical Manifestations

Acute Respiratory Alkalosis

When pCO$_2$ is lowered acutely, paresthesias of lower extremities, circumoral numbness, tingling of the hands and mouth, and a feeling of chest tightness occur. Headache, light-headedness, confusion, and disorientation are also common. Severe alkalosis may precipitate seizures and cardiac arrhythmias. These manifestations are related to the central nervous system (CNS), cardiovascular, and metabolic effects.

Table 33.2 Causes of respiratory alkalosis

Direct stimulation of medullary respiratory center
Voluntary or psychogenic hyperventilation
Stroke
CNS infection, tumor, or trauma
Gram-negative sepsis
Liver failure
Pregnancy
Hypermetabolic state (fever, thyrotoxicosis)
Drugs (salicylates, progesterone, nicotine, xanthine derivatives, catecholamines, antipsychotic drug quetiapine)
Pain
Hypoxemic stimulation of medullary respiratory center
Pulmonary diseases (pneumonia, asthma, pulmonary edema, pulmonary embolus, interstitial lung disease, high altitude, hypotension, severe anemia)
Mechanical ventilation
High minute ventilation

CNS Effects

Acute hypocapnia causes sudden decrease in brain blood flow due to cerebral vaso-constriction. This results in a decrease in intracranial and intraocular pressures.

- Light-headedness, confusion, and other manifestations are related to decreased cerebral perfusion.
- Electroencephalogram (EEG) changes such as slowing and high-voltage wave forms also occur.
- Acid–base changes are similar in both cerebrospinal fluid (CSF) and systemic blood during acute hypocapnia.
- Acral paresthesias are due to decreased blood flow to the skin.

Cardiovascular Effects

Acute hypocapnia decreases myocardial blood flow and O_2 supply.

- Cardiac output is decreased.
- Coronary vasoconstriction and chest pain occur.
- Cardiac arrhythmias are common with severe hypocapnia.

Metabolic Effects

Lactate production is increased.

- A decrease in plasma volume is observed.
- Acute hypocalcemia due to increased binding of Ca^{2+} to albumin can occur with precipitation of tetany and perioral tingling.
- Mild hyponatremia, hypokalemia, and hypophosphatemia may be present due to cellular shift.

Chronic Respiratory Alkalosis

Individuals with chronic respiratory alkalosis are generally less symptomatic than subjects with acute respiratory alkalosis. Hyperventilation is subtle in many patients, and it is not even recognized by patients and clinicians. However, certain CNS, cardiovascular, and metabolic effects do occur in patients with chronic respiratory alkalosis.

CNS Effects

- CSF pH rises when pCO_2 is sufficiently low.
- CSF lactate levels may be high (alkalosis-induced).
- Light-headedness may be common.

Cardiovascular Effects

Common in individuals who climb mountains and live at high altitudes. These effects are:

- Initially, cardiac output increases due to a decrease in peripheral vascular resistance.
- Heart rate goes up.
- Blood pressure remains normal secondary to decreased peripheral vascular resistance.
- Cardiac output returns to baseline 1–6 weeks after exposure to high altitude, but heart rate remains elevated.
- Blood flow to the kidneys and skin is reduced.
- Both blood and plasma volumes are reduced due to renal Na^+ loss; however, after several days of high-altitude exposure, only blood volume returns to normal due to an increase in hemoglobin and hematocrit.
- All of the above manifestations are related to hypoxemia.

Metabolic Effects

In addition to low plasma volume, hyponatremia, hypokalemia, and hypophosphatemia due to cellular shifts are common. Decreased ionized Ca^{2+} is also common, causing tetany and Chvostek's and Trousseau's signs.

Diagnosis

History and physical examination can provide useful information about the causes of both acute and chronic respiratory alkaloses.

History of pain, anxiety, drug use, or pregnancy can easily be obtained. Pulmonary causes of respiratory alkalosis should be addressed. Hyperventilation in patients on ventilators can be recognized from settings of the ventilators.

Pertinent physical examination findings are summarized in Table 33.3.

Laboratory results:

Table 33.3 Physical examination and possible cause of respiratory alkalosis

Examination	Clinical cause (clue)
Vital signs	
Hypotension	Hypoxemia
↑ heart rate	Fever, anxiety
Orthostatic changes	↓ plasma volume
↑ temperature	Infection or sepsis
Tachypnea	Arrhythmias, hypoxemia, pulmonary disease
Lungs	
Inspiratory crackles	Pulmonary edema
Inspiratory ronchi and crackles	Pulmonary fibrosis
Tachypnea, pulmonary rub	Pulmonary embolism
Prolonged expiratory wheezing	Asthma
Heart	
Irregular rhythm	Arrhythmia
↑ P_2, palpable P_2, right ventricular heave	Pulmonary hypertension
Abdomen	
Ascites, asterixis	Liver disease
Gravid uterus	Pregnancy
Extremities	
Cyanosis	Hypoxemia
Neurologic	
Tremor, paresthesias	Anxiety, low blood flow to skin
Muscle weakness	Hypokalemia, hypophosphatemia
Chvostek's and Trousseau's signs	Low ionized Ca^{2+}

Arterial Blood Gas (ABG)

- Respiratory alkalosis is characterized by low pCO_2, low serum $[HCO_3^-]$, and high pH. In acute respiratory alkalosis, serum $[HCO_3^-]$ is around 20 mEq/L, because the secondary response to hypocapnia of 20 mmHg is a decrease of 4 mEq/L from normal $[HCO_3^-]$ of 24 mEq/L (Table 33.1)
- On the other hand, the serum $[HCO_3^-]$ from normal level of 24 mEq/L drops to 16 mEq/L in chronic respiratory alkalosis for the same hypocapnia of 20 mmHg.
- Note that without pH, it is sometimes difficult to differentiate between hyperchloremic metabolic acidosis from chronic respiratory alkalosis, because both of them have hyperchloremia.

Serum Chemistry

- Persistent hyponatremia, hypokalemia, hypophosphatemia, and low ionized Ca^{2+}—suggestive of chronic respiratory alkalosis
- ↑ WBC—suggestive of infectious process
- ↓ Hemoglobin—suggestive of anemia

Table 33.4 Treatment of respiratory alkalosis

Cause	Treatment options
Anxiety-hyperventilation syndromes	Rebreathing into a paper or plastic bag, mild sedation and reassurance
Hypoxia	O_2
Salicylates	Urinary alkalinization, forced diuresis, dialysis
Sepsis	Antibiotics
Hyperthyroidism	β-Blockers, antithyroid medications
Asthma	Bronchodilators, corticosteroids
Pneumonia	Antibiotics
Pulmonary edema	Diuretics, improvement in CHF
Pulmonary embolism	O_2, anticoagulation
Cardiac arrhythmias	Lower pH <7.50, acetazolamide, rebreather
High altitude, climbing	O_2, acetazolamide
Mechanical ventilation	↓ Ventilatory rate and tidal volume, ↑ dead space, mild sedation without skeletal muscle paralysis

- ↑ Hematocrit—suggestive of exposure to high altitude
- Abnormal liver function tests—liver disease
- ↑ T_3 and T_4 and low TSH—suggestive of hyperthyroidism
- When both respiratory alkalosis and high AG metabolic acidosis are present—suspect salicylate intake
- Positive urine β-human chorionic hormone—pregnancy

Other Tests

- Chest X-ray
- Blood cultures

Treatment

- Respiratory alkalosis is not benign and no longer self-limited. Treatment is, therefore, warranted.
- Correction of the primary disorder of the respiratory alkalosis is extremely important.
- Table 33.4 shows the cause-specific treatment of respiratory alkalosis.

Study Questions

Case 1 A 24-year-old woman with asthma is seen in the Emergency Department (ED) for acute exacerbation due to upper respiratory tract infection. Prior to bronchodilator and corticosteroid therapy, laboratory results show:

Serum	ABG
Na$^+$ = 139 mEq/L	pH = 7.55
K$^+$ = 3.4 mEq/L	pCO$_2$ = 22 mmHg
Cl$^-$ = 96 mEq/L	pO$_2$ = 88 mmHg
HCO$_3^-$ = 21 mEq/L	HCO$_3^-$ = 20 mEq/L
Creatinine = 0.6 mg/dL	
BUN = 18 mg/dL	
Glucose = 92 mg/dL	

Question 1 What is the acid–base disturbance?

Answer Based on alkaline pH, low HCO$_3^-$, and low pCO$_2$, the acid–base disturbance is respiratory alkalosis.

Question 2 Is it acute or chronic respiratory alkalosis?

Answer It is acute respiratory alkalosis, as the decrease in serum [HCO$_3^-$] from 24 to 21 mEq/L (for each mmHg decrease in pCO$_2$, HCO$_3^-$ decreases by 0.2 mEq/L) is consistent with uncomplicated acute respiratory alkalosis. Hypocapnia due to hyperventilation is common during exacerbation of asthma.

Case 2 A 66-year-old man with chronic obstructive pulmonary disease is admitted for increasing shortness of breath and swollen legs for 10 days. He is on bronchodilators and furosemide. Physical examination reveals crackles and an S$_3$, and 2+ pitting edema in lower extremities. The patient receives IV furosemide 60 mg Q12H for 3 days, and his shortness of breath and edema improved. Electrocardiography is normal. Laboratory results:

Serum electrolytes and ABG—on admission	Serum electrolytes and ABG—on the fourth day
Na$^+$ = 136 mEq/L	Na$^+$ = 134 mEq/L
K$^+$ = 3.3 mEq/L	K$^+$ = 3.2 mEq/L
Cl$^-$ = 104 mEq/L	Cl$^-$ = 96 mEq/L
HCO$_3^-$ = 18 mEq/L	HCO$_3^-$ = 21 mEq/L
Creatinine = 1.1 mg/dL	Creatinine = 1.2 mg/dL
BUN = 28 mg/dL	BUN = 38 mg/dL
Glucose = 102 mg/dL	Glucose = 112 mg/dL
ABG	
pH = 7.45	pH = 7.48
pCO$_2$ = 26 mmHg	pCO$_2$ = 28 mmHg
pO$_2$ = 90 mmHg	pO$_2$ = 92 mmHg
HCO$_3^-$ = 17 mEq/L	HCO$_3^-$ = 20 mEq/L

Question 1 What is the acid–base disturbance on admission?

Answer Based on alkaline pH, low serum [HCO$_3^-$], and pCO$_2$, the acid–base disturbance is respiratory alkalosis. The expected serum [HCO$_3^-$] from secondary response for acute respiratory alkalosis is 21 mEq/L (24–3 = 21 mEq/L). For chronic respiratory alkalosis, the expected serum [HCO_3^-] from secondary response is 18 (24–6 = 18 mEq/L). Therefore, the patient has uncomplicated chronic respiratory alkalosis.

Question 2   What is the acid–base disorder on the fourth day?

Answer   Although the patient had chronic respiratory alkalosis on admission, the pH, serum [HCO_3^-], and pCO_2 are elevated following treatment, suggesting super-imposed metabolic alkalosis caused by administration of furosemide. The induction of metabolic alkalosis due to loop diuretics is not uncommon in patients with con-gestive heart failure and edema.

Suggested Reading

1. Adrogué HJ, Madias NE. Management of life-threatening acid-base disorders [1 of 2 parts]. N Engl J Med. 1998;338:26–34.
2. Elliott CG, Morris AH. Clinical syndromes of respiratory acidosis and alkalosis. In: Seldin DW, Giebisch G, editors. The regulation of acid-base balance. New York: Raven Press; 1989. p. 483–521.
3. Laffey JG, Kavanagh BP. Hypocapnia. N Engl J Med. 2002;347:43–53.
4. Krapf R, Hulter HN. Respiratory alkalosis. In: Gennari FJ, Adrogué HJ, Galla JH, Madias NE, editors. Acid-base disorders and their treatment. Boca Raton: Taylor & Francis; 2005. p. 641–79.

Mixed Acid–Base Disorders

34

A mixed acid–base disorder is defined as the coexistence of two or three primary disorders in the same patient. These disorders can occur simultaneously or at different times. Two groups of patients are at risk for mixed acid–base disturbances: the critically ill patients in the intensive care units and the elderly. Also, diabetic or alcoholic subjects may present to the emergency department with a double or triple acid–base disturbance.

In general, the critically ill patients have multiple medical conditions that can elicit a mixed acid–base disturbance. For example, a septic or liver failure patient can present initially with a respiratory alkalosis and subsequently develop a high anion gap (AG) metabolic acidosis due to hypotension. The other group of patients, the elderly, may have a chronic disease such as chronic obstructive pulmonary disease (COPD) with respiratory acidosis and subsequent development of metabolic alkalosis due to a thiazide or loop diuretic for treatment of cor pulmonale.

Recognition of a mixed acid–base disorder by the clinician is extremely important for appropriate care of the patient. For example, failure to recognize the metabolic alkalosis superimposed on chronic respiratory acidosis may aggravate hypoxemia because both disorders are associated with an increase in pCO_2. Also, vigorous saline administration may improve the underlying metabolic alkalosis while lowering the pH to a dangerous level. To avoid these changes, it is extremely important to recognize both disorders and treat them simultaneously so that the patient's condition would ultimately improve.

Furthermore, identification of a mixed acid–base disorder may provide a clue to the onset of a new condition, particularly in a critically ill patient. For example, a patient with severe pneumonia and respiratory alkalosis may start developing an increase in AG within a few hours of admission. This suggests that the patient may be generating lactic acid due to septic shock.

© Springer Science+Business Media LLC 2018
A.S. Reddi, *Fluid, Electrolyte and Acid-Base Disorders*,
DOI 10.1007/978-3-319-60167-0_34

Analysis of Mixed Acid–Base Disorders

Mixed acid–base disorders should be suspected whenever (see also Chap. 27):

1. There is no compensatory response or overcompensation for a primary simple acid–base disorder.
2. The pH and [HCO_3^-] are normal, but the AG is high (mixed metabolic acidosis and metabolic alkalosis).
3. The pH is near normal, but [HCO_3^-] is low (mixed metabolic acidosis and respiratory alkalosis).
4. The pH is low (<7.40), but [HCO_3^-] is normal or slightly low (mixed metabolic acidosis and respiratory acidosis).
5. The pH is near normal, but [HCO_3^-] is high (mixed metabolic alkalosis and respiratory acidosis).
6. The pH is high (>7.40), but [HCO_3^-] is normal (mixed metabolic alkalosis and respiratory alkalosis).

Several factors should be taken into consideration in analyzing a mixed acid–base disorder. Such factors include:

1. Medical and clinical settings: stable or unstable, intubation, sepsis, hypotension, nasogastric suction, ketoacidosis, etc.
2. Drug administration: sedation
3. Evaluation of pH: lower than before (additive), normal (counterbalancing), or high (additive)
4. AG: normal or high
5. Time course of pH changes: acute or chronic disturbance

The following discussion will focus on the clinical settings in which a common mixed acid–base disorder occurs with characteristic electrolyte and arterial blood gas (ABG) values. Note that these laboratory values vary depending on the presence of dominant disturbance and the duration of the coexisting disorder. Table 34.1 summarizes the most frequently observed mixed acid–base disorders in hospitalized patients.

Table 34.1 Common mixed acid–base disorders, pH, and electrolyte profiles

Acid–base disorder	Clinical setting	pH	pCO$_2$[a]	Na$^+$	K$^+$	Cl$^-$	HCO$_3^{-a}$	AG
Double acid–base disorders								
Metabolic acidosis and metabolic alkalosis	Renal failure (CKD 4 and 5), diabetic ketoacidosis, lactic acidosis with vomiting, or diuretics	N	N	N/↓	N↓	N↓	~N	↑
Metabolic acidosis and respiratory alkalosis	Renal failure (CKD 4 and 5) with sepsis or salicylate intoxication or pulmonary embolus	~N	↓↓	N	N	N/↑	↓↓	↑ or N[b]
Metabolic acidosis and respiratory acidosis	Cardiac arrest or renal failure with emphysema or sedatives or narcotics	↓↓	N/↑	N	N	N	N/↓	↑ or N[b]
Metabolic alkalosis and respiratory alkalosis	Vomiting, diuretics with pneumonia, hepatic failure, pregnancy	↑↑	N/↓	~ N	↓	N	N/↑	Slight↑
Metabolic alkalosis and respiratory acidosis	Vomiting or diuretics with emphysema or sedatives	N/↑	↑↑	N/↓	N/↓	N	↑↑	N
Triple acid–base disorders								
Metabolic acidosis, metabolic alkalosis, and respiratory alkalosis	Ketoacidosis with vomiting and abdominal pain or pneumonia	↑	↓	N	N/↓	N/↓	Slight↓	↑
Metabolic acidosis, metabolic alkalosis, and respiratory acidosis	Ketoacidosis with vomiting, sedative, or COPD	↓↓	↓	N	N	N	↓↓	↑

AG anion gap, *COPD* chronic obstructive pulmonary disease, *CKD* chronic kidney disease
[a]Concentrations of these vary depending on the severity of the dominant acid–base disorder
[b]AG depends on the etiology of metabolic acidosis

Metabolic Acidosis and Metabolic Alkalosis

This disorder can be seen in two clinical settings:

1. Metabolic acidosis due to chronic kidney disease (CKD) stages 4 and 5 (renal failure), ketoacidosis, or lactic acidosis with a superimposed metabolic alkalosis due to vomiting or nasogastric suction. The most compatible electrolyte and ABG values are as follows:

Serum	ABG
Na^+ = 138 mEq/L	pH = 7.39
K^+ = 3.6 mEq/L	pCO_2 = 39 mmHg
Cl^- = 96 mEq/L	pO_2 = 92 mmHg
HCO_3^- = 23 mEq/L	HCO_3^- = 22 mEq/L
Creatinine = 4.6 mg/dL	
BUN = 48 mg/dL	
AG = 19	

   ABG arterial blood gas, *AG* anion gap, *BUN* blood urea nitrogen

2. Metabolic alkalosis due to loop or thiazide diuretic use with a superimposed metabolic acidosis due to ketoacidosis or renal failure. Compatible laboratory results are:

Serum	ABG
Na^+ = 130 mEq/L	pH = 7.41
K^+ = 3.2 mEq/L	pCO_2 = 41 mmHg
Cl^- = 86 mEq/L	pO_2 = 92 mmHg
HCO_3^- = 25 mEq/L	HCO_3^- = 24 mEq/L
Creatinine = 1.4 mg/dL	
BUN = 28 mg/dL	
AG = 19	

   ABG arterial blood gas, *AG* anion gap, *BUN* blood urea nitrogen

Note that electrolyte and ABG values vary depending on the dominant acid–base disorder. The effect on pH by these acid–base disorders is to bring it to near normal (counterbalancing). One consistent abnormality is serum AG, which is elevated. If diarrhea is the cause for metabolic acidosis, the AG may not be that high.

Metabolic Acidosis and Respiratory Alkalosis

The clinical setting is usually renal failure, ketoacidosis, or lactic acidosis with sepsis. Salicylate overdose or pulmonary embolism can produce both metabolic acidosis and respiratory alkalosis. The representative electrolyte and ABG are shown in the following table. The AG is elevated. The effect on pH is counterbalancing, so that the pH is brought to near normal, but the fall in pCO_2 is greater with both disorders. In salicylate overdose, the initial acid–base disorder is respiratory alkalosis due to direct central nervous system (CNS) stimulation followed by the development of metabolic acidosis. The presence of dominant disorder can be identified by calculation of appropriate secondary response. For example, if metabolic acidosis is the dominant acid–base disorder, the superimposed respiratory alkalosis can be diagnosed by a greater fall in pCO_2 than expected for a simple metabolic acidosis. If respiratory alkalosis is the dominant disturbance, a coexisting metabolic acidosis can be identified by a greater fall in serum $[HCO_3^-]$ than expected for a simple respiratory alkalosis.

The laboratory values shown in the following table indicate that metabolic acidosis is the dominant acid–base disturbance. The expected pCO_2 should be 26 ± 2 mmHg ($1.5 \times$ serum $HCO_3^- + 8 \pm 2 = 18 + 8 = 26 \pm 2$). Instead, the reported pCO_2 is 22 mmHg, indicating that the patient is more hypocapnic than expected. Thus, respiratory alkalosis is superimposed on metabolic acidosis.

Serum	ABG
Na^+ = 129 mEq/L	pH = 7.36
K^+ = 3.4 mEq/L	pCO_2 = 22 mmHg
Cl^- = 92 mEq/L	pO_2 = 90 mmHg
HCO_3^- = 12 mEq/L	HCO_3^- = 11 mEq/L
Creatinine = 8.6 mg/dL	
BUN = 68 mg/dL	
AG = 25	

ABG arterial blood gas, *AG* anion gap, *BUN* blood urea nitrogen

Metabolic Acidosis and Respiratory Acidosis

This acid–base disorder occurs in the clinical setting of cardiac arrest, renal failure, lactic acidosis with sedatives or narcotics, or COPD. The effect on pH is additive, as both acid–base disorders lower pH. The electrolyte pattern and ABG (see table below) suggest that the primary acid–base disorder is chronic respiratory acidosis and the coexisting disturbance is metabolic acidosis due to lactic acidosis. The AG is high. The AG may be normal, if the cause of metabolic acidosis is diarrhea or renal tubular defect.

Serum	ABG
Na^+ = 136 mEq/L	pH = 7.27
K^+ = 3.9 mEq/L	pCO_2 = 44 mmHg
Cl^- = 100 mEq/L	pO_2 = 88 mmHg
HCO_3^- = 20 mEq/L	HCO_3^- = 19 mEq/L
Creatinine = 1.0 mg/dL	
BUN = 24 mg/dL	
AG = 16	

ABG arterial blood gas, *AG* anion gap, *BUN* blood urea nitrogen

Metabolic Alkalosis and Respiratory Alkalosis

The conditions that predispose to this mixed acid–base disorder are vomiting or diuretic therapy with metabolic alkalosis complicated by respiratory alkalosis due to pneumonia or hepatic failure. Pregnant individuals usually have respiratory alkalosis because of progesterone and elevated diaphragm; however, when they develop profuse vomiting, a superimposed metabolic alkalosis develops.

When patients on mechanical ventilator develop respiratory alkalosis because of increased respiratory rate, they are predisposed to metabolic alkalosis, if nasogastric suction is applied. The effect on pH is additive. The following electrolyte and ABG pattern was observed in a patient with alkali ingestion and pneumonia:

Serum	ABG
Na^+ = 146 mEq/L	pH = 7.60
K^+ = 2.8 mEq/L	pCO_2 = 45 mmHg
Cl^- = 80 mEq/L	pO_2 = 68 mmHg
HCO_3^- = 52 mEq/L	HCO_3^- = 51 mEq/L
Creatinine = 1.6 mg/dL	
BUN = 24 mg/dL	
AG = 14	

ABG arterial blood gas, *AG* anion gap, *BUN* blood urea nitrogen

The AG is elevated because of alkalosis-induced lactate production.

Metabolic Alkalosis and Respiratory Acidosis

The clinical setting in patients with mixed metabolic alkalosis and respiratory acidosis is vomiting, diuretic use with COPD, sedatives, or narcotics that inhibit the medullary respiratory center. This disorder is commonly seen in patients with COPD, hypertension, and congestive heart failure (CHF), who are treated with either loop or thiazide diuretics. The effect on pH is counterbalancing. The following electrolytes and ABG are consistent in a patient with chronic respiratory acidosis and diuretic therapy for hypertension.

Serum	ABG
Na^+ = 134 mEq/L	pH = 7.42
K^+ = 3.6 mEq/L	pCO_2 = 59 mmHg
Cl^- = 91 mEq/L	pO_2 = 62 mmHg
HCO_3^- = 37 mEq/L	HCO_3^- = 36 mEq/L
Creatinine = 1.3 mg/dL	
BUN = 18 mg/dL	

ABG arterial blood gas, *AG* anion gap, *BUN* blood urea nitrogen

Two other mixed acid–base disorders are seen clinically but infrequently. They are:

1. Hyperchloremic (non-AG) metabolic acidosis and high AG metabolic acidosis
   The clinical setting is a patient with profuse diarrhea who subsequently develops hypotension and lactic acidosis. The effect on pH is additive. Typical laboratory results are as follows:

$$pH = 7.10$$
$$pCO_2 = 18 \, mmHg$$
$$pO_2 = 86 \, mmHg$$
$$Serum \left[HCO_3^- \right] = 6 \, mEq/L$$
$$Calculated \left[HCO_3^- \right] = 5 \, mEq/L$$
$$AG = elevated$$

2. Acute respiratory acidosis and chronic respiratory acidosis

The clinical setting is a COPD patient with chronic respiratory acidosis, who develops deterioration in his/her lung disease, or application of a sedative or high inspired O_2. The effect on pH is additive. Typical laboratory results are as follows:

$$pH = 7.31$$
$$pCO_2 = 80 \, mmHg$$
$$pO_2 = 70 \, mmHg$$
$$Serum \left[HCO_3^- \right] = 39 \, mEq/L$$
$$Calculated \left[HCO_3^- \right] = 38 \, mEq/L$$
$$AG = normal$$

The ABG suggests respiratory acidosis. However, the observed HCO_3^- is higher than for both acute (expected $HCO_3^- = 28$ mEq/L) and chronic (expected $HCO_3^- = 36$ mEq/L) respiratory acidosis, suggesting acute superimposed on chronic respiratory acidosis. Metabolic alkalosis also increases both pCO_2 and HCO_3^-, but the pH also is elevated. The typical pH in patients with acute respiratory acidosis superimposed on chronic respiratory acidosis is much lower than that of a patient with chronic respiratory acidosis, which is usually >7.34. The pCO_2 of 80 mmHg is not consistent with chronic respiratory acidosis alone.

Triple Acid–Base Disorders

Although rare, triple acid–base disorders can be seen in certain ill patients. For example, a patient with ketoacidosis with vomiting and abdominal pain can present with high AG metabolic acidosis, metabolic alkalosis, and respiratory alkalosis (see Case 2).

Similarly, a patient with lactic acidosis, who is on a ventilator with low tidal volume and low respiratory rate and nasogastric suction, typically develops high AG metabolic acidosis, metabolic alkalosis, and respiratory acidosis (see Case 3).

Treatment

Treatment of a mixed acid–base disorder is difficult compared to that of a simple acid–base disorder. Identification of a dominant acid–base disorder and its cause is extremely important. Furthermore, treatment is guided by attention to the blood pH, because therapy of one aspect of mixed acid–base disorder may not aggravate the other coexisting disturbance. Treatment of common mixed disturbances is outlined in the following sections.

Metabolic Acidosis and Metabolic Alkalosis

- Normal (0.9%) saline improves Cl^--responsive metabolic alkalosis. If metabolic acidosis is due to diabetic ketoacidosis, insulin and normal (or 0.45%) NaCl improve ketoacidosis. If ketoacidosis is related to starvation or alcohol, glucose infusion (D5W) is sufficient. For lactic acidosis and metabolic alkalosis, normal saline is effective. In patients with renal failure, metabolic acidosis can be improved by renal replacement therapies.

Metabolic Acidosis and Respiratory Alkalosis

- Correcting the cause of both disorders improves the acid–base disturbance. Administration of $NaHCO_3$ may not be helpful all the time, because it may worsen alkalemia. Rebreather may alleviate respiratory alkalosis.
- Renal replacement therapy improves both acidosis and alkalosis.

Metabolic Acidosis and Respiratory Acidosis

- Both disorders lower pH below 7.1. The cause for respiratory failure should be addressed, and if necessary, intubation should be considered. Hyperventilation and lowering pCO_2 judiciously improve pH. The goal pH is 7.20–7.28.

Metabolic Alkalosis and Respiratory Alkalosis

- Both disorders increase pH above 7.50. If respiratory alkalosis is new, the cause such as sepsis or unrecognized pulmonary embolus should be addressed. A patient on ventilator and nasogastric suction can be managed efficiently to improve both disorders.
- $NaHCO_3$ therapy should be avoided.
- Normal saline or KCl or both can improve Cl^--responsive metabolic alkalosis.

Metabolic Alkalosis and Respiratory Acidosis

- Cl^--responsive metabolic alkalosis responds to normal saline and/or KCl. This treatment promotes renal excretion of HCO_3^- and lowers pH.
- Lowering pCO_2 too much worsens alkalemia. Also, vigorous saline administration lowers pH. In order to maintain reasonable pH and pCO_2, it is important to identify the dominant disorder and treat that disorder appropriately. Addressing the other disorder, if necessary, results in proper management of this mixed acid–base disturbance.
- Patients with chronic respiratory acidosis depend on acidemia for ventilatory drive; rapid increase in their pH should be avoided.

Study Questions

Case 1   For each set of laboratory data, select the appropriate acid–base disturbance:

Option	Na$^+$ (mEq/L)	Cl$^-$ (mEq/L)	HCO$_3^-$ (mEq/L)	pH	pCO$_2$ (mmHg)	HCO$_3^{-a}$ (mEq/L)
A	130	95	10	7.34	19	9
B	136	94	24	7.39	39	23
C	130	85	29	7.50	36	28
D	140	100	20	7.27	44	19
E	142	100	32	7.41	52	31

^{a}Calculated HCO$_3^-$

1. Metabolic alkalosis and respiratory acidosis
2. Metabolic acidosis and respiratory alkalosis
3. Metabolic acidosis and respiratory acidosis
4. Metabolic acidosis and metabolic alkalosis
5. Metabolic alkalosis and respiratory alkalosis

Answers   A = 2; B = 4; C = 3; D = 5; E = 1 or (1 = E; 2 = A; 3 = D; 4 = B; 5 = C)

To answer these questions, it is important to calculate the AG. The AG and an understanding of the pathogenesis of previously mentioned mixed acid–base disorders provide important clues for their identification. The AG for options A–E are 25, 18, 16, 20, and 10 mEq/L, respectively. Regarding the pathogenesis of the acid–base disorder in Answer 1, either vomiting or diuretic (thiazide or loop diuretic) use generally causes metabolic alkalosis, and emphysema or any disorder causing retention of CO_2 results in respiratory acidosis. Laboratory data shown in option E are consistent with metabolic alkalosis and respiratory acidosis. The combination of both disorders has a normal to high pH, elevated HCO_3^-, and pCO_2. The AG is usually normal or slightly elevated, if metabolic alkalosis predominates.

The acid–base disturbance given in Answer 2 may be caused by diseases such as renal failure, lactic acidosis, and ketoacidosis or ingestion of toxins such as methanol or ethylene glycol, which lower serum [HCO_3^-] and elevate AG. The appropriate response for metabolic acidosis is hyperventilation. This results in low pCO_2. Data shown in option A are consistent with metabolic acidosis and respiratory alkalosis. Metabolic acidosis may exist alone (pure) or may exist with another primary disorder (mixed). In order to distinguish between the two disorders, the expected PCO_2 should be calculated, as shown under the discussion of mixed metabolic acidosis and respiratory alkalosis. If the ABG values shown in option A were pure metabolic acidosis, the pCO_2 would have been between 21 and 25 mmHg. Instead, the pCO_2 is 19 mmHg. Therefore, respiratory alkalosis is superimposed on metabolic acidosis.

The acid–base disturbance given in Answer 3 is generally caused by a condition that generates lactic acid acutely, such as sudden cardiac arrest, seizures, or severe hypotension superimposed on a patient with underlying emphysema with CO_2 retention. The combination of metabolic acidosis and respiratory acidosis lowers pH below 7.40 and [HCO_3^-] below 24 mEq/L with normal to slightly elevated pCO_2. The AG is usually elevated because of accumulation of lactic acid or a similar anion. Laboratory data shown in option D are consistent with both metabolic and respiratory acidosis.

The acid–base disorder given in Answer 4 occurs in a patient with renal failure who develops vomiting or on a thiazide or loop diuretic. Renal failure causes high AG metabolic acidosis with low pH, low [HCO_3^-], and low pCO_2. On the other hand, metabolic alkalosis results in a high pH, elevated [HCO_3^-], and a high pCO_2 due to hypoventilation. When both disorders coexist, the pH, [HCO_3^-], and pCO_2 may appear normal. The only clue to this acid–base disorder is elevated AG, because both metabolic acidosis and metabolic alkalosis cause elevated AG. However, metabolic acidosis due to diarrhea or renal tubular acidosis does not elevate AG. The combination of normal AG metabolic acidosis and metabolic alkalosis generally causes slight elevation in AG because of the latter acid–base disorder. Laboratory data shown in option B are consistent with metabolic acidosis and metabolic alkalosis.

The acid–base disturbance given in Answer 5 is seen in a patient who has liver failure with hyperventilation. This causes respiratory alkalosis. If this patient is also being treated with a diuretic, such as furosemide, or has experienced vomiting, the patient develops metabolic alkalosis. In such a patient, the pH is usually >7.40, the [HCO_3^-] is normal to high, and pCO_2 is normal to slightly low. Laboratory data shown in option C are consistent with respiratory and metabolic alkalosis. A similar acid–base disorder can be seen in a normal pregnant woman with severe vomiting.

Case 2 A 38-year-old man with history of type 1 diabetes and pancreatitis is admitted for nausea, vomiting, and severe abdominal pain for the last 4 days. He did not take insulin because of poor oral intake. Laboratory results are as follows:

Serum	ABG
Na^+ = 120 mEq/L	pH = 7.47
K^+ = 3.9 mEq/L	pCO_2 = 23 mmHg
Cl^- = 60 mEq/L	pO_2 = 109 mmHg
HCO_3^- = 17 mEq/L	HCO_3^- = 16 mEq/L
Creatinine = 3.1 mg/dL	
BUN = 88 mg/dL	
Glucose = 776 mg/dL	
Ketones = positive	

Question 1 Characterize the acid–base disturbance.

Answer Using the Henderson equation, the [H^+] is 32, which corresponds to a pH of 7.48 and close to the patient's pH. From the ABG values, the initial disturbance is respiratory alkalosis, and calculation of secondary response suggests that it is chronic rather than acute respiratory alkalosis. Hyperventilation due to abdominal pain accounts for this acid–base disturbance.

The calculated AG is 43, which is not due to alkalosis but entirely due to the presence of metabolic acidosis. Insulin withdrawal and subsequent generation of ketoacids (ketones positive) account for this high AG metabolic acidosis.

Assuming the normal AG of 10, this patient has an excess of 33 (43–10 = 33; ΔAG = 33) anions. If 1 H^+ is buffered by 1 HCO_3^-, the patient should not have any measurable HCO_3^- in the serum. However, his measured HCO_3^- is 17 mEq/L, suggesting that he had a high level of serum HCO_3^- before the development of metabolic acidosis. Thus, he had metabolic alkalosis prior to the development of metabolic acidosis. This was confirmed by the patient that his vomiting started before he withdrew insulin injections. Thus, the patient has a triple acid–base disorder of *chronic respiratory alkalosis, high AG metabolic acidosis, and metabolic alkalosis*.

Question 2 Does Na^+ need to be corrected for hyperglycemia to calculate AG?

Answer No. From Chap. 27, it is clear that Na^+ correction for hyperglycemia is not needed to calculate the AG.

Question 3 Is $\Delta AG/\Delta HCO_3^-$ useful in the analysis of ABG?

Answer Yes. The $\Delta AG/\Delta HCO_3^-$ ratio of >2 is indicative of metabolic alkalosis. In this patient, the $\Delta AG/\Delta HCO_3^-$ ratio is 4.71 (ΔAG = 33; ΔHCO_3^- = 7 (24–17); ratio = 33/7 = 4.71). However, it is not necessary to depend on $\Delta AG/\Delta HCO_3^-$ ratio all the time. For example, this patient's serum [HCO_3^-] is disproportionately high compared to the increase in AG, suggesting an underlying metabolic alkalosis.

Case 3 A 31-year-old woman with alcohol abuse and pancreatitis is admitted for shortness of breath, confusion, profuse vomiting, and abdominal pain. She is electively intubated and sedated. The following laboratory results are obtained:

Serum	ABG
Na^+ = 136 mEq/L	pH = 7.01
K^+ = 4.9 mEq/L	pCO_2 = 26 mmHg
Cl^- = 87 mEq/L	pO_2 = 67 mmHg
HCO_3^- = 7 mEq/L	HCO_3^- = 6 mEq/L
Creatinine = 4.1 mg/dL	
BUN = 7 mg/dL	
Glucose = 72 mg/dL	
Ketones = positive	

ABG Arterial blood gas, *BUN* blood urea nitrogen

Question 1 Characterize the acid–base disturbance.

Answer Based on low pH and serum [HCO_3^-] and the AG of 42, the patient has a high AG metabolic acidosis due to alcoholic ketoacidosis.

Since the expected pCO_2 for this degree of acidemia is 18.5 mmHg (range 16.5–20.5), the patient has respiratory acidosis (hypercapnia), which is due to the sedative.

As in Case 2, there is a disproportionate relationship between the increase in AG and decrease in HCO_3^-, suggesting an underlying metabolic alkalosis. This is evident from low serum [Cl^-], which is due to vomiting. The $\Delta AG/\Delta HCO_3^-$ ratio is 1.9 (ΔAG = 42–10=32; ΔHCO_3^-=24–7=17; ratio 32/17=1.9), which also supports the underlying metabolic alkalosis.

Thus, the acid–base disorder is a *high AG metabolic acidosis*, *respiratory acidosis*, and *metabolic alkalosis*.

Question 2 What would be her pH, if her pCO_2 is lowered to 18 mmHg?

Answer Her pH would be ~7.18, if her pCO_2 is lowered by increasing the respiratory rate. This pH is obtained by using the Henderson equation:

$$\left[H^+\right] = 24 \times \frac{pCO_2}{HCO_3^-}$$

$$\left[H^+\right] = 24 \times \frac{18}{7} = 62 = pH = 7.18$$

Case 4 A 60-year-old woman with HIV/AIDS is admitted for diarrhea and poly-substance abuse. She is hypotensive (systolic blood pressure of 90 mmHg) with heart rate of 112 beats per minute. Laboratory results are as follows:

Serum	ABG
Na^+ = 130 mEq/L	pH = 7.06
K^+ = 5.5 mEq/L	pCO_2 = 28 mmHg
Cl^- = 112 mEq/L	pO_2 = 84 mmHg
HCO_3^- = 9 mEq/L	HCO_3^- = 8 mEq/L
Creatinine = 1.5 mg/dL	
BUN = 38 mg/dL	
Glucose = 80 mg/dL	
Albumin = 2.3 g/dL	
Urine toxicology: positive for cocaine and heroin	

Question 1 Which one of the following describes the BEST of her acid–base status?

(A) Metabolic acidosis and metabolic alkalosis
(B) Metabolic alkalosis and respiratory alkalosis
(C) Metabolic acidosis and respiratory acidosis
(D) Respiratory acidosis, metabolic alkalosis and metabolic acidosis
(E) Metabolic acidosis, respiratory alkalosis and metabolic alkalosis

The answer is C The patient has a high AG metabolic acidosis and respiratory acidosis. Her AG is 14 when corrected for normal albumin level of 4.3 g/dL. Note that the AG decreases by 2.5 for each gram decrease in serum albumin from normal values of 4–4.5 g/dL. The superimposed respiratory acidosis is caused by her illicit drug use, which inhibits the medullary respiratory center. The high AG seems to be due to lactic acid production (hypotension) and acute kidney injury.

Question 2 Does $\Delta AG/\Delta HCO_3^-$ ratio have any significance in this patient?

Answer Yes. In diarrhea, the $\Delta AG/\Delta HCO_3^-$ ratio is usually <1 (see Chap. 27). In this patient, this ratio is 0.3 (ΔAG = 14–10=4; ΔHCO_3^- = 24–9=15; ratio 4/15=0.3). The $\Delta AG/\Delta HCO_3^-$ ratio of <1 is suggestive of diarrhea as a cause of abnormal ABG in a patient who does not give adequate history of diarrhea.

Suggested Reading

1. Adrogué HJ, Madias NE. Respiratory acidosis, respiratory alkalosis, 2 mixed disorders. In: Floege J, Johnson RJ, Feehally J, editors. Comprehensive clinical nephrology. 4th ed. St. Louis: Elsevier/Saunders; 2010. p. 176–89.
2. Emmett M, Narins RG. Mixed acid–base disorders. In: Narins RG, editor. Maxwell & Kleeman's clinical disorders of fluid and electrolyte metabolism. 5th ed. New York: McGraw-Hill; 1994. p. 991–1107.
3. Kraut JA, Kurtz I. Mixed acid–base disorders. In: Mount DB, Sayegh MH, Singh AJ, editors. Core concepts in the disorders of fluid, electrolytes and acid–base balance. New York: Springer; 2013. p. 307–26.
4. Rastegar A. Mixed acid–base disorders. In: Gennari FJ, Adrogué HJ, Galla JH, Madias NE, editors. Acid–base disorders and their treatment. Boca Raton: Taylor & Francis; 2005. p. 681–96.

Drug-Induced Acid–Base Disorders

35

In Chaps. 28, 29, 30, 31, 32, and 33, we discussed various systemic and drug-induced causes of acid–base disorders. Since drug-induced acid–base disorders are rather common in daily clinical practice, this chapter summarizes the iatrogenic causes of the four primary acid–base disorders. The pathophysiology of systemic and drug-induced primary acid–base disorders is discussed in the above chapters.

Metabolic Acidosis

Drugs that cause metabolic acidosis fall into three groups:

1. Drugs that generate endogenous acid (Table 35.1)
2. Drugs that cause loss of HCO_3^- from the GI tract or kidney (Table 35.2)
3. Drugs that impair renal tubular function (Tables 35.3, 35.4, and 35.5)

Table 35.1 Common drugs that generate acids with high AG

Drug	Major acid generated
Metformin	Lactic acid
Antiretrovirals (didanosine, zidovudine, stavudine, zalcitabine, tenofovir, abacavir)	Lactic acid
Linezolid	Lactic acid
Propofol	Lactic acid
Cyanide poisoning	Lactic acid
Propylene glycol	Lactic acid
Salicylate	Ketoacid
Ethanol	Ketoacid
Methanol	Formic acid
Ethylene glycol	Oxalic acid
Toluene	Hippuric acid
Acetaminophen, netilmicin, flucloxacillin, vigabatrin	Pyroglutamic acid

© Springer Science+Business Media LLC 2018
A.S. Reddi, *Fluid, Electrolyte and Acid-Base Disorders*,
DOI 10.1007/978-3-319-60167-0_35

Table 35.2 Drugs that cause loss of HCO_3^- from the GI tract or kidney with normal AG

Drug	Source of loss
Acetazolamide	Kidney
Topiramate	Kidney
Cholestyramine	GI tract
Sevelamer HCl	GI tract
Calcium chloride	GI tract

Table 35.3 Drugs that cause proximal RTA with hypokalemia and normal AG

CA inhibitors (acetazolamide, topiramate)
Anticancer drugs (ifosfamide, cisplatin, carboplatin, streptozotocin, azacitidine, suramin, mercaptopurine)
Antibacterial drugs (outdated tetracyclines, aminoglycosides)
Anticonvulsants (valproic acid, topiramate)
Antiviral agents (DDI, adefovir, cidofovir, tenofovir)
Others (fumarate, ranitidine, salicylates, alcohol, cadmium)

Table 35.4 Drugs that cause distal RTA with hypokalemia and normal AG

Amphotericin B
Toluene
Foscarnet
Vanadate (?)
Lithium
Analgesics
Cyclamate

Table 35.5 Drugs that cause distal RTA with hyperkalemia and normal AG

Drugs causing low renin and low aldosterone
NSAIDs
β-blockers
Cyclosporine
Tacrolimus
Drugs causing high renin and low aldosterone
ACE inhibitors
Angiotensin II receptor blockers
Ketoconazole
Heparin
ENaC inhibitors
Amiloride
Trimethoprim
Pentamidine
Triamterene
Na/K-ATPase inhibitors/activation of Na/Cl cotransporter
Cyclosporine
Tacrolimus
Aldosterone blockers
Spironolactone
Eplerenone

Metabolic Alkalosis

The following table (Table 35.6) shows the drugs that cause metabolic alkalosis.

Respiratory Acidosis

Drugs that cause respiratory acidosis are shown in Table 35.7.

Respiratory Alkalosis

Table 35.8 shows drugs that cause respiratory alkalosis.

Table 35.6 Drugs causing metabolic alkalosis

Loop diuretics
Thiazide diuretics
Poorly reabsorbable anions (carbenicillin, other penicillins, phosphate, sulfate)
`Gentamicin
$NaHCO_3$ (baking soda)
Sodium citrate, lactate, gluconate, acetate
Antacids
Licorice, chewing tobacco, carbenoxolone
Fludrocortisone
Laxatives

Table 35.7 Drugs that cause respiratory acidosis

Anesthetics (Diprivan, Ketalar, Pentothal, etc.)
Sedatives (pentobarbital, diazepam, clonazepam, etc.)
Opiates (morphine, codeine, heroin, etc.)
Succinylcholine
Curare
Aminoglycosides

Table 35.8 Drugs that cause respiratory alkalosis

Salicylates
Progesterone
Nicotine
Xanthine derivatives (caffeine, theophylline, pentoxifylline, etc.)
Antipsychotic drug (quetiapine)
Epinephrine

Suggested Reading

1. Kitterer D, Schwab M, Dominik M, et al. Drug-induced acid-base disorders. Pediatr Nephrol. 2015;30:1407–23.
2. Pham AQT, Xu LHR, Moe OW. Drug-induced metabolic acidosis. F1000Research 2015; 1–13.
3. Wiener SM. Toxicologic acid-base disorders. Emerg Med Clin N Am. 2014;32:149–65.

Part II

Fluid, Electrolyte and Acid-Base Disorders in Special Conditions

Acute Kidney Injury 36

Definition

Before 2004, at least 60 different definitions of acute kidney injury (AKI) have been reported in the literature, which were not validated or standardized. In 2004, the RIFLE (Risk, Injury, Failure, Loss, End-stage kidney disease) classification (Table 36.1) of AKI was introduced by the Acute Dialysis Quality Initiative (ADQI) group, which was subsequently validated.

- The RIFLE classification of AKI was further refined by the AKIN (Acute Kidney Injury Network) investigators. In this classification, AKI was categorized into three stages, and L and E from RIFLE classification were eliminated. Both classifications are based on serum creatinine and urine output. Table 36.1 shows both the RIFLE and AKIN classifications (criteria) of AKI.
- AKI can be nonoliguric (urine output >500 mL/day), oliguric (100–500 mL/day), or anuric (<100 mL/day).
- AKI is usually of sudden onset without warning, and there is not enough time for any adaptive mechanisms. Therefore, fluid, electrolyte, and acid–base imbalances are rather severe in AKI.

Fluid and Sodium (Na) Imbalances

- In patients with AKI, free water excretion is reduced. Fluid retention occurs in anuric or oliguric patients, if their oral intake of water exceeds 1 L/day unless they have fever or GI losses. For example, if anuric patient received >600 mL/day (<100 mL urine and 500 mL insensible loss), fluid is retained, and hypoosmolality (hyponatremia) develops.

© Springer Science+Business Media LLC 2018
A.S. Reddi, *Fluid, Electrolyte and Acid-Base Disorders*,
DOI 10.1007/978-3-319-60167-0_36

Table 36.1   RIFLE and AKIN classifications of AKI

RIFLE (criteria)	Serum creatinine (mg/dL)	Urine output[a] (mL/kg/h)	AKIN criteria (stages)	Serum creatinine (mg/dL)
R (risk)	↑in creatinine × 1.5 times or GFR ↓ >25%	<0.5 mL/k/h for >6 h	1	↑in creatinine × 1.5 to 2 from baseline or ↑in creatinine ≥0.3 mg/dL
I (injury)	Creatinine × 2 or GFR decreased >50%	<0.5 mL/k/h for >12 h	2	↑in creatinine × 2–3 from baseline
F (failure)	Creatinine × 3 or creatinine >4 mg/dL or GFR decreased >75%	<0.3 mL/kg/h for 24 h or anuria for 12 h	3	↑in creatinine × >3 from baseline or creatinine ≥4.0 mg/dL or ↑in creatinine ≥0.5 mg/dL from baseline creatinine of >4 mg/dL or RRT
L (loss)	Complete loss of renal function >4 weeks			
E (end-stage kidney disease)	ESKD >3 months			

RRT renal replacement therapy
[a]Applies to both RIFLE and AKIN classifications

- In nonoliguric or during recovery (diuretic) phase of AKI, fluid retention does not usually occur as the patients have good urine output. In these conditions, tubule dysfunction with resistance to ADH develops, resulting in excess free water loss. Hyperosmolality (hypernatremia) develops due to free water loss.
- Na balance is altered in AKI depending on the urine output. Anuric patients are more likely to retain Na than oliguric or nonoliguric patients. In general, Na retention occurs due to abrupt reduction in both GFR and Na excretion. Na intake should be restricted until diuretic phase of AKI.

Potassium (K) Imbalance

- K retention is rather common in AKI due to reduced GFR and decreased urine production. Hyperkalemia is seen more frequently in anuric and oliguric than nonoliguric patients.
- Nonoliguric AKI due to rhabdomyolysis or tumor lysis syndrome can present with severe hyperkalemia due to increased K release from cells.
- K should be restricted until diuretic phase of AKI.

Calcium (Ca) Imbalance

- Generally serum [Ca^{2+}] is reduced in AKI. Severe hypocalcemia is seen in patients with rhabdomyolysis because of hyperphosphatemia as well as skeletal resistance to PTH. Also, hypocalcemia in rhabdomyolysis is related to deposition of Ca in the injured muscle tissue.
- Severe hypocalcemia is seen in postoperative patients and in ethylene glycol poisoning due to complexing of Ca with oxalate to form Ca oxalate crystals.
- Hypercalcemia is observed during recovery phase of AKI, particularly in patients with rhabdomyolysis. This hypercalcemia is related to (1) improvement in hyperphosphatemia, (2) release of Ca from recovering injured muscles, and (3) improved skeletal resistance to PTH action.
- At times hypercalciuria is seen at presentation of AKI. This should alert the physician of some predisposing conditions such as multiple myeloma, or granulomatous disease, or Ca-containing medications, including vitamin D compounds.

Phosphate Imbalance

- Hyperphosphatemia is usually observed in anuric and oliguric AKI patients, which is due to reduced GFR and also related to cell lysis in conditions such as rhabdomyolysis and tumor lysis syndrome.
- Phosphate binders and/or renal replacement therapy are required in some patients.

Magnesium (Mg) Imbalance

- Mild elevation in serum [Mg^{2+}] is usually present in patients with AKI, which is due to reduced GFR and also Mg-containing products. Hypermagnesemia resolves following recovery phase of AKI.

Acid–Base Changes

- Metabolic acidosis with high anion gap (AG) is seen in most of the patients with anuric and oliguric AKI. This type of acidosis results from decreased excretion of H^+ that are generated from protein intake and endogenous generation of anions.
- $NaHCO_3$ (650 mg twice a day) or renal replacement therapy for severe acidosis may be required in some patients.

- Combined metabolic acidosis and respiratory alkalosis are commonly seen in patients with AKI.
- Metabolic alkalosis is sometimes observed following vomiting or nasogastric suction.

Suggested Reading

1. Franklin SS, Klein KL. Acute renal failure: fluid and electrolyte and acid-base complications. In: Narins RG, editor. Maxwell & Kleeman's clinical disorders of fluid and electrolyte metabolism. 5th ed. New York: McGraw-Hill, Inc; 1995. p. 1175–94.
2. Singbartl K, Joannidis M. Short-term effects of acute kidney injury. Crit Care Clin. 2015;31:751–62.
3. Swartz RD. Fluid, electrolyte, and acid-base changes during renal failure. In: Kokko JP, Tannen RL, editors. Fluids and electrolytes. 3rd ed. Philadelphia: WB. Saunders Company; 1996. p. 487–532.

Chronic Kidney Disease

37

Definition

Chronic kidney disease (CKD) is defined as abnormalities of the kidney structure or function present for >3 months with implications for health. These abnormalities include: GFR <60 mL/min, hematuria, proteinuria, and abnormal kidney structure. The following table (Table 37.1) shows the KDIGO (Kidney Disease Improving Global Outcomes) recommendations for CKD definition

Depending on GFR, CKD is classified into various stages, as shown below (Table 37.2).

Table 37.1 Criteria for CKD (either of the following present for >3 months)

Criterion	Recommendation
Markers of kidney damage (one or more)	Albuminuria (AER ≥30 mg/24 h; ACR ≥30 mg/g [≥3 mg/mmol]
	Urine sediment abnormalities
	Electrolyte and other abnormalities due to tubular disorders
	Abnormalities detected by histology
	Structural abnormalities detected by imaging
	History of kidney transplantation
Decreased GFR	GFR <60 mL/min/1.73 m^2 (GFR categories G3a-G5)

AER albumin excretion rate, *ACR* albumin/creatinine ratio, *GFR* glomerular filtration rate

© Springer Science+Business Media LLC 2018
A.S. Reddi, *Fluid, Electrolyte and Acid-Base Disorders*,
DOI 10.1007/978-3-319-60167-0_37

Table 37.2 CKD stages and their prevalence

Stage	GFR (mL/min)	Description	Prevalence in millions (%)
1[a]	≥90	Kidney damage with normal or increased GFR	3.6 (1.80%)
2	60–89	Kidney damage with mildly decreased GFR	6.5 (3.20%)
3[b]	30–59	Moderately decreased GFR	15.5 (7.70%)
4	15–29	Severely decreased GFR	0.7 (0.35%)
5	<15 or dialysis	Kidney failure	0.4 (0.20%)

Adapted from Coresh et al. [6]
[a]CKD is mostly recognized by either albuminuria or structural renal abnormality or eGFR <60 mL/min for >3 months
[b]CKD 3 is subdivided into CKD 3a (eGFR 45–59 mL/min) and CKD 3b (eGFR 30–44 mL/min)

Sodium (Na) Imbalance

- Na retention occurs once GFR is severely reduced and Na intake is unchanged.
- In CKD 2–3, Na balance is maintained by increasing its excretion by the surviving nephrons. This renal adaptation continues until the GFR falls to 10–15 mL/min.
- Several renal adaptive mechanisms have been implicated. A few examples of such adaptive mechanisms include natriuretic factors, volume expansion, decreased aldosterone activity, insulin resistance, glomerular hyperfiltration, and metabolic acidosis.
- Na restriction is necessary when renal function slowly deteriorates in order to prevent Na accumulation and volume-dependent hypertension.
- Generally Na is restricted in the diet to 1 g Na or 5 g salt, which equals 88 mEq. In clinical practice less than this amount of salt restriction is unpalatable and adherence is limited. Salt substitutes are not recommended, as they contain K. Na restriction may potentiate the action of ACE inhibitors. Na excretion is reduced with salt restriction.
- Some patients with renal dysfunction develop renal wasting of Na. They are usually hypotensive and may benefit from liberalization of salt in their diet.

Water Imbalance

- Normally the kidney maintains water balance by conserving water in water-deprived conditions and excretes free water during conditions of water excess. This water balance is lost in CKD 4–5.
- Normal kidneys have the ability to dilute urine and lower its osmolality to 50 mOsm/kg H_2O (mOsm), and they have the ability to concentrate with an osmolality of 1,200 mOsm. A typical American diet contains a minimum of 600 mOsm. These osmoles can be excreted in 12 L of urine with an osmolality of 50 mOsm (600/50 = 12 L) or in 0.5 L with an osmolality of 1,200 mOsm (600/1,200 = 0.5 L).

- Free water excretion is reduced, particularly in CKD 4–5. Both maximum concentrating and diluting abilities are impaired, and the urine osmolality is fixed at 300 mOsm (isosthenuria) at lower GFRs. In order to excrete 600 mOsm from diet, the CKD patient with lower GFRs (10 mL/min) should excrete at least 2 L (600/300 = 2 L) of urine. Since excretion of 2 L of urine daily in a patient with severe reduction in GFR is limited, intake of water >2 L may cause water retention with resultant hyponatremia. On the other hand, if water intake is <2 L/day, hypernatremia may develop.
- Loss of concentrating ability of urine occurs much earlier than loss of diluting ability in CKD. Impaired concentrating ability in CKD is related to several factors: (1) decreased tubular response to ADH, (2) decreased medullary hypertonicity due to impaired countercurrent mechanism, and (3) decreased urea recycling in the loop of Henle.
- Dilution of urine depends on several factors: (1) delivery of adequate filtrate to the diluting segment, (2) the diluting segment must reabsorb Na so that the urine is adequately diluted, and (3) ADH levels must be sufficiently suppressed. All of these factors are impaired in CKD.
- Because of the above impaired concentrating and diluting abilities in CKD 4–5, the urine osmolality is fixed at 300 mOsm.
- In order to prevent fluid retention in CKD 4–5 patients, restriction of both water and solute (protein restriction of <1 g/kg/day) is recommended. This would also prevent the development of hyponatremia and metabolic acidosis. In CKD 2–3, water restriction is generally not indicated.

Potassium (K) Imbalance

- Normal serum K^+ levels are maintained in CKD patients until GFR is 20–15 mL/min. Thus, normokalemia is maintained in CKD 2–4. At least three protective mechanisms operate to maintain normokalemia or prevent hyperkalemia. These include cellular shift (ECF to ICF), increased renal excretion, and increased colonic secretion of K. Enhanced colonic secretion of K is due to upregulation of angiotensin II receptors in the colon.
- Hyperkalemia develops once GFR is <20–15 mL/min because of ineffective protective mechanisms. Another important cause for hyperkalemia is decreased delivery of filtrate to cortical collecting duct.
- High dietary intake of K is another cause for hyperkalemia in CKD 5 patients. Also, medications such as ACE inhibitors and K-sparing diuretics, NSAIDs, hyperosmolality, and heparin can contribute to hyperkalemia. Blockade of epithelial Na channel (ENaC) by drugs (amiloride, trimethoprim) and inhibition of Na/K-ATPase activity cause hyperkalemia.
- Constipation also causes hyperkalemia because it inhibits colonic secretion of K.
- Treatment of hyperkalemia is outlined in Chap. 16. Restriction of K to 40 mEq/day is suggested for patients on dialysis.

Calcium (Ca) Imbalance

- Ca along with phosphate, PTH, fibroblast growth factor-23 (FGF-23), and active vitamin D_3 (calcitriol) plays an important role in mineral bone disorder in CKD patients. Hypocalcemia (serum Ca^{2+} level <8.4 mg/dL) is more common than hypercalcemia.
- Serum Ca^{2+} levels are low only in CKD 4–5 patients because of (1) decreased intestinal absorption, (2) decreased production of calcitriol, and (3) skeletal resistance to PTH despite high circulating levels of this hormone. Additionally, hypocalcemia may result from phosphate-restricted diet that is low in Ca. Another cause for hypocalcemia is hyperphosphatemia which inhibits the production of calcitriol. Also high phosphate levels bind to Ca in the intestine and prevent its absorption.
- A study showed that serum Ca^{2+} levels <8.4 mg/dL and >9.2 mg/dL are associated with all-cause mortality. Therefore, serum Ca^{2+} levels above 8.5 mg/dL need to be maintained in CKD 4–5 patients.
- PTH and FGF-23 have opposite effects on calcitriol production. PTH stimulates whereas FGF-23 inhibits calcitriol production. In addition, FGF-23 promotes calcitriol degradation.
- Hypercalcemia due to renal failure is rather uncommon except in those CKD patients who are on Ca-containing phosphate binders.
- Therapy of hypocalcemia includes vitamin D supplementation with calcitriol, which not only improves serum Ca^{2+} levels but also suppresses PTH production. Correction of hyperphosphatemia also improves Ca^{2+} levels.

Phosphate Imbalance

- Serum phosphate levels are usually within normal limits in CKD 2–4, and higher in CKD 5. These normal levels are maintained because of an early increase in both PTH and FGF-23, which are phosphaturic. As a result, FE_{PO4} increases in CKD 2–4.
- In CKD 5 (or dialysis-dependent patients), both PTH and FGF-23 levels are elevated as well. However, these hormones lose their effectiveness on phosphate excretion. Because of reduced PTH action, an increase in bone resorption of phosphate occurs. This increase in bone resorption together with decreased excretion precipitates hyperphosphatemia in CKD 5 (predialysis and dialysis) patients.
- Frank hyperphosphatemia (>5.5 mg/dL) is an independent risk factor for all-cause or cardiovascular mortality. Even upper limits of normal phosphate levels were found to be associated with vascular calcification.
- In CKD 2–3, restriction of dietary phosphate stimulates the production of calcitriol, which may improve not only serum Ca^{2+} levels but also delay the development of secondary hyperparathyroidism.

- In CKD 3–4, dietary restriction of phosphate and phosphate binders and correction of nutritional deficiency of vitamin D by cholecalciferol (400–1,000 U per day), ergocalciferol (400–1,000 U per day), or calcifediol (20–50 µg 3 × a week or once a day) should be started to improve mineral bone disorder.
- In CKD 5 (predialysis and dialysis patients), use of calcitriol and calcimimetic agent (cinacalcet) improves mineral bone disorder by lowering mainly PTH levels. In addition, dietary restriction of phosphate is indicated.

Magnesium (Mg) Imbalance

- In CKD 2–3, Mg balance is maintained by increasing its excretion in the urine. This results in the maintenance of normal serum Mg^{2+} levels.
- When GFR is <20–30 mL/min (CKD 4–5), Mg retention occurs due to (1) reduced filtration of Mg, (2) reduced GI absorption, and (3) decreased calcitriol levels. The net result is a positive Mg balance, and most of the Mg is stored either in cells or bone or both.
- Despite positive Mg balance, serum Mg^{2+} levels are slightly elevated (<4 mg/dL). However, signs and symptoms of hypermagnesemia are not evident in most of the patients.
- Restriction of Mg-containing compounds is usually recommended to improve serum Mg^{2+} levels. Dialysis is necessary in patients with serum Mg^{2+} levels >5 mg/dL.

Acid–Base Changes

- A normal subject generates 1 mEq/kg/day of nonvolatile acid (H^+) from dietary protein and endogenous catabolism. These H^+ need to be excreted by the kidneys as titratable acidity and NH_4^+ in order to maintain normal blood pH of 7.4. Both anion gap (AG) and non-AG metabolic acid–base disorders may develop in CKD patients.
- In progressive renal failure, the nonvolatile acid load is not excreted, and H^+ are retained with development of metabolic acidosis.
- One of the mechanisms for acid retention is decreased production of NH_4^+ and reduced HCO_3^- regeneration. Also, some bicarbonaturia occurs with progressive renal failure, which may contribute to the development of metabolic acidosis. The usual response for metabolic acidosis is hyperventilation.
- AG metabolic acidosis does not develop until GFR is <20–30 mL/min. The AG is usually 18–20 mEq/L in CKD 5 unless there is superimposed organic acidosis.
- Hyperchloremic (non-AG) metabolic acidosis develops during the development of CKD, which is due to HCO_3^- wasting. This non-AG metabolic acidosis persists with progression of renal disease, and it is not uncommon to see both AG

and non-AG metabolic acid–base disorders in some patients with GFR 20–30 mL/min.
- Renal tubular acidosis (type IV) with moderate renal failure can be observed in patients with such diseases as diabetes, hypertension, and urinary tract obstruction.
- Proximal RTA is reported in patients with tubular defects.
- Chronic metabolic acidosis has several adverse effects, including bone disease, impaired growth, muscle wasting, and reduced albumin synthesis.
- Chronic metabolic acidosis should be treated to prevent the adverse effects. The initial treatment includes $NaHCO_3$ (650 mg twice daily) and low protein diet (<1 g/kg/day). A few studies have shown that ad libitum intake of base-inducing fruits (oranges, apples, apricots, peaches, pears, strawberries, raisins) and vegetables (potatoes, tomatoes, carrots, cauliflower, eggplant, lettuce, spinach) raised serum $[HCO_3^-]$ and improved metabolic acidosis after 1 year of treatment. Serum $[K^+]$ was not affected. Thus, fruit and vegetable diet improves metabolic acidosis and reduces kidney damage in CKD 4 patients without producing hyperkalemia.
- Dialysis improves metabolic acidosis in those with GFR <10 mL/min because the dialysate contains bicarbonate.

Suggested Reading

1. Bigger P, Rothe H, Keltler M. Epidemiology of calcium, phosphate, and parathyroid hormone disturbances in chronic kidney disease. In: Turner NN, et al., editors. Oxford textbook of clinical nephrology. 4th ed. Oxford: Oxford University Press; 2016. p. 869–76.
2. Combs S, Berl T. Dysnatremias in patients with kidney disease. Am J Kidney Dis. 2014;63:294–303.
3. Khan S, Floris M, Pani A, et al. Sodium and volume disorders in advanced chronic kidney disease. Adv Chron Kidney Dis. 2016;23:240–6.
4. Kurtz I, Madias NE. Metabolic acidosis of CKD: an update. Am J Kidney Dis. 2016;67:307–17.
5. Qi Qian TD. Electrolyte and acid-base disorders in chronic kidney disease and end-stage kidney failure. Blood Purif. 2017;43:179–88.
6. Coresh J, Selvin E, Stevens LA, et al. Prevalence of chronic kidney disease in the United States. JAMA. 2007;298:2038–47.

Kidney Transplantation

38

Kidney or renal transplantation is the best modality of treatment for renal failure patients. Kidney transplantation is associated with fluid, electrolyte, and acid–base changes due to the allograft itself or exogenous administration of immunosuppressive drugs.

Volume Changes

- Posttransplant diuresis is common and is seen immediately after vascular anastomosis. Up to 14–24 L of urine volume has been reported in 24 h. Diuresis and polyuria peak 12 h after surgery. This type of diuresis is documented particularly in cases of living donor transplants.
- Mechanisms for extensive diuresis include (1) expansion of ECF volume and increased sodium (Na) excretion, (2) urea-induced osmotic diuresis, (3) renal denervation, (4) proximal tubular dysfunction, (5) medullary ischemia, and (6) resetting of tubuloglomerular feedback.
- Increased natriuresis, glucosuria, and aminoaciduria have been reported during polyuric condition due to proximal tubular dysfunction.
- Diuresis and polyuria are less observed in cadaveric transplant due to delayed graft function.
- The initial treatment includes administration of hypotonic solutions to match urinary losses to prevent volume depletion.

Electrolyte Abnormalities

- Hypotonic hyponatremia has been reported during posttransplant ATN, rejection, and proteinuria conditions.

© Springer Science+Business Media LLC 2018
A.S. Reddi, *Fluid, Electrolyte and Acid-Base Disorders*,
DOI 10.1007/978-3-319-60167-0_38

- Hypervolemic hyponatremia has been observed during posttransplant development of diabetes.
- Hypernatremia is rather rare but is reported in the immediate posttransplant period possibly due to urea-induced diuresis.
- Hyperkalemia is rather common due to allograft dysfunction and administration of immunosuppressive drugs (cyclosporine, tacrolimus, azathioprine).
- Occasionally supplementation of potassium (K) may also be a reason for hyperkalemia during peri-and postoperative periods.
- Conventional treatment for hyperkalemia is recommended. A 12-lead EKG may suggest the need for immediate treatment.
- Changes in mineral (Ca, phosphate, and Mg) metabolism are frequently seen in long-term transplant recipients.
- Hypercalcemia is more common than hypocalcemia. Mechanisms for hypercalcemia include (1) persistent secondary hyperparathyroidism, (2) release of Ca from metastatic calcification, (3) increased calcitriol synthesis, (4) increased bone resorption possibly due to cyclosporine, and (5) vitamin D supplementation and Ca-containing antacids. There is some evidence that rapamycin may cause hypercalcemia in the presence of secondary hyperparathyroidism.
- Hypercalcemia due to tertiary hyperparathyroidism is seen in some patients after several months of transplantation.
- Hypercalcemia is usually present in three patterns: (1) early posttransplant hypercalcemia (present initially or few weeks posttransplant), (2) transient posttransplant hypercalcemia (onset is from 1.5 months to several months posttransplant), and (3) persistent posttransplant hypercalcemia (hypercalcemia persists for >1 year).
- Hypocalcemia is less frequent than hypercalcemia due to (1) posttransplant hypoalbuminemia, (2) posttransplant hyperphosphatemia, (3) posttransplant hypomagnesemia, and (4) posttransplant proximal tubular dysfunction.
- Hypophosphatemia is more common than hyperphosphatemia and is the most reported electrolyte abnormality following transplantation. Hypophosphatemia may persist for >10 years.
- Mechanisms for hypophosphatemia include (1) persistent elevations of PTH, (2) relative deficiency of calcitriol, (3) steroid use, (4) antacid use, and (5) most importantly elevated FGF-23 levels.
- Depending on the severity of hypophosphatemia, either intravenous or oral phosphate can be given. Neutra Phos (250 mg/packet) can be given until serum phosphate level reaches ≥2.5 mg/dL. Neutra Phos promotes net acid excretion and may improve metabolic acidosis as well.
- Hypomagnesemia is more frequent than hypermagnesemia, which is attributed to hypercalcemia, hypophosphatemia, and tubular leak with high urinary excretion. Cyclosporine use is associated with persistent hypomagnesemia during late transplant period. Steroid and diuretic use may cause and precipitate hypomagnesemia.

- Hyperuricemia is another laboratory abnormality with gout in 2–13% of renal transplant patients. Use of diuretics for fluid overload (edema) and hypertension is an important cause of hyperuricemia.
- Another risk factor for hyperuricemia is the use of cyclosporine and tacrolimus. These drugs seem to interfere with handling of uric acid by the transplanted kidney.

Acid-Base Changes

- Among various types of acid–base disorders, renal tubular acidosis (RTA) is the most frequently encountered disorder in renal transplant recipients.
- Proximal RTA (type II) develops in approximately 19% of cases during the first 3 months of transplantation and then resolves spontaneously. This acid–base disorder is due to HCO_3^- wasting caused by ischemic tubular necrosis that is partially attributed to the harvest procedure.
- If proximal RTA develops after 2 years following transplantation, chronic rejection should be suspected.
- Distal RTA (type I) is rather common. It may develop as early as the first 3 months and may last up to 9 years. Causes for its development include chronic rejection and calcineurin inhibitors (cyclosporine or tacrolimus).
- Both proximal and distal RTAs can occur early after transplantation with spontaneous resolution of proximal RTA. Distal RTA can persist for a long period of time (up to 9 years). Alkali therapy is indicated for patients with distal RTA.
- Type IV RTA is seen most frequently with cyclosporine use and other drugs that lower aldosterone levels.

Suggested Reading

1. Ambühl PM. Posttransplant metabolic acidosis: a neglected factor in renal transplantation? Curr Opin Nephrol Hypertens. 2007;16:379–87.
2. Helderman JH, Schaefer H, Langone AJ, et al. Homeostasis of solute and water by the transplanted kidney. In: Alpern RJ, Moe OW, Caplan M, editors. Seldin and Giebisch's the kidney. Physiology and pathophysiology. 5th ed. San Diego: Academic Press (Elsevier); 2013. p. 3151–83.

Liver Disease

39

Fluid, electrolyte, and acid–base disorders in cirrhosis are functional and not related to renal pathologic abnormalities.

Fluid Imbalance

- Sodium (Na) retention is the earliest renal abnormality seen in cirrhotic patients before and after formation of ascites. It is mostly due to impaired excretion.
- Na balance is determined by its intake and excretion in the urine. If urinary excretion of Na is less than its intake, Na is retained with resultant ascites and edema formation.
- Retention of Na in cirrhotic patients without renal failure is due to an increase in its reabsorption in the proximal tubule and in the cortical collecting duct. In the latter segment, the expression of ENaC is enhanced, and spironolactone inhibits the activity of this channel.
- Na retention is more in patients with renal failure than in those without renal failure.
- With Na, water is reabsorbed isosmotically. As a result, the extracellular volume is increased with subsequent development of edema and ascites.
- In addition to peripheral edema, pleural and/or pericardial effusions can occur due to Na retention. These effusions occur independent of cardiac or pulmonary disease.
- Determination of urinary Na is extremely important in cirrhotic patients with ascites, because it helps the physician in two ways: (1) to have an understanding of the extent of Na retention, and (2) to make a therapeutic decision of diuretic use.
- For example, if the patient is on 2 g (88 mEq) Na diet and the urinary excretion of Na is <10 mEq/L, the patient is retaining approximately 58 mEq of Na/day, assuming stool Na of 20 mEq and urine output of 1 L/day or simply:

© Springer Science+Business Media LLC 2018
A.S. Reddi, *Fluid, Electrolyte and Acid-Base Disorders*,
DOI 10.1007/978-3-319-60167-0_39

Na retention = Na intake – (urinary Na + stool Na)
Na retention in the above example is:

$$88 - (10 + 20) = 58 \, \text{mEq} / \text{day}$$

- Cirrhotic patients with urine Na <10 mEq/L have poor prognosis (survival). Such patients should benefit from high doses of spironolactone (100–200 mg per day) with or without furosemide (40–80 mg per day).
- Patients with urine Na >10 mEq/L will have better prognosis. These patients may require low dose of spironolactone (25–100 mg/day). Large doses of diuretics in these patients may induce hypovolemia, orthostasis, and prerenal azotemia.
- Management of edema and ascites is discussed in Chap. 8. Also, clinical use and complications of diuretics are presented in Chap. 5.

Water Imbalance

- As mentioned previously, water is reabsorbed isosmotically with Na reabsorption. This causes impaired water excretion and expansion of plasma volume.
- Free water clearance decreases because of decreased delivery of glomerular filtrate to the diluting segment.
- The result of plasma volume expansion is hypervolemic hyponatremia, which is defined in cirrhosis as serum [Na$^+$] <130 mEq/L (conventionally hyponatremia is defined as serum [Na$^+$] <135 mEq/L).
- Patients with hyponatremia and ascites are at increased risk for hepatorenal syndrome.
- Patients also develop hypovolemic hyponatremia with orthostatic blood pressure and pulse changes following diuretic therapy.
- Treatment of hypervolemic hyponatremia is fluid restriction and diuretic, if necessary. The following formula can be used to restrict fluid intake:

$$\text{Urine} \left[Na^+ + K^+ \right] / \text{plasma} \left[Na^+ \right]$$

If the ratio is >1, restrict fluid to <500 mL/day. For a ratio of 1, restriction from 800–700 mL/day is required. If the ration is <1, fluid restriction of 1 L/day is adequate to improve serum [Na$^+$].

- Normal saline or 5% albumin is recommended to treat hypovolemic hyponatremia.
- Symptomatic hyponatremia should be corrected carefully in cirrhotic patients with malnutrition because they are at risk for osmotic demyelination syndrome following rapid correction of hyponatremia. Correction of serum [Na$^+$] should not exceed >6 mEq in 24 h (see Chap. 12).

- Some patients with chronic hyponatremia may respond to V_2 receptor antagonists (tolvaptan), but their use in cirrhosis is not recommended because of abnormal liver function tests, increased thirst, polyuria, and no mortality advantage.
- Use of demeclocycline should be avoided in cirrhotics to prevent acute kidney injury.
- Hypernatremia is occasionally seen in cirrhotic patients, which may be due to excess water loss (urine and insensible loss) caused by diuretics or infections.
- Another important cause of hypernatremia is the use of lactulose in the management of hepatic encephalopathy. Patients on lactulose lose more water than electrolytes in the stool (osmotic diarrhea).

Potassium (K) Imbalance

- Serum [K^+] varies widely in cirrhotic patients. Both hypokalemia and hyperkalemia have been reported.
- Hypokalemia is caused by (1) poor dietary intake; (2) shift from ECF to ICF compartment due to alkalosis; (3) renal loss due to diuretics, hyperaldosteronism, hypomagnesemia, vomiting, and RTA; and (4) GI loss due to diarrhea.
- Hyperkalemia is mostly caused by K-sparing diuretics, particularly spironolactone. Also rhabdomyolysis and severe renal failure can cause hyperkalemia.
- Treatment of hypo- and hyperkalemia is similar to that of noncirrhotic patient, as outlined in Chaps. 15 and 16.

Calcium Imbalance

- Hypocalcemia is rather common than hypercalcemia.
- Hypocalcemia may be related to several factors, including poor dietary intake, vitamin D deficiency ($25(OH)D_3$), hypomagnesemia, low albumin levels, subclinical pancreatitis, and fat malabsorption.
- Hypercalcemia, as stated previously, is uncommon. If present, granulomatous diseases rather than primary hyperparathyroidism or malignancy need to be explored. Also, Ca-containing medications need to be considered.
- Treatment with vitamin D supplementation and correction of hypoalbuminemia and hypomagnesemia may prevent signs and symptoms of hypocalcemia (see Chap. 18).

Phosphate Imbalance

- Hypophosphatemia is extremely common in chronic alcoholism and is also present in patients with liver disease.
- Important causes of hypophosphatemia include poor dietary intake, respiratory alkalosis, renal and GI losses, and intestinal malabsorption.
- Dietary phosphate intake with milk supplementation improves serum phosphate levels.
- Hyperphosphatemia, when present, is suggestive of decreased renal excretion, exogenous phosphate load, or release from cell lysis.

Magnesium (Mg) Imbalance

- Hypomagnesemia is a frequently seen electrolyte abnormality in a cirrhotic patient.
- Common causes of hypomagnesemia include poor dietary intake, GI losses from diarrhea, and starvation ketosis-induced renal loss.
- Hypomagnesemia is usually associated with hypokalemia and hypocalcemia. Mg supplementation corrects all of these electrolyte abnormalities.

Acid–Base Changes

- Most frequently seen acid–base disorders are respiratory alkalosis, metabolic alkalosis, and hyperchloremic metabolic acidosis.
- Respiratory alkalosis is the frequently seen acid–base disorder in patients with liver disease and ascites. Factors that contribute to respiratory alkalosis include hypoxemia, NH_3, progesterone, and elevation of diaphragms by ascites as well as pleural effusions.
- Rapid lowering of pH in patients with liver disease is not advisable, as treatment with 5% CO_2 inhalation or acetazolamide worsened neurologic changes despite a decrease in NH_3 levels in the brain.
- Metabolic alkalosis is commonly seen in patients on thiazide and loop diuretics. Vomiting is also a frequent cause of this acid–base disorder.
- Hyperchloremic metabolic acidosis is also seen following diarrhea, RTA, and spironolactone use. In one study, serum HCO_3^- level decreased from 18 to 11 mEq/L in patients treated with spironolactone.
- AG metabolic acidosis due to lactic acid production and ingestion of toxic alcohols is seen occasionally in patients with liver disease.

Suggested Reading

1. Anderson RJ. Electrolyte, water, mineral, and acid-base disorders in liver disease. In: Narins RG, editor. Maxwell & Kleeman's clinical disorders of fluid and electrolyte metabolism. 5th ed. New York: McGraw-Hill, Inc; 1995. p. 1153–73.
2. Gińes P, Cardenas A, Sola E, et al. Liver disease and the kidney. In: Coffman TM, et al., editors. Schrier's diseases of the kidney. 9th ed. Philadelphia: Lippincott Williams & Wilkins; 2013. p. 1965–96.
3. Sinha VK, Ko B. Hyponatremia in cirrhosis – pathogenesis, treatment, and prognostic significance. Adv Chron Kidney Dis. 2015;22:361–7.

Pregnancy

40

Pregnancy is associated with several hemodynamic, fluid, electrolyte, and acid–base disorders.

Hemodynamic Changes

- In early pregnancy, cardiac output increases by 30–40% as compared with non-pregnant women. This increase in cardiac output is primarily due to a decrease in peripheral vascular resistance with resultant vasodilation. In some women, significant increase in peripheral vasodilation occurs, which manifests clinically as palmar erythema and spider telangiectasia.
- Blood pressure is low because of systemic vasodilation. Several hormones are involved in systemic vasodilation. One of the hormones is human chorionic gonadotropin-induced relaxin. Also, a blunted vascular response to vasoconstrictors has been observed during pregnancy.
- Renal function changes have also been observed in normal pregnancy. These include an increase in GFR and renal plasma flow. Elevations in both GFR and renal plasma flow are maintained until term and return to baseline 3 months after delivery. Glomerular hyperfiltration due to decreased renal vascular resistance has been implicated in the elevation of GFR. Progesterone, relaxin, and vasodilatory prostaglandins have been implicated in the elevated GFR and renal plasma flow. Serum creatinine and BUN are relatively low in pregnancy.

Volume Changes

- Generally, retention of fluid up to 12 L and accumulation of sodium (Na) up to 900 mEq has been reported during normal pregnancy. This causes an increase in plasma volume with a resultant decrease in plasma osmolality by about 10 mOsm/kg H_2O. This fall in osmolality (hypoosmolality) is related to changes in the

© Springer Science+Business Media LLC 2018
A.S. Reddi, *Fluid, Electrolyte and Acid-Base Disorders*,
DOI 10.1007/978-3-319-60167-0_40

osmoregulation of ADH. Normally, ADH is secreted once plasma osmolality exceeds 285 mOsm/kg H_2O. However, in pregnancy ADH is secreted when plasma osmolality exceeds 278 mOsm/kg H_2O. Thus, the threshold or set point for ADH release is decreased in pregnancy. In addition to decrease in threshold for ADH release, increased thirst also contributes to hypoosmolality. Hemoglobin and hematocrit also decrease due to plasma volume expansion.

Electrolyte Abnormalities

- Hyponatremia due to volume expansion is common in pregnancy. There is at least 5 mEq/L decrease in serum [Na^+]. An imbalance in natriuretic factors (ANP, progesterone, elevated GFR) and antinatriuretic factors (aldosterone, Na/K-ATPase) and changes in osmoregulation of ADH seem to be responsible for hyponatremia. Urinary excretion of Na is increased due to dominant action of natriuretic factors during pregnancy.
- Hypernatremia can occasionally be observed during late pregnancy due to transient diabetes insipidus (DI). DI is caused by increased production of vasopressinase by the placenta, which degrades vasopressin (ADH). Thus, ADH, which is suppressed by volume expansion, is further lowered by vasopressinase. Desmopressin, which is not degraded by vasopressinase, is the treatment of choice for DI. However, resistance to desmopressin has been reported in some women, suggesting that these women may have developed nephrogenic DI.
- Serum [K^+] is usually normal, but a decrease of 0.2–0.3 mEq/L has been reported during 10–28 weeks of pregnancy.
- Despite normal serum [K^+], there is a cumulative retention of approximately 350 mEq of K during pregnancy. This excess K is stored in the products of conception and reproductive organs.
- The retention of K occurs despite high Na delivery to the distal nephron and elevated levels of aldosterone. Increased progesterone, which antagonizes aldosterone, has been implicated in K retention.
- Approximately 25–30 g of calcium (Ca) is retained during pregnancy due to an increase in placental production and increased intestinal absorption.
- Total serum Ca^{2+} levels are usually normal, but they fall by 0.5 mg/dL only during the third trimester, which is due to a decrease in serum albumin. In some pregnant women, both bound and ionized Ca^{2+} levels were found to be decreased compared to nonpregnant women.
- Urinary Ca excretion is increased during normal pregnancy which parallels the increase in GFR. Those who are high Ca excretors are prone to develop calcium stones. Low Ca excretion was reported in preeclamptic women.

- Serum Mg^{2+} levels usually fall by 5–9% during pregnancy, which may be due to plasma volume expansion and decreased protein binding. However, urinary Mg excretion is normal.

Acid–Base Changes

- Compensatory respiratory alkalosis is commonly present in pregnant women. This acid–base disorder is related to increased progesterone level, which causes hyperventilation. Also, elevated diaphragms cause hyperventilation.
- Metabolic alkalosis superimposed on respiratory alkalosis may be seen in those with vomiting of any etiology.

Others

- Uric acid is low because of increased secretion. Also, glucosuria and aminoaciduria can be seen in some due to increased filtration and decreased reabsorption (Table 40.1).
- The following table shows some important lab values in a normal pregnant woman.

Table 40.1 Some important lab values in pregnancy

Labs	Pregnancy	Reference values
Serum		
Na^+ (mEq/L)	130–135	140
K^+ (mEq/L)	3.0–4.0	4.5
HCO_3^- (mEq/L)	18–22	24
BUN (mg/dL)	7–10	12
Creatinine (mg/dL)	0.4–0.6	0.8–1.2
Albumin (g/dL)	3.0–4.0	3.5–4.5
Uric acid (mg/dL)	2.5–4.0	4.5
Hematocrit (g/dL)	30–33	40
Urine		
Glucose	High	Absent
Amino acids	High	Normal
Protein	Normal	Normal (<150 mg/day)
Calcium	High	Normal
Others		
ABG	pH = 7.43; pCO_2 = 31 mmHg; HCO_3^-= 19 mEq/L	pH = 7.40; pCO_2 = 40 mmHg; HCO_3^-= 24 mEq/L
BP	105/60 mmHg	115/70 mmHg

Suggested Reading

1. Conrad KP, Karumanchi A. Renal physiology and disease in pregnancy. In: Alpern RJ, Moe OW, Caplan M, editors. Seldin and Giebisch's the kidney. Physiology and pathophysiology. 5th ed. San Diego: Academic Press (Elsevier); 2013. p. 2689–761.
2. Pallar MS, Ferris TP. Fluid and electrolyte metabolism during pregnancy. In: Narins RG, editor. Maxwell & Kleeman's clinical disorders of fluid and electrolyte metabolism. 5th ed. New York: McGraw-Hill, Inc; 1995. p. 1121–36.

Index

© Springer Science+Business Media LLC 2018
A.S. Reddi, *Fluid, Electrolyte and Acid-Base Disorders,*
DOI 10.1007/978-3-319-60167-0